Diagnosis and Treatment of Breast Cancer

Diagnosis and Treatment of Breast Cancer

Edited by **Sandra Lekin**

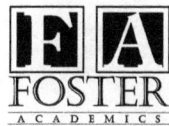

FOSTER ACADEMICS

New Jersey

Published by Foster Academics,
61 Van Reypen Street,
Jersey City, NJ 07306, USA
www.fosteracademics.com

Diagnosis and Treatment of Breast Cancer
Edited by Sandra Lekin

© 2016 Foster Academics

International Standard Book Number: 978-1-63242-429-7(Hardback)

Contents

Preface

This book is a valuable compilation of topics, ranging from the basic to the most complex advancements in the field of diagnosis and treatment of breast cancer. Breast cancer is one of the most common cancers found in women and also one of the most common reasons for female deaths. Therefore, its diagnosis and treatment is an extensive field of study. This book is compiled in such a manner, that it provides in-depth knowledge about the theory and practice related to this field. It discusses the classifications of breast cancer, its various diagnostic methods and its diverse forms of treatments. It includes contributions of experts and scientists which will provide innovative insights into this field. Thus, it will prove to be a valuable asset for students and experts alike.

This book is the end result of constructive efforts and intensive research done by experts in this field. The aim of this book is to enlighten the readers with recent information in this area of research. The information provided in this profound book would serve as a valuable reference to students and researchers in this field.

At the end, I would like to thank all the authors for devoting their precious time and providing their valuable contributions to this book. I would also like to express my gratitude to my fellow colleagues who encouraged me throughout the process.

Editor

An Evaluation of FaHRAS Computer Programmes' Utility in Family History Triage of Breast Cancer

Áine Gorman, Michael Sugrue*, Zuhair Ahmed, Alison Johnston

Donegal Clinical and Research Academy, Breast Centre North West, Letterkenny Hospital, Donegal, Ireland
Email: *michael.sugrue@hse.ie

Abstract

Introduction: Rapid and appropriate family risk assessment and triage of patients are essential for patients presenting to a symptomatic breast unit and international criteria for review are well established. Family History Risk Assessment Software (FaHRAS) is a computerized program, involving different modalities of risk assessment, which is available but has not been widely assessed. Aims: This study evaluated the FaHRAS software scoring of family history risk. Its analysis was compared to multi-tool family history risk assessment models in a cohort of 353 patients on a historic family history waiting list. Methods: A recent published pilot study assessed and categorized family history risk in 353 patients on a historic family history waiting list, according to international guidelines including NICE criteria, Gail and IBIS risk estimates. The current study involved a reassessment of all 353 patients using the FaHRAS software program to determine its accuracy and ease of use. Patient demographics and time required to perform the analysis were documented. Results: FaHRAS identified 73 (20.7%) patients had an IBIS family history score of 17% or greater and 89 (25.2%) patients met the NICE guidelines criteria for management beyond primary care. In the previous study, this was 79 (22.4%) and 112 (31.7%) respectively. Using the largest denominator (NICE guidelines), 264/353 (74.8%) patients could be discharged to primary care using FaHRAS. Using this largest denominator, FaHRAS also identified a total of 28 (7.9%) patients requiring referral to tertiary care while the previous study identified 3 (0.8%). Conclusion: This is one of the first studies to validate FaHRAS, which is accurate and easy to use. FaHRAS system can enable clinicians to become more efficient gatekeepers to genetic services.

Keywords

Breast Cancer, Risk Assessment, Family History

---

*Corresponding author.

1. Introduction

Health care initiatives relating to early detection and management of breast cancer have highlighted awareness of breast cancer as a public health issue [1]. This has resulted in increased referral to symptomatic breast services nationally and internationally [2]. Anxiety and fear relating to inappropriate risk assessment, breast cancer diagnosis and its management can confound a rational approach to its management [3].

One of the main reasons for this increased referral is the fact that an individual's relative(s) may have previously been diagnosed with breast cancer which they perceive to put them at increased risk of the disease. Family history is key to risk classification of breast cancer and indeed a positive family history can significantly influence a woman's risk for breast cancer depending on such issues as number and age of the affected relative(s) [4].

However, risk factors relating to family history are not universally well understood [5]. 20 - 30 percent of women with breast cancer have at least one relative with the disease, but only 5 to 10 percent have a true hereditary predisposition [6]. Triaging patients' appropriate family history risk is important to identify those needing increased surveillance and those who can be maintained in family care [7] [8].

NICE has recently updated its Familial Breast Cancer Guidelines and two of its recommendations are that tools such as family history questionnaires and computer packages exist that can aid accurate collection of family history information and they should be made available. In addition the Guidelines state that when accessible in secondary care, a credible carrier probability calculation method should be used as well as family history to determine who should be offered referral to a specialist genetic clinic [9]. Computerized family history risk assessment programs have been available for some time, but have not been widely assessed in symptomatic breast units [10]. In a previous clinical audit of family history risk assessment, a significant number of inappropriate family history referrals and reviews were occurring [11]. A subsequent study showed that the appropriate referrals had increased from 45% to 78% but there was still room for improvement [12]. This risk assessment was cumbersome and time consuming and newer computer programs have been developed to aid in triage. FaHRAS®[1] is a sophisticated evidence-based software system which enables a user to build and store a family history and to run a variety of analyses against their family history to quantify their risk of developing breast cancer.

This study evaluated FaHRAS software ability to triage family history risk referrals and compare its analysis to that previously undertaken using multi-tool family history risk assessment models.

2. Methods

An ethically approved study was undertaken at Letterkenny Hospitals' Breast Unit as a two stage evaluation of family history risk assessment. Letterkenny Hospital Breast Unit, established in 1998 as a satellite to its parent centre 250 km away in Galway University Hospital, is a designated breast cancer service under the National Cancer Control Programme in Ireland [13]. The Breast Unit treats almost 80 new cancer patients per annum, in addition 1800 new patients and 1500 review patients currently attend the Breast Unit. The Unit had a historical family history recall review waiting list of 353 patients. This had built up over a period of 8 years serviced by three different locum breast surgeons.

The first stage of this study reviewed the medical charts of 353 patients on a family history recall list. Risk stratification was objectively assessed using the NICE guidelines, Gail model and modified Tyrer-Cuzick (IBIS) risk assessment tools [9] [14] [15]. The 353 patients were then triaged into GP review or breast clinic review [11].

The second stage of the study, reported in this paper, re-evaluated the data on these 353 patients utilizing the FaHRAS software program. The software was donated from the University of Nottingham spinout company FaHRAS, where it has been developed. The FaHRAS software had been beta tested in two specialist familial breast cancer units before being released. Risk assessment models used included the NICE Guidelines as used by the NHS, IBIS (Tyrer-Cuzick) and BOADICEA Model Risk Assessments [16]. Patient history, including a family history evaluation, was entered into the FaHRAS programme. Their lifetime risk and ten-year risk for the development of breast cancer was documented and the risk of gene defect BCRA 1 and 2 were calculated using the FaHRAS programme. **Table 1** outlines the criteria for referral to primary, secondary and tertiary care utilizing existing best practice guidelines [9]. The accuracy of the software's risk assessment was evaluated by completing a risk assessment on the 353 patients and making a comparison with the risk assessment already com-

[1]FaHRAS Ltd 1, Pines Way, Harlow Wood, Mansfield, Notts England. NG184UU.

Table 1. Criteria for risk stratification into primary, secondary and tertiary care.

	Primary Care	Secondary Care	Tertiary Care
Lifetime risk of breast cancer	<17%	≥17% - <30%	≥30%
Risk of a BRCA1 or BRCA2 mutation	-	-	>20%

pleted on the same 353 patients by clinicians during the above mentioned clinical audit. Further evaluation involved assessing whether the management recommendations of FaHRAS for primary and secondary care would correlate with the triage recommendations which were manually assessed in the clinical audit. The length of time taken to input the data, plot the family tree and to complete the three risk assessments was recorded for the 353 patients.

3. Results

A total of 353 patients' family history and risk factors were assessed using the FaHRAS programme. Mean age of patients assessed was 49.1 ± 11.5 years (range 21 - 76). The distribution of patients reaching the criteria for family history triage review in the first and second stage of this study is shown in **Table 2**.

Using FaHRAS, 73 (20.7%) patients had an IBIS score of 17% or greater. In the first stage 79 (22.4%) reached this threshold value in the audit conducted. Review of the 6 discordant cases identified incorrect data entry relating to age, menopausal status and family history.

In addition 89 (25.2%) patients met the NICE guidelines criteria for management beyond primary care compared with 112 (31.7%) patients meeting the NICE guidelines for referral during the initial clinical audit. **Table 3** demonstrates how FaHRAS changed the triage code from clinical assessment alone, reducing the number referred to secondary care from 109 to 61. It did increase the number referred to tertiary care.

Using BOADICEA risk assessment, 2 (0.25%) patients reached the criteria as high risk for a BRCA1 or BRCA2 mutation and referral to tertiary care was recommended.

The mean length of time taken to complete the risk assessment was 3.9 ± 0.6 minutes, with a range of 3-6 minutes. With increasing experience of using the FaHRAS system, the length of time needed to input the data decreased. The mean length of time taken to input data for the first 100 patients was 4.7 ± 0.5 minutes. In comparison, the mean length of time taken to input data for the final 100 patients was 3.1 ± 0.2 minutes.

4. Discussion

FaHRAS provided an acceptable and reliable means for assessing patients' risk of breast cancer. The study suggested that, using the largest denominator (NICE guidelines) slightly less patients needed review beyond primary care however 7.1% more needed review in tertiary care than the initial reported audit recommended. The differences in triage recommendations highlight the difficulties that can arise in risk stratification of patient with a family history.

There are several reasons why FaHRAS risk assessment using IBIS could be more efficient than the modified Tyrer-Cuzick internet based risk assessment tool which was used in the previous audit. The FaHRAS enables the user to input with systematic thoroughness. The FAHRAS software programme enabled users to obtain a three generation or greater family history of not just breast cancer but many types of cancer and allows updates of family history. The Tyrer-Cuzick risk assessment tool allows users to obtain a three generation family history pedigree which can lead to an underestimated cancer risk as it only allows for a family history of breast cancer to be taken into account [17].

The FaHRAS programme was significantly better at interpreting the NICE criteria for referral to specialist genetic services than the clinician based assessment performed during the audit. It highlights what has been shown in previous studies that computer programmes for interpreting family history of breast and ovarian cancer can produce more appropriate management decisions in comparison to other methods [18]. This study shows that computer based software such as FaHRAS can provide accurate risk assessment and could enable clinicians to be more effective gatekeepers to genetic services [17]. Even following regional education programs initiated in our area referral systems without routine computer aided systems will result in 22% inappropriate referrals [12].

Table 2. Risk stratification of patients based on each risk assessment tool.

	Clinical Audit n = 353			FaHRAS n = 353		
	Primary Care	Secondary Care	Tertiary Care	Primary Care	Secondary Care	Tertiary Care
IBIS	274	79	0	280	71	2
Gail	296	57	0	-	-	-
NICE	241	109	3	264	61	28
BOADICEA	-	-	-	351	0	2

Table 3. Summary of NICE Recommendations in the previous audit and using the FaHRAS programme.

NICE Recommendation	Clinician n = 353	FaHRAS n = 353
Refer to Primary Care	241	264
Manage in Secondary Care	109	61
Offer referral to specialist genetics surveillance	3	28

Although the BOADIECA risk assessment tool was not used in the previous audit, the FaHRAS programme enabled the probability of detecting a BRCA1 or BRCA2 mutations [16]. Previous studies using the BOADIECA model have shown that BOADIECA in comparison to other models can accurately predict the overall number of mutation detected [19]. Two women in this study were classed as "high risk" for a BRCA mutation using the BOADIECA risk assessment. The identification of women who are high risk for a BRCA 1 or BRCA 2 mutation is important as genetic testing can be targeted towards individual patients who are more likely to test positive [20].

The mean length of time taken to input the data into the FaHRAS system does require time which would result in longer consultation times. The mean time to complete a risk assessment was 3.9 minutes over the whole study. This ranged from a mean time of 4.7 minutes for the first hundred patients to 3.1 minutes for the final 100 patients. The FaHRAS programme compares favorably to other computer based programmes which can take up to 15 minutes to input all the relevant data [17]. If computer based programs are used it enables pedigrees to be generated and for family history information to be stored. FaHRAS is therefore ideal in a well resourced breast system and could be completed by trained breast nurses.

This study shows the important role that computer based programmes such as FaHRAS could have in the assessment of patients with a family history of breast cancer. The FaHRAS system could enable clinicians to become more efficient gatekeepers to genetic services and reassure clinicians in their classification of women as low risk who can be managed in primary care. It has facilitated a major restructuring of the manner we undertake our risk assessment, triage and referral process. FaHRAS helped identify that 264/353 (74.8%) at our clinic could have been cared for in primary care. However further development of the FaHRAS could be undertaken to reduce the time required to complete for each patient and have linkages with hospital based computer systems and those in primary care.

References

[1] Linsell, L., *et al.* (2009) A Randomised Controlled Trial of an Intervention to Promote Early Presentation of Breast Cancer in Older Women: Effect on Breast Cancer Awareness. *British Journal of Cancer*, **101**, 40-S48. http://dx.doi.org/10.1038/sj.bjc.6605389

[2] Watson, E., Austoker, J. and Lucassen, A. (2001) A Study of GP Referrals to a Family Cancer Clinic for Breast/Ovarian Cancer. *Family Practice*, **18**, 131-134. http://dx.doi.org/10.1093/fampra/18.2.131

[3] Welch, H.G., Schwartz, L.M. and Woloshin, S. (2011) Overdiagnosed: Making People Sick in the Pursuit of Health. Beacon Press, Boston.

[4] Collaborative Group on Hormonal Factors in Breast Cancer (2001) Familial Breast Cancer: Collaborative Reanalysis of Individual Data from 52 Epidemiological Studies including 58209 Women with Breast Cancer and 101 986 Women without the Disease. *Lancet*, **358**, 1389-1399. http://dx.doi.org/10.1016/S0140-6736(01)06524-2

[5]   Rose, P., *et al.* (2001) Referral of Patients with a Family History of Breast/Ovarian Cancer—GPs' Knowledge and Expectations. *Family Practice*, **18**, 487-490. http://dx.doi.org/10.1093/fampra/18.5.487

[6]   Carter, R.F. (2001) BRCA1, BRCA2 and Breast Cancer: A Concise Clinical Review. *Clinical & Investigative Medicine*, **243**, 147-157.

[7]   Lakhani, N.S., Weir, J., Alford, A., Kai, J. and Barwell, J.G. (2009-2011)Could Triaging Family History of Cancer during Palliative Care Enable Earlier Genetic Counselling Interventions for Families at High Risk? Tipping Points Project (2009-2011).

[8]   Maurice, A., *et al.* (2006) Screening Younger Women with a Family History of Breast Cancer—Does Early Detection Improve Outcome? *European Journal of Cancer*, **42**, 1385-1390. http://dx.doi.org/10.1016/j.ejca.2006.01.055

[9]   National Institute for Health and Care Excellence (2013) Familial Breast Cancer: Classification and Care of People at Risk of Familial Breast Cancer and Management of Breast Cancer and Related Risks in People with a Family History of Breast Cancer. Update of Clinical Guideline 14 and 41. (Clinical Guideline 164.).
http://guidance.nice.org.uk/CG164

[10] Guerra, C.E., Sherman, M. and Armstrong, K. (2009) Diffusion of Breast Cancer Risk Assessment in Primary Care. *The Journal of the American Board of Family Medicine*, **22**, 272-279. http://dx.doi.org/10.3122/jabfm.2009.03.080153

[11] Ahmed, Z., Shields, G., Momin, M., Curran, S. and Sugrue, M. (2010) Breast Cancer Family History Risk Assessment, Fact or Fantasy? *Irish Journal of Medical Sciences*, **179**, S331-S373.

[12] Thomas, J., Sugrue, M., Curran, S., Furey, M. and Sugrue, R. (2013) Are Family Doctors Compliant with Breast Family History Guidelines? *Advances in Breast Cancer Research*, **2**, 149-153. http://dx.doi.org/10.4236/abcr.2013.24024

[13] National Cancer Control Programme. http://www.hse.ie/eng/services/list/5/nccp/

[14] Gail, M., *et al.* (1989) Projecting Individualized Probabilities of Developing Breast Cancer for White Females Who Are Being Examined Annually. *Journal of the National Cancer Institute*, **81**, 1879-1886.
http://dx.doi.org/10.1093/jnci/81.24.1879

[15] IBIS Software Tyrer-Cuzick Computerised Model V6 (2008) http://www.ems-trials.org/riskevaluator/

[16] Antoniou, A.C., *et al.* (2006) BRCA1 and BRCA2 Mutation Predictions Using the BOADICEA and BRCAPRO Models and Penetrance Estimation in High-Risk French-Canadian Families. *Breast Cancer Research*, **8**, R3.
http://dx.doi.org/10.1186/bcr1365

[17] Amir, E.O., Freedman, C., Evans, D.G. and Seruga, B. (2010) Assessing Women at High Risk of Breast Cancer: A Review of Risk Assessment Models. *Journal of the National Cancer Institute*, **102**, 680-691.
http://dx.doi.org/10.1093/jnci/djq088

[18] Emery, J.R., *et al.* (2000) Computer Support for Interpreting Family Histories of Breast and Ovarian Cancer in Primary Care: Comparative Study with Simulated Cases. *British Medical Journal*, **321**, 28-32.
http://dx.doi.org/10.1136/bmj.321.7252.28

[19] Parmigiani, G.S., *et al.* (2007) Validity of Models for Predicting BRCA1 and BRCA2 Mutations. *Annals of Internal Medicine*, **147**, 441-450. http://dx.doi.org/10.7326/0003-4819-147-7-200710020-00002

[20] Antoniou, A.P., Pharoah, P., Smith, P. and Easton, D.F. (2004) The BOADICEA Model of Genetic Susceptibility to Breast and Ovarian Cancer. *British Journal of Cancer*, **91**, 1580-1590.

2

Social Support Provided to Women Undergoing Breast Cancer Treatment: A Study Review

Ana Fátima Fernandes*, Amanda Cruz, Camila Moreira, Míria Conceição Santos, Tiago Silva

Department of Nursing, Federal University of Ceará, Fortaleza, Brazil
Email: *afcana@ufc.br

Abstract

Breast cancer treatment may have implications for women's quality of life and social support, which refers to mechanisms through which interpersonal relationships protect people from the detrimental effects of stress. This study's objective was to analyze evidence available in the literature concerning social support provided to women with breast cancer undergoing chemotherapy. The Latin American and Caribbean Literature on Health Sciences (LILACS), PubMed, Web of Science, Psycinfo and Cumulative Index to Nursing and Allied Health Literature (CINAHL) databases were used to select the studies. The papers were pre-selected after reading titles and abstracts and ten papers were ultimately selected after fully reading the texts. The studies were summarized, while their methodological designs and results were noted. The analysis of the studies shows that social support can be provided to women with breast cancer, such as emotional, instrumental and informational support. It is apparent that emotional and instrumental support is provided in the first phase of the treatment. The main sources of support include the spouses, family members and friends. Spouses provide emotional support, but mainly provide instrumental support, while family members and friends are the most important source of emotional support. The conclusion is that emotional support greatly contributes to the health-disease continuum, favoring treatment adherence and creating opportunities for women to express their feelings, positively influencing the treatment.

Keywords

Breast Cancer, Oncological Treatment, Social Support

---

*Corresponding author.

1. Introduction

Breast cancer is the most common type of cancer affecting women around the world. There are approximately 1000 new cases every year and it accounts for a significant number of deaths among adult women, thus is a severe public health problem [1].

The most common therapeutic modality for this type of cancer is mastectomy with extraction of the compromised breast. In some women, only parts of the breast are removed: quadrantectomy (removal of one quarter of the breast) and lumpectomy (removal of only the tumor and a small surrounding region), producing good results in terms of survival and a better aesthetic effect, since the breast is largely retained. In more advanced cases, radiotherapy and chemotherapy are the indicated treatments. The choice for the most appropriate therapeutic method depends on various factors, such as age, the site of the tumor, financial availability, analysis of mammography, and the manner in which the patient deals with the affected breast [2].

In addition to treatment-related implications, one should also consider the deleterious effects of the disease (fear of death, of rejection, of being stigmatized, of mutilation, relapse, the effects of the chemotherapy, uncertainty concerning the future and others), which are representations that concern health professionals involved with the quality of life of these patients [2].

Patients with breast cancer have many needs, including a need for strategies to cope with associated stress, both during and after treatment. The creation and/or utilization of social support has been a strategy to reduce the deleterious effect of stressful events related to the treatment of breast cancer [3]. Social support or social networks are structures consisting of family, friends, neighbors, and other individuals who inter-relate and provide reciprocal support. It refers to mechanisms through which interpersonal relationships protect people from the detrimental effects of stress. Social support is a key for any individual's emotional safety because every individual has a need to feel part of a family or group of friends [4].

Given the previous discussion, we note that the breast cancer treatment leads to many situations that may threaten the psychosocial integrity of those affected by the disease. The social behavior of women is affected, leading to restrictions on their social lives and changes in daily life activities, facts that may contribute to depressive behavior and social isolation.

This study's objective was to analyze evidence available in the literature regarding the social support provided to women with breast cancer who are undergoing chemotherapy.

2. Materials and Methods

In order to accomplish this study's objective, we conducted an integrative literature review, which is a technique that compiles and synthesizes scientific information by analyzing the results reported by studies. This review followed five distinct stages to meet the same methodological rigor of any conventional study [5].

The initial phase comprised the identification of the problem under study, after which a guiding question was asked and inclusion and exclusion criteria were established. Having well-delineated criteria facilitates the other stages of the review, especially the differentiation of information concerning data collection [5]. Therefore, the following guiding question was chosen: "What is the scientific knowledge available regarding social support provided to women with breast cancer undergoing treatment?

The databases chosen for a comprehensive search and selection of studies included: PubMed, digital files created by the National Library of Medicine (USA) in the biosciences field; Web of Science, encompassing a set of databases (Science Citation Index, Social Science Citation Index, Arts and Humanities Citation Index, Current Chemical Reactions and Index Chemicus) compiled by the Institute for Scientific Information (ISI); CINAHL (Cumulative Index of Nursing and Allied Health Literature), which encompasses the main scientific studies in the nursing field; PsycINFO, a reference source for the psychology, behavioral and education sciences; and LILACS, which gathers scientific studies in the health field in Latin America and the Caribbean.

In this context, inclusion criteria were primary studies published in English, Spanish or Portuguese addressing some type of social support provided to women with breast cancer; studies in which social support was the main focus and object of study; and studies in which women with breast cancer were undergoing treatment or up to 24 months after the beginning of treatment.

Exclusion criteria were studies the subjects of which were younger than 18 years old or elderly individuals because social support, in these cases, would include other issues not strictly related to chemotherapy. Studies addressing other types of cancer were also excluded.

The search terms included social support, family, and breast neoplasms, which were used in different combinations to increase the number of potential references.

First, the titles of papers were analyzed to verify their adequacy to answer the guiding question. The papers were then further checked by reading the abstracts. The full texts of those studies that were preselected were then read to make sure they met the inclusion criteria previously established.

Following the established strategies, the final sample was composed of ten papers, three of which were found in the PubMed database, two in the Web of Science, three in CINAHL, and another two in PsycInfo (**Figure 1**).

2.1. Categorization of the Studies

An adapted instrument was used to collect and summarize data concerning the selected studies, which included information concerning the identification of studies, introduction and aims, methodology, description of results, conclusion, and level of evidence [6]. The instrument was subjected to a pretest to establish its goodness of fit with the aims of the study and to ensure rigor. Two articles meeting the inclusion criteria were used to identify the most appropriate manner to use the instrument and to verify the validity of its content.

2.2. Analysis of Studies

Following categorization, the relevant aspects concerning the identification of the data from the studies and their content concerning introduction, methods, results, and conclusions were analyzed. Synthesis of information is presented in a descriptive manner and tables are used to summarize data, as well as the main findings of this study.

2.3. Interpretation of Results

Data are discussed and compared to theoretical knowledge addressing the implications resulting from this study.

2.4. Presentation of the Integrative Review

The review presents relevant and detailed information on procedures and findings and contributes to a critical analysis and a more thorough understanding of the subject under study.

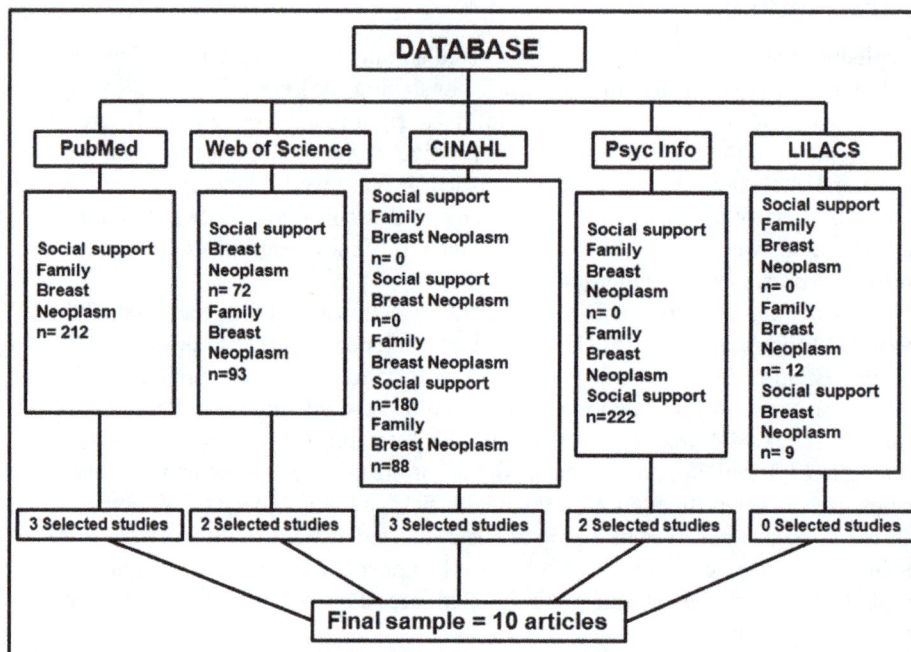

Figure 1. References resulting from the combination of the search terms using the PUBMED, WEB OF SCIENCE, CINAHL, PSYCINFO and LILACS databases.

3. Results

Ten articles were selected for full-text analysis. Their data were extracted and analyzed for categorization based on the data collection instrument that was used in this review. Each paper and corresponding data collection instrument was given an identification number to generate an organized information structure. **Table 1** lists details of the studies included in this review.

All ten papers included in the sample were published in English. Six of them originated in the United States [7]-[10] [14] [15]; one paper was published in Canada [12], another one in England [13], one in Holland [11], and one paper was published in Israel [16].

An analysis of the database showed that three papers were found in PubMed [7]-[9], another two in Web of Sciences [10] [11], three in CINALH [12]-[14], and two in PsycInfo [15] [16]. In regard to the studies' methodological design, one consisted of a randomized clinical trial [13] and nine were descriptive studies [7]-[12] [14]-[16].

We verified that researchers from the nursing field wrote four of the papers and only one study was conducted in partnership with other professionals, such as physicians. In regard to the year of publication, the papers were published between 1989 and 2011. The United States accounted for the highest number of publications and, even though some studies had other countries of origin, English predominated. In regard to characteristics concerning the types of studies, of the ten studies included in this review, one used a quantitative methodological approach, a randomized clinical trial with evidence level II [13]. The other nine studies used a qualitative methodological approach and were all descriptive studies with level of evidence IV [7]-[12] [14]-[16].

4. Discussion

The results are consistent with existing literature addressing the need for support of women undergoing breast cancer treatment. Women undergoing treatment require greater support and are, in fact, more likely to receive it. This review shows that individuals undergoing treatment experience more problems concerning psychological, social, sexual and emotional issues and usually obtain the support and help necessary to overcome these side effects.

Additionally, emotional support influences the decisions women make to adhere to treatment, which also agrees with one study reporting that emotional support can influence and/or facilitate decisions concerning treatment adherence and post-treatment care, contributing to health promotion [17].

Studies suggest there is a source of discomfort within the patient/spouse dyad due to changes in roles imposed by the disease and, as a result, the support provided is no longer a protective factor against distress [18]. No studies were found addressing a lack of balance between couples facing breast cancer. Even though patients facing such an important stressor related to health do benefit from support provided by the spouses, these benefits are also extended to the spouses themselves. Women with breast cancer may benefit their spouses with intimacy and

Table 1. Details of the studies included in this review.

Study	Experimental design	Year/Country
Belcher, *et al.* [7]	Descriptive	2011/United States
Budin [8]	Descriptive	1998/United States
Walsh [9]	Descriptive	2005/United States
Lepore *et al.* [10]	Descriptive	2008/United States
Oudsten *et al.* [11]	Descriptive	2009/Holland
Zemore, Shepel [12]	Descriptive	1989/Canada
Gellaitry *et al.* [13]	Randomized controlled clinical trial	2009/England
Makabe, Hull [14]	Descriptive	2000/United States
Alferi *et al.* [15]	Descriptive	2001/United States
Feigin *et al.* [16]	Descriptive	2000/Israel

provide support. The daily relationship between couples may benefit the patient's wellbeing and provide a sense of connection through receiving and providing daily support to each other [7].

Women with breast cancer perceive that less social support is provided over time. Some report that a lack of balance is perceived when support requested is not provided or when the support provided was not the support sought. One should take into account that perception of social support may be influenced by personality factors along with one's psychological state [11].

One study reports that women receive high levels of support but that it decreases over time [17]. This perception of decreased support may be related to lower availability of support or a lower quality of support, when available. The author speculates there are three explanations for these results: first, ongoing support affects the one providing it and may result in exhaustion; second, women acquire skills to deal with the disease over time, thereby the need for support provided by family, friends and others may decrease; and third, this perception of reduced support may be related to a certain incompatibility between the patient's real needs and the support provided.

Patients experiencing greater psychological distress may view the supply of support as a sign of personal incompetence or loss or need for a previous level of independence. This may occur when the social support provided does not agree with one's needs or desires. Likewise, it may occur when there is a lack of clear communication between suppliers and recipients of support, while such a lack of communication results in members of the social network being ill-informed regarding the patient's situation. When support emphasizes the vulnerability of the recipients of care, their dependency or inequality, or when the recipient does not feel able to reciprocate, patients may feel more distress over support. Reciprocity attenuates the relationship between support supply and self-esteem or between support and distress among Japanese women. In this women's cultural norm, giving back kindness received is the key to avoiding a sense of guilt and shame in their social interactions. If they cannot reciprocate, the support provided may become a negative and interfere in their self-esteem [17].

This review's findings indicate that distress and depression related to treatment side effects, together with social support, affect a patient's psychosocial adjustment to breast cancer and are consistent with the literature. This situation occurs in a greater proportion of patients in chemotherapy in which women under treatment experience significantly greater distress and experience problems regarding psychosocial adjustment. High levels of anxiety and distress and low affability tend to reduce as one's perception of social support due to psychosocial changes are experienced by women undergoing breast cancer treatment.

Compared to older women, younger women with breast cancer are more likely to experience adverse psychosocial outcomes. This study found an inverse relationship between age and discomfort, indicating that older participants experience less distress [19].

Single women report not being affected by the lack of a husband, though they were surrounded by family members and friends who provided support. Women with partners tend to have better mental health compared to single women. Among various types of instrumental and emotional support provided by other significant people, only emotional support provided by spouses, such as listening to concerns and instrumental support when helping at home, are predictors of less depressive symptoms [20].

Different types of social support are tightly connected with quality of life. Attitudes such as involving the partner and the family in treatment so they become aware of the problems women with breast cancer face, educating women concerning the importance of social support, teaching them to ask for help and discuss their needs, are exercises of social support. During treatment, women often suffer from distress and social support may be provided when these actions are implemented, leading them to experience better quality of life.

Other types of support that influence quality of life include: support groups and expressive writing. Given the stress accruing from experiencing cancer, a support group is essential to maintaining patients' hope and wellbeing. Women participating in support groups acquire more acknowledgment, awareness and management practices to deal with their treatment.

The direct effect of religious support was not found in the analyzed studies. This is inconsistent with the results of some previous studies specifically addressing positive effects of religion and, at the same time, is consistent with other studies suggesting that religion does not have a significant impact on the survival of breast cancer patients [21]. These relationships may be discussed in light of recent literature. Seeking support in religion through ritual practices or by invoking God in a situation of disease is an easily accessible strategy [22]. Religiosity may be both a negative and positive coping strategy. Individuals dealing with stress may become dependent on religious resources or question their own religion [23]. Additionally, people facing great hardships may seek comfort in religion.

Support during treatment comprises a complex balance among family, social well-being, psychosocial adjustment and quality of life. Finally, the success of treatment is not determined only by the cure of the disease, but mainly by how the patient perceives quality of life, one aspect of which is social support.

5. Conclusions

Women with breast cancer undergoing treatment have a real need for support. Providing social support is a part of integral care provided by nurses. Emotional support was the most beneficial in the adjustment of women with breast cancer, generating opportunities for them to express feelings and favoring treatment adherence. The main sources are the spouse, family and friends, while the spouse is the most important emotional support and the main source of instrumental support.

Over time, women may perceive a decrease in emotional support, which may be related to personality factors or to one's psychological state. In some cases, women may even interpret the reception of support as personal incompetence.

Distress and depression accruing from the side effects of treatment together with perceived support may affect the psychosocial adjustment of women with breast cancer. Religiosity does not directly influence quality of life, though social support provided by support groups and ways to express feelings such as writing, may influence quality of life.

6. Relevance to Clinical Practice

Health professionals should assess women's social networks, observing sources of support, the type of support provided and whether the needs of patients are being met by the support provided. Information needs of women should be assessed and acknowledged by nurses and other health workers, highlighting not only the importance of emotional and instrumental support but also of informational support. Support may be provided during treatment in environments where women have the opportunity to express their needs, feelings, and share their experiences with the disease.

Even though the experience of the women addressed in these studies probably does not represent the experience of the entire population of women with breast cancer, the knowledge acquired from these papers can be used by professionals around the world to explore the needs of women undergoing treatment in their own configurations for support, considering the context of practice of each professional, their competencies and skills and the preferences of women under their care.

Conflict of Interest

The authors do not have any conflict of interest.

References

[1]   Urban, C.A., Lima, R.S., Schunemann Junior, E., Hakimneto, C.A., Yamada, A. and Torres, L.F.B. (2001)Linfonodo Sentinela: Um Novo Conceito no Tratamento Cirúrgico do Câncer de Mama. *Revista do Colégio Brasileiro de Cirurgiões*, **28**,1-7. http://dx.doi.org/10.1590/S0100-69912001000300011

[2]   Moura, F.M.J.S.P., Silva, M.G., Oliveira, S.C. and Moura, L.J.S.P. (2010) Os Sentimentos das Mulheres Pós-Mastectomizadas.*Revista Escola de Enfermagem Anna Nery*, **14**, 477-484. http://dx.doi.org/10.1590/S1414-81452010000300007

[3]   Moreira, C.B., Fernandes, A.F.C., Gomes, A.M.F., Silva, A.M.L. and Santos, M.C.L. (2013) Educational Strategy Experimented with Mastectomized Women: Experience Report. *Journal of Nursing UFPE on Line*, **7**, 302-305. http://dx.doi.org/10.5205/reuol.3049-24704-1-LE.0701201339

[4]   Tilden, V.P. and Weinert, C. (1987) Social Support and the Chronically Ill Individual. *Nursing Clinics of North America*, **22**, 613-620.

[5]   Whittemore, R. and Knalf, K. (2005) The Integrative Review: Update Methodology. *Journal of Advanced Nursing*, **52**, 546-553. http://dx.doi.org/10.1111/j.1365-2648.2005.03621.x

[6]   Ursi, E.S. and Gavão, C.M. (2006). Prevenção de Lesões de Pele no Perioperatório: Revisão Integrativa da Literatura. *Revista Latino-Americana de Enfermagem*, **14**, 124-131. http://dx.doi.org/10.1590/S0104-11692006000100017

[7]   Belcher, A.J., Laurenceau, J.P., Graber, E.C., Cohen, L.H. and Dasch, K.B. (2011) Daily Support in Couples Coping with Early Stage Breast Cancer: Maintaining Intimacy during Adversity. *Health Psychology*, **30**, 665-673. http://dx.doi.org/10.1037/a0024705

[8]   Budin, W.C. (1998) Psychosocial Adjustment to Breast Cancer in Unmarried Women. *Research in Nursing & Health*, **21**, 155-166. http://dx.doi.org/10.1002/(SICI)1098-240X(199804)21:2<155::AID-NUR6>3.0.CO;2-I

[9]   Walsh, J.M. (2005) Social Support as a Mediator between Symptom Distress and Quality of Life in Women with Breast Cancer. *Journal of Obstetric, Gynecologic, & Neonatal Nursing*, **34**, 482-493. http://dx.doi.org/10.1177/0884217505278310

[10]   Lepore, S.J., Glaser, D.B. and Roberts, K.J. (2008) On the Positive Relation between Received Social Support and Negative Affect: A Test of Triage and Self-Esteem Threat Models in Women with Breast Cancer. *Psycho-Oncology*, **17**, 1210-1215. http://dx.doi.org/10.1002/pon.1347

[11]   Oudsten, B.L.D., Heck, G.L.V., Van der Steeg, A.F.W., Roukema, J.A. and Vries, J.D. (2009) Personality Predicts Perceived Availability of Social Support and Satisfaction with Social Support in Women with Early Stage Breast Cancer. *Supportive Care in Cancer*, **18**, 499-508. http://dx.doi.org/10.1007/s00520-009-0714-3

[12]   Zemore, R. and Shepel, L.F. (1989) Effects of Breast Cancer and Mastectomy on Emotional Support and Adjustment. *Social Science & Medicine*, **28**, 19-27. http://dx.doi.org/10.1016/0277-9536(89)90302-X

[13]   Gellaitry, G., Peters, K., Bloomfield, D. and Horne, R. (2009) Narrowing the Gap: The Effects of an Expressive Writing Intervention on Perceptions of Actual and Ideal Emotional Support in Women Who Have Completed Treatment for Early Stage Breast Cancer. *Psycho-Oncology*, **19**, 77-84. http://dx.doi.org/10.1002/pon.1532

[14]   Makabe, R. and Hull, M.M. (2000) Components of Social Support among Japanese Women with Breast Cancer. *Oncology Nursing Forum*, **27**, 1381-1390.

[15]   Alferi, S.M., Carver, C.S., Antoni, M.H., Weiss, S. and Durán, R.E. (2001) An Exploratory Study of Social Support, Distress, and Life Disruption among Low-Income Hispanic Women under Treatment for Early Stage Breast Cancer. *Health Psychology*, **20**, 41-46. http://dx.doi.org/10.1037/0278-6133.20.1.41

[16]   Feigin, R., Greenberg, A., Ras, H., Hardan, Y., Rizel, S., Efraim, T.B. and Stemmer, S.M. (2000) The Psychosocial Experience of Women Treated for Breast Cancer by High-Dose Chemotherapy Supported by Autologous Stem Cell Transplant: A Qualitative Analysis of Support Groups. *Psycho-Oncology*, **9**, 57-68. http://dx.doi.org/10.1002/(SICI)1099-1611(200001/02)9:1<57::AID-PON434>3.0.CO;2-C

[17]   Arora, N.K., Rutten, L.J.F., Gustafson, D.H., Moser, R. and Hawkins, R.P. (2007) Perceived Helpfulness and Impact of Social Support Provided by Family, Friends, and Health Care Providers to Women Newly Diagnosed with Breast Cancer. *Psycho-Oncology*, **16**, 474-486. http://dx.doi.org/10.1002/pon.1084

[18]   Soler-Vila, H., Kasl, S.V. and Jones, B.A. (2003) Prognostic Significance of Psychosocial Factors in African-American and White Breast Cancer Patients. *Cancer*, **98**, 1299-1308. http://dx.doi.org/10.1002/cncr.11670

[19]   Nausheen, B. and Kamal, A. (2007) Familial Social Support and Depression in Breast Cancer: An Exploratory Study on a Pakistani Sample. *Psycho-Oncology*, **16**, 859-862. http://dx.doi.org/10.1002/pon.1136

[20]   Maly, R.C., Umezawa, Y., Leak, B. and Silliman, R.A. (2005) Mental Health Outcomes in Older Women with Breast Cancer: Impact of Perceived Family Support and Adjustment. *Psycho-Oncology*, **14**, 535-545. http://dx.doi.org/10.1002/pon.869

[21]   Tominaga, K., Andow, J., Koyama, Y., Numao, S., Kurokawa, E., Ojima, M. and Nagai, M. (1998) Family Envairoment, Hobbies and Habits as Psychosocial Predictors of Survival for Surgically Treated Patients with Breast Cancer. *Japanese Journal of Clinical Oncology*, **28**, 36-41.

[22]   Fernandes, A.F.C., Bonfim, I.M., Araújo, I.M.A., Silva, R.M., Barbosa, I.C.F.J. and Santos, M.C.L. (2012) Significado do cuidado familiar à mulher mastectomizada. *Escola Anna Nery*, **16**, 27-33. http://dx.doi.org/10.1590/S1414-81452012000100004

[23]   Hasson-Ohayon, I., Goldzweig, G., Braun, M. and Galinsky, D. (2010) Women with Advanced Breast Cancer and Their Spouses: Diversity of Support and Psychological Distress. *Psycho-Oncology*, **19**, 1195-1204. http://dx.doi.org/10.1002/pon.1678

3

Patient with Metastatic Breast Cancer Achieves Stable Disease for 5 Years on Graviola and Xeloda after Progressing on Multiple Lines of Therapy

Damien Mikael Hansra, Orlando Silva, Ashwin Mehta, Eugene Ahn

Department of Hematology and Oncology, Sylvester Comprehensive Cancer Center at the University of Miami, Miami, USA
Email: dmhansra@med.miami.edu

Abstract

Breast cancer (BC) is the most common malignancy in women and is second to lung cancer in terms of cancer mortality. Treatment of BC remains a challenge as current therapies are limited by toxicity and drug resistance. Graviola (*Annona muricata*) is a tree that grows in the tropics of North and South America. Traditionally, the leaves and stems from the graviola tree have been used for a wide range of human diseases including cancer. *In vitro* and *in vivo* studies demonstrate anticancer activity in BC however clinical studies are lacking. We present the first case demonstrating clinical benefit without side effects using graviola in a patient with BC whose disease was refractory to multiple lines of chemotherapy including anthracyclines and taxanes.

Keywords

Breast Cancer, Graviola, Therapy

1. Introduction

Breast cancer (BC) is the most common malignancy in women and treatment of BC remains challenge as current therapies are limited secondary to toxicity and drug resistance. New integrative treatment strategies should be explored. Graviola (*Annona muricata*) is an Amazon fruit tree that grows in the tropics of North and South America and has been used for a wide range of human diseases including inflammatory conditions, rheumatism, neuralgia, diabetes, hypertension, insomnia, cystitis, parasitic infections, and cancer. Despite graviola being used for centuries, research on its health benefits has been extremely limited. To date there are no published reports on outcomes using graviola in cancer patients.

2. Methods

A retrospective chart review of one patient diagnosed with BC from 1999-2012. Detailed clinical history was obtained including age at diagnosis, stage at diagnosis, therapy (chemotherapy, hormone, graviola) and response to therapy. Review of laboratory data was performed including liver function testing and tumor markers. Finally imaging with FDG PET CT was reviewed from diagnosis to end of study.

3. Results

A 66-year-old female diagnosed with estrogen and progesterone receptor positive human epidermal growth factor receptor negative pT2N1M0 stage IIb of the left breast cancer diagnosed in 1998 status post lumpectomy, adjuvant anthracycline & taxane based chemotherapy followed by breast radiation completed in 1999. She subsequently presented with biopsy proven lung metastasis in 2002. She was started on hormonal therapy and progressed on Femara, Tamoxifen, and Faslodex. Chemotherapy with Navelbine was initiated from March 2005 until February 2006, Abraxane, Avastin, Gemcitabine (AAG) from Feburary 2006 to May 2007, Doxil from May 2007 to September 2007. Unfortunately the patient was found to have new liver metastases and she was started on Xeloda 2500 mg PO daily (2 weeks on 1 week off) at that time. The patient also started using graviola 10 - 12 dry leaves boiled in water for 5 - 7 minutes, 8 oz. PO daily at that time. Tumor markers at time of initiation of graviola and Xeloda were CEA 12.5 ng/ml (0.0 - 3.4 ng/mL), CA 15-3 1249.0 U/ml (0.0 - 25.0 U/mL), CA 27-29 1295 U/ml (<38 U/mL). Tumor markers in April 2008 were: CEA 5.9 ng/ml, CA 15-3 68.6 U/ml, CA 27-29 113 U/ml. Patient moved to Alaska and continued her regimen, then returned in December 2011 and autonomously discontinued graviola at that time. Labs in March 2012 showed AST 75 U/L (15 - 46 U/L) ALT 84 U/L (9 - 52 U/L), CEA 4.3 ng/ml, CA 15-3 25.7 U/ml, CA 27.29 35 U/ml. Also, PET-CT at that time demonstrated worsening left upper lung disease. Graviola was re-initiated at this point and labs in November 2012 showed AST 43 U/L, ALT 50 U/L, CEA 2.9, CA 27-29 32 U/ml, CA 15-3 20.7 U/ml. Re-imaging with PET/CT in November 2012 showed stable disease. So far, patient has had stable disease and experienced no side effects from therapy for over 5 years.

4. Discussion

Breast cancer (BC) is the most common malignancy in women and is second to lung cancer in terms of cancer mortality. An estimated 234,580 Americans will be diagnosed with BC and 40,030 will die of the disease in the United States in 2013 [1]. Treatment of BC remains a challenge as current therapies are limited secondary to toxicity and drug resistance and alternative treatment strategies should be explored. Furthermore the incidence of breast cancer has been steadily increasing over the past few decades [2] necessitating development of greater preventative strategies. It is well established that increased consumption of fruits and vegetables is associated with a reduced risk of most cancers [3]. The beneficial effect is partly due to the fact that fruits and vegetables contain antioxidants, fiber, and other potentially antineoplastic compounds. For this reason, natural products have been investigated as potential anticancer agents with the most attractive feature of these agents being limited side effect profiles as compared to conventional chemotherapeutic drugs. Specific bioactive compounds in foods, notably sulfur-containing gluconsinolates and green tea polyphenols are associated with reduced risk of BC risk [4] [5]. Graviola (*Annonaceous muricata* L.) is an Amazon fruit tree that grows in the tropics of North and South America and is also known as soursop and guanabana. Traditionally, the leaves and stems from the graviola tree have been used for a wide range of human diseases including inflammatory conditions, rheumatism, neuralgia, diabetes, hypertension, insomnia, cystitis, parasitic infections, and cancer [6] [7]. Graviola has been widely consumed by indigenous people for centuries however research on its health benefits are extremely limited. To date there are no published reports on outcomes using graviola in cancer patients. We present the first case demonstrating clinical benefit using graviola in a patient with BC. Arguably, the patient was taking single agent chemotherapy however the median progression free survival on single agent Xeloda in the metastatic setting is only a few months [8]. Also, the patient's liver function tests were elevated off graviola in the absence of other non-metastatic causes of hepatic injury and then normalized once graviola was resumed. This further supports the notion that graviola stabilized our patient's disease. The exact mechanism of graviola in cancer cells is under investigation. Annonaceous acetogenins, the major bioactive components in graviola, are derivatives of long chain fatty acids that are selectively toxic to cancer cells, including multidrug resistant cancer cell lines [9]-[13] [14]. One study found that graviola inhibited tumorgenicity and metastasis in pancreatic cancer cells *in vitro* and *in vivo* by inhibiting multiple signaling pathways that regulate metabolism, cell cycle, survival, and metastatic properties in pancreatic cells [15]. Another study demonstrated that graviola induced growth inhibition of human breast cancer cells *in vitro* and *in vivo* through a mechanism involving the EGFR/ERK signaling pathway [16]. In terms of toxicity, graviola may cause movement disorders and myeloneuropathy with symptoms mimicking Parkinson's disease [17]. Our patient did not suffer any significant side effects. Further clinical research is required to determine the efficacy, effective dose, potential drug interactions and toxicity so this plant-derived extract could potentially gain approval for usage in breast cancer patients.

References

[1]   American Cancer Society (2012) Cancer Facts and Figures 2012. Atlanta GACS.

[2]   Siegel, R., Ward, E., Brawley, O. and Jemal, A. (2011) Cancer Statistics 2011: The Impact of Eliminating Socioeconomic and Racial Disparities on Premature Cancer Deaths. *CA: A Cancer Journal for Clinicians*, **61**, 212-236. http://dx.doi.org/10.3322/caac.20121

[3]   Chakraborty, S., Baine, M.J., Sasson, A.R. and Batra, S.K. (2011) Current Status of Molecular Markers for Early Detection of Sporadic Pancreatic Cancer. *Biochimica et Biophysica Acta (BBA)*, **1815**, 44-64

[4]   Duffy, C. and Cyr, M. (2003) Phytoestrogens: Potential Benefits and Implications for Breast Cancer Survivors. *Journal of Women's Health*, **12**, 617-631.

[5]   Mukhtar, H. and Ahmad, N. (2000) Tea Polyphenols: Prevention of Cancer and Optimizing Health. *The American Journal of Clinical Nutrition*, **71**, 1698-1702.

[6]   Taylor, L. (2002) Technical Data Report for Graviola: *Annona muricata*. Sage Press, Inc., Herbal Secrets of the Rainforest second ed.

[7]   Adewole, S.O. and Caxton-Martins, E.A. (2006) Morphological Changes and Hypoglycemic Effects of *Annona muricata* Linn. (Annonaceae) Leaf Aqueous Extract on Pancreatic B-Cells of Streptozotocin-Treated Diabetic Rats. *African Journal of Biomedical Research*, **9**, 173-187.

[8]   Bajetta, E., Procopio, G., Celio, L., *et al.* (2005) Safety and Efficacy of Two Different Doses of Capecitabine in the Treatment of Advanced Breast Cancer in the Treatment of Advanced Breast Cancer in Older Women. *Journal of Clinical Oncology*, **23**, 2155-2161. http://dx.doi.org/10.1200/JCO.2005.02.167

[9]   Oberlies, N.H., Jones, J.L., Corbett, T.H., Fotopoulos, S.S. and McLaughlin, J.L. (1995) Tumor Cell Growth Inhibition by Several Annonaceous Acetogenins in an *in vitro* Disk Diffusion Assay. *Cancer Letters*, **96**, 55-62. http://dx.doi.org/10.1016/0304-3835(95)92759-7

[10]   McLaughlin, J.L. (2008) Paw Paw and Cancer: Annonaceous Acetogenins from Discovery to Commercial Products. *Journal of Natural Products*, **71**, 1311-1321. http://dx.doi.org/10.1021/np800191t

[11]   Tormo, J.R., Royo, I., Gallardo, T., Zafra-Polo, M.C., Hernandez, P., Cortes, D. and Pelaez, F. (2003) *In Vitro* Antitumor Structure-Activity Relationships of Threo/Trans/Threo Mono-Tetrahydrofuranicacetogenins: Correlations with Their Inhibition of Mitochondrial Complex I. *Oncology Research*, **14**, 147-154.

[12]   Chang, F.R. and Wu, Y.C. (2001) Novel Cytotoxic Annonaceous Acetogenins from *Annona muricata*. *Journal of Natural Products*, **64**, 925-931. http://dx.doi.org/10.1021/np010035s

[13]   Liaw, C.C., Chang, F.R., Lin, C.Y., Chou, C.J., Chiu, H.F., Wu, M.J. and Wu, Y.C. (2002) New Cytotoxic Monotetrahydrofuran Annonaceous Acetogenins from *Annona muricata*. *Journal of Natural Products*, **65**, 470-475. http://dx.doi.org/10.1021/np0105578

[14]   Oberlies, H.N., Chang, C.J. and McLaughlin, J.L. (1997) Structure-Activity Relationships of Diverse Annonaceous Acetogenins against Multidrug Resistant Human Mammary Adenocarcinomas (MCF-7/Adr) Cells. *Journal of Medicinal Chemistry*, **40**, 2102-2106. http://dx.doi.org/10.1021/jm9700169

[15]   Torres, M.P., *et al.* (2012) Graviola: A Novel Promising Natural Derived Drug That Inhibits Tumorgenicity and Metastasis of Pancreatic Cancer Cells *in Vitro* and *in Vivo* through Altering Cell Metabolism. *Cancer Letters*, **323**, 29-40. http://dx.doi.org/10.1016/j.canlet.2012.03.031

[16]   Yumin, D., Hogan, S., Schmelz, E.M., Young, H.J., Canning, C. and Zhou, K. (2011) Selective Growth Inhibition of Human Breast Cancer Cells by Graviola Fruit Extract *in Vitro* and *in Vivo* Involving Downregulation of EGFR Expression. *Nutrition and Cancer*, **63**, 795-801. http://dx.doi.org/10.1080/01635581.2011.563027

[17] Lannuzel, A., Michel, P.P., Caparros-Lefebvre, D., Abaul, J., Hocquemiller, R. and Ruberg, M. (2002) Toxicity of Annonaceae for Dopaminergic Neurons: Potential Role in Atypical Parkinsonism in Guadeloupe. *Movement Disorders*, **17**, 84-90. http://dx.doi.org/10.1002/mds.1246

4

Influence of Surgical Technique on Overall Survival, Disease Free Interval and New Lesion Development Interval in Dogs with Mammary Tumors

Rodrigo dos Santos Horta[1]*, Gleidice Eunice Lavalle[1], Rúbia Monteiro de Castro Cunha[1], Larissa Layara de Moura[1], Roberto Baracat de Araújo[1], Geovanni Dantas Cassali[2]

[1]Veterinary School, Universidade Federal de Minas Gerais-UFMG, Belo Horizonte, Brazil
[2]Biological Sciences Institute, Universidade Federal de Minas Gerais-UFMG, Belo Horizonte, Brazil
Email: *rodrigohvet@gmail.com

Abstract

The best surgical technique for the treatment of mammary tumors in female dogs has been exhaustively debated among the scientific community. Despite biological knowledge of these tumors, some authors have suggested aggressive procedures, without any clinical advantage. The aim of this study was to evaluate the influence of surgical procedure on the overall survival, disease-free interval and new lesion development interval in dogs with mammary tumors treated according to established prognostic factors. This prospective study included 143 intact female dogs that underwent surgery for mammary neoplasms and were followed up for about 738.5 days. Each animal represented a repetition. Each surgical technique represented a group: lumpectomy (P1), mammectomy (P2), regional mastectomy without cranial abdominal gland involvement (P3), regional mastectomy with cranial abdominal gland involvement (P4), and radical mastectomy (P5). Considering only the first surgical event, 84.6% of animals had more than one mammary tumor, and tumors were identified in two mammary chains in 52.5%. There was no difference in ipsilateral and contralateral tumor development when surgical techniques were compared. Only 33 dogs developed new lesions in remaining mammary tissue, without correlation with primary lesion. Surgical technique had no effect on the overall survival, disease-free interval and new lesion development interval in patients on this study, which respected oncological surgery principles and established prognostic factors for mammary gland tumors in dogs.

---

*Corresponding author.

Keywords

Female Dog, Mammary Neoplasms, Mastectomy

1. Introduction

Mammary gland tumors represent 42% of all tumors in the female dog [1]. Although there are numerous studies about disease development and progression, some questions concerning the surgical treatment remain unanswered [2].

Similar to human mammary neoplams [3], lymphatic system represents the main route of metastasis of mammary malignant pathologies of dogs and cats [4]-[6]. In the dog, cranial and caudal thoracic glands drain to axillary lymph nodes, whilst inguinal and caudal abdominal glands drain to inguinal lymph nodes. Cranial abdominal gland, however, may drain to either axillary or inguinal lymph nodes [4] [7]. Axillary lymph nodes are rarely related to mammary cancer in the dog and must be removed with caution, in selected cases. The inguinal lymph node, which is intimately associated with the ipsilateral inguinal gland, should be removed whenever this gland is surgically removed [5]. Connections between glands on different sides and between other mammary glands are rare, but may exist [7]. Pereira *et al.* (2003) [8] reported that neoplastic lesions may induce the development of lymphatic anastomoses, modifying the natural drainage of mammary tissue.

Surgery is the basic treatment of canine mammary tumors and is the most effective for disease regional control [4]. Many surgical techniques may be used for the treatment of canine mammary tumors [5] [9] and similar to Medicine [10] [11]. The advantages and disadvantages of each procedure have been extensively discussed [12]. Radical surgeries were thoroughly performed on women with mammary tumors between 1910 and 1964, without any clinical benefits [13] [14]. As from the 1950's, Halsted's mastectomy started to be questioned [11], however, the lack of clinical benefits of the radical mastectomy was only proved by the end of the 1970's [10]. When studying the biological behavior of canine mammary tumors, Gilbertson *et al.* (1983) [15] indicated the radical mastectomy as the best surgical option. In the same year, Brodey *et al.* (1983) [16] advocated individual treatments, in which surgical procedure should respect known lymphatic connections and base itself on tumor location, number and size of lesions and existence of skin or muscular adherences. Similar to Medicine, a prospective study conducted by MacEwen *et al.* (1985) [17], with 144 dogs, did not find any difference between the recurrence rate and the survival time when the single mastectomy was compared to chain mastectomy.

A greater understanding about the canine mammary pathology and new therapeutic modalities made the definition of distinct groups regarding prognosis and treatment possible [6]. Aggressive surgical procedures for the treatment of localized lesions may reduce the risk of developing new lesions in a small number of dogs, especially in young intact bitches [5]. Stratmann *et al.* (2008) [2] also indicated radical mastectomy as the best surgical option, regardless of the number and the size of lesions. Authors reported a greater probability of new tumor growth ipsilateral to the first surgery, although statistical significance was not assessed.

The purpose of this study is to evaluate the influence of surgical procedure on the survival time, disease free interval and new lesion development interval in dogs with mammary tumors treated according to the biological behavior of these lesions.

2. Materials and Methods

2.1. Inclusion Criteria

Intact bitches were submitted to surgery for the treatment of mammary tumors. Patients that had malignancies with compromised surgical margins (accessed by histopathological evaluation) and/or dogs submitted to targeted adjuvant therapies with the usage of cyclooxygenase inhibitors or ovariohisterectomy during the follow-up were excluded. Adjuvant chemotherapy was performed in selected patients. Candidates to chemotherapy were those with lymph node or distant metastasis and patients with guarded to poor prognostic tumor diagnoses including: micropapilar carcinoma, high degree tubular carcinoma, mucinous, secretory or lipid-rich carcinoma, solid carcinoma, malignant myoepithelioma, carcinosarcoma and other sarcomas [6].

Prior to surgery, all animals went through a complete clinical exam, abdominal ultrasound and two-view thoracic radiographs were taken for metastasis evaluation. Lymph nodes with size, shape or consistency alterations were removed during surgery, but were primarily submitted to fine-needle aspiration cytology for metastasis evaluation.

The ethics committee on animal experiments approved this study (023/2011).

2.2. Choosing the Surgical Technique

The removal of mammary tumors was performed through the simplest and less invasive surgical procedure necessary to the complete removal of all tumors and main known lymphatic connections between affected glands, as suggested by Brodey *et al.* (1983) [16] and Sorenmo *et al.* (2013) [5].

It was not possible to separate the surgical technique used from the type and stage of disease, once the surgical technique was chosen according to number of lesions and site, respecting lymphatic drainage and established prognostic factors such as lesions size and existence of skin or muscular adherences.

Lumpectomy was considered for the removal of single solid superficial non-adherent tumors less than two centimeter wide. Lesions larger than two centimeters implied the need to remove the entire gland. Mammectomy or simple mastectomy was indicated for lesions up to three centimeters, affecting only one gland whilst regional mastectomy was indicated for the removal of lymphatic connections of glands affected by lesions larger than three centimeters. The removal of cranial abdominal gland during regional mastectomy was sometimes necessary to obtain adequate surgical margins or for lesions between one and three centimeters in this gland. Radical mastectomy was the removal of a unilateral mammary chain, when lesions larger than three centimeters affected the cranial abdominal gland. Regional and radical mastectomies were also performed on multiple lesions, of one to three centimeters, to obtain a single surgical wound through a single incision and resection of mammary tissue.

The inguinal lymph nodes were resected in bloc with the inguinal mammary gland whenever this gland was removed or, by the same way as axillary lymph nodes, when changes in their shape, volume or consistency were observed.

The surgically removed tumors were submitted to surgical margin analyses, histopathological evaluation and classification, as proposed by Cassali *et al.* (2011) [6].

2.3. Clinical Follow-Up

Throughout clinical follow up, dogs were examined, including abdominal ultrasound and thoracic radiographic exams, in intervals from three to six months or sooner, in case the owner recognized changes on the mammary chain or in case the patient was submitted to adjuvant chemotherapy. Subsequent surgery was indicated and performed in dogs that developed recurrences or new tumors on the remaining mammary tissue.

The survival time was defined as the time (in days) from the first surgery until death related to the disease. Disease free interval was defined as the time (in months) from the first surgery until development of local recurrence or distant metastatic disease. New mammary lesion development interval was defined as time (in months) from the first surgery until development of subsequent lesions in the remaining mammary tissue.

2.4. Experimental Design and Statistical Analysis

Each animal represented a repetition. Each surgical technique represented a group: lumpectomy (P1), mammectomy (P2), regional mastectomy without cranial abdominal gland involvement (P3), regional mastectomy with cranial abdominal gland involvement (P4), and radical mastectomy (P5).

After the descriptive analysis of data and the determination of malignant lesion frequency according to the surgical technique, the groups were compared with chi-squared test.

The Spearmann's test was used to determine the correlation between the number of lesions and the number of histological diagnoses in dogs that presented multiple mammary lesions at initial diagnoses or that underwent new surgical procedures, due to the development of new lesions in the remaining mammary tissue.

The Spearman's correlation was used to access the association between surgical technique and patient staging. The ages of animals in each surgical technique group were submitted to analysis of variance and the median values were compared with Fisher exact test and Tukey's post-test.

New tumor development can only happen on the same gland of dogs treated by lumpectomy. Radical mastectomy precludes new ipsilateral tumor development. Therefore, new contralateral and ipsilateral mammary lesion development in each surgical technique (with the exception of ipsilateral lesions frequency evaluation for radical mastectomy) was compared by the usage of a chi-squared analysis.

The overall survival, disease free interval and new mammary lesion development interval (unrelated to primary tumor) were estimated by Kaplan-Meier product limit method. The Longrank statistics of Cox-Mantel was used to compare groups. Some cases were censored for analysis whenever follow-up was lost or death was not related to the disease.

Statistical significance for all testing procedures was set at 5%.

3. Results

143 patients were included in this study. Adjuvant chemotherapy was performed with carboplatin (n = 23), carboplatin and doxorubicin (n = 6) or gencitabin and carboplatin (n = 2). Median follow-up was of 738.5 days. The dogs ages ranged from three to 16 years (mean 9.2 ± 2.3 years). There were 23 mixed breed dogs (16%) with the other 120 dogs representing 25 breeds. Poodle was the most common breed (n = 52; 36.4%), followed by Cocker Spaniel (n = 11; 7.7%) and Yorkshire terrier (n = 10; 7%) (**Table 1**).

Considering only the first surgical procedure, 121 (84.6%) of 143 dogs had more than one mammary lesion, and 52.5% of animals had tumors on both mammary chains. Histopathological diagnosis were established for 391 lesions, and 219 (56%) were classified as malignant neoplasms, 121 (31%) were benign neoplasms and 49 (12.5%) were non-neoplastic lesions. Histological types, in each surgical technique, are demonstrated on **Table 2**. Benign mixed tumor represented 56.2% of benign neoplasms, followed by papilloma (23.1%) and adenomas (17.4%). Carcinoma in mixed tumor was the most frequent mammary cancer (47.5%), followed by malignant lesions "*in situ*" (23.3%) and papillary carcinoma (7.7%).

There were no significant differences between surgical techniques with regard to malignant lesion frequency (p > 0.05), however, there was a correlation between patient staging and surgical technique (p < 0.0001; rs = 0.409) and between staging and patient age (p < 0.002; rs = 0.247). The number of animals submitted to each technique and mean age in each group are demonstrated on **Table 3**. Dogs submitted to lumpectomy (P1) were younger than dogs on other groups, and so were animals submitted to regional mastectomy without removal of cranial abdominal gland (P3) compared with those submitted to radical mastectomy (P5) (p < 0.0001).

There was no significant correlation between lesions, but there was a strong association between number of mammary tumors and histological diagnoses variety (p < 0.0001; rs = 0.833), as shown on **Table 4**. Thirty-three (24.8%) dogs developed new tumors on the remaining mammary tissue. The number and percentage of animals that developed new tumors on the same gland where the first tumor was removed (only for lumpectomies), the ipsilateral chain adjacent mammary gland or not adjacent (except for radical mastectomy) or the contralateral mammary chain, according to surgical technique, is shown on **Table 5**. New lesions were not observed in 30%, 72.7%, 72.7%, 71.4% and 90.2% of dogs in groups P1, P2, P3, P4 and P5, respectively. There was no significant

Table 1. Breeds from the 143 dogs submitted to surgical treatment for the removal of mammary tumors.

	Number	Percentage
Poodle	52	36.4%
Cocker Spaniel	11	7.7%
Yorkshire Terrier	10	7.0%
Dachshund	7	4.9%
Pinscher	6	4.2%
German Shepherd	6	4.2%
Bichon frise	4	2.8%
Others	24	16.8%
Crossbreed	23	16.1%
Total	143	100%

Table 2. Histopathological exams results and number of lesions found for each tumor type for each surgical technique on 143 dogs.

Malignant neoplasms	Surgical technique					
	P1	P2	P3	P4	P5	TOTAL
Carcinoma in mixed tumor	6	5	25	12	56	104
"*in situ*" carcinoma	1	2	6	13	29	51
Papillary carcinoma	0	1	2	4	10	17
Tubular carcinoma	0	0	0	1	10	11
Solid carcinoma	0	0	0	5	4	9
Tubulopapillary carcinoma	1	0	4	0	3	8
Carcinosarcoma	0	0	1	1	4	6
Complex carcinoma	0	0	2	1	0	3
Mucinous, secretory or lipid-rich carcinoma	0	0	0	0	3	3
Malignant myoepithelioma	0	0	0	0	2	2
Hemangiosarcoma	0	1	1	0	0	2
Sarcoma in mixed tumor	0	0	0	0	1	1
Osteosarcoma	0	0	0	0	1	1
Micropapillary carcinoma	0	0	0	0	1	1
TOTAL	8	9	41	37	124	219
Malignant neoplasms						
Benign mixed tumor	3	4	16	19	26	68
Papilloma	1	5	5	5	12	28
Simple, basaloid and complex adenoma	0	2	2	6	11	21
Adenomioepitelioma	0	0	1	0	0	1
Lipoma	0	0	1	0	0	1
Hemangioma	0	0	0	0	1	1
Fibroadenoma	0	0	0	0	1	1
TOTAL	4	11	25	30	51	121
Malignant neoplasms						
Ductaland lobular hyperplasia	1	0	7	5	19	32
Mastitis	0	0	2	6	7	15
Columnar cell lesion	0	0	0	0	2	2
TOTAL	1	0	9	11	28	49

P1—Lumpectomy; P2—Mammectomy; P3—Regional mastectomy without involvement of cranial abdominal gland; P4—Regional mastectomy with involvement of cranial abdominal gland; P5—Radical mastectomy.

difference between development of tumors ipsilaterally or contralaterally in regard to surgical technique (p > 0.05).

During follow-up, only fifteen, of 33 animals that developed new mammary lesions on the remaining tissue after the first surgery were submitted to subsequent surgery. There was no correlation between lesions (p > 0.05), and only five dogs (33.3%) had the same histological type on both procedures.

Table 3. Number of animals, mean of age and standard deviation in each group, by surgical technique.

	Number	Age ($x \pm s^2$)
Lumpectomy	10	6.2 ± 2.2
Mammectomy	11	10.0 ± 2.3
Regional mastectomy without involvement of cranial abdominal gland	33	8.9 ± 2.2
Regional mastectomy with involvement of cranial abdominal gland	28	10.2 ± 2.5
Radical mastectomy	61	10.5 ± 2.2
Total	143	9.7 ± 2.3

Table 4. Number of lesions and mean of distinct diagnoses on 143 dogs.

	Number of patients	Mean of distinct diagnosis
One lesion	33	1.00
Two lesions	43	1.74
Three lesions	31	2.45
Four lesions	24	2.96
Five lesions	4	3.50
Six lesions	3	4.00
Seven lesions	4	4.75
13 lesions	1	6.00
Total	143	2.14

Table 5. Number and percentage of animals that developed new tumors by surgical technique.

	Same mammary gland	Ipsilateral mammary chain adjacent gland	Ipsilateral mammary chain non adjacent gland	Contralateral mammary chain
Lumpectomy	4 (40%)	2 (20%)	1 (10%)	3 (30%)
Mammectomy	-	0 (0%)	2 (18.2%)	2 (18.2%)
Regional mastectomy without involvement of cranial abdominal gland	-	2 (6.1%)	4 (12.2%)	5 (15.2%)
Regional mastectomy with involvement of cranial abdominal gland	-	0 (0%)	2 (7.1%)	7 (25%)
Radical mastectomy	-	-	-	6 (9.8%)

None of the patients submitted to lumpectomy and mammectomy died due to the disease or developed signs of the disease during follow-up. It was observed greater survival (p < 0.03) and disease free interval (p < 0.05) in patients of groups P1 and P2, when compared with P5, as shown in **Figure 1** and **Figure 2**, respectively. New lesion development interval (**Figure 3**) was random and there was no evidence of reducing the interval of development of new lesions by using of a more extensive surgical technique (p > 0.05).

4. Discussion

The mean age of dogs diagnosed with mammary tumors and the search for veterinary assistance were in accordance with earlier reports [4] [18]-[20]. The high incidence of crossbreeds, Poodles and Cocker spaniels may be related to population profile. However, in a study by Zatloukal et al. (2005) [20], of 214 dogs, Poodles and Cocker spaniels had a statistically significant higher relative risk of developing mammary gland neoplasms.

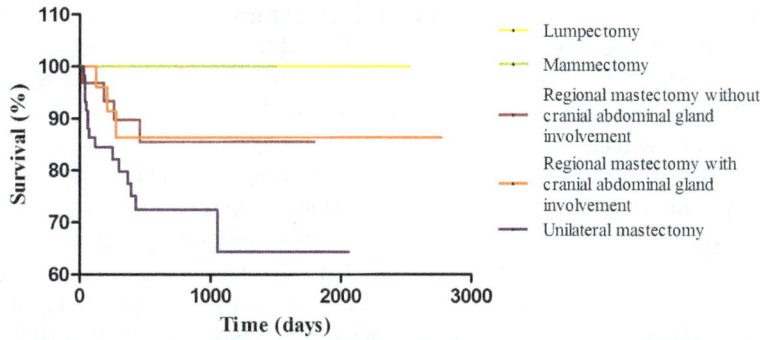

Figure 1. Graphical representation (Kaplan-Meier curve) of survival evaluation of 143 dogs with mammary tumors, by surgical technique.

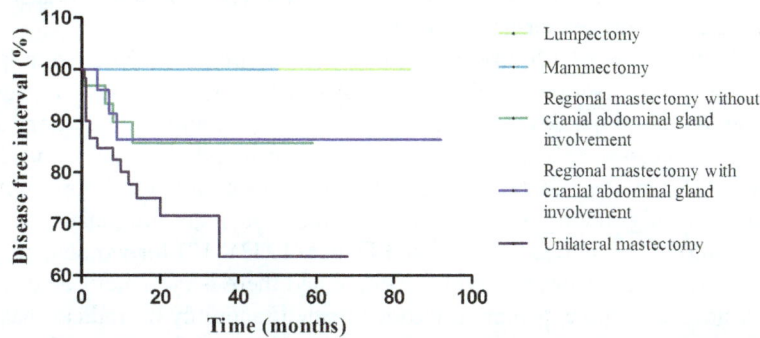

Figure 2. Graphical representation (Kaplan-Meier curve) of disease free interval evaluation of 143 dogs with mammary tumors, by surgical technique.

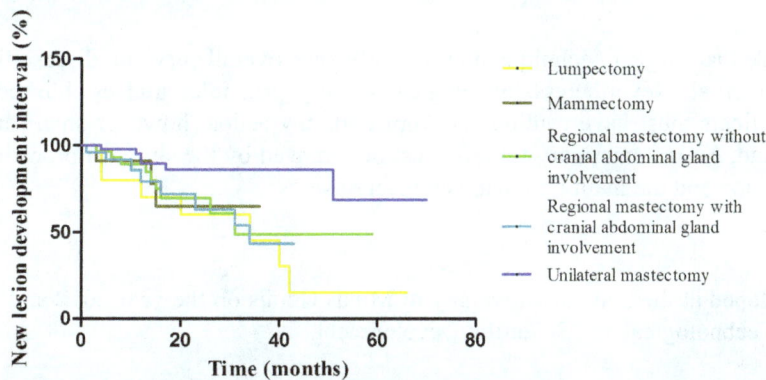

Figure 3. Graphical representation (Kaplan-Meier curve) of new lesion development interval evaluation of 143 dogs with mammary tumors, by surgical technique.

Multiple mammary tumors, seen in 84.6% of animals in this study, are not related with the possibility of multicentric disease and do not imply a worse prognosis [4]. Fowler *et al.* (1974) [21] and Benjamin *et al.* (1999) [22] described multiple lesions in over 60% of the cases, and each tumor should be examined separately, because there is a great possibility of distinct histopathological diagnoses. The strong correlation between number of lesions and distinct diagnoses, which occurred in 83.3% of the study population, is in accordance with Fowler *et al.* (1974) [21] and Cassali *et al.* (2011) [6].

In this study, malignant neoplasm frequency of 56% was superior to the 50% ratio reported by Sorenmo (2003) [4] and Sorenmo *et al.* (2013) [5]. However, De Nardi *et al.* (2002) [19] and Filho *et al.* (2010) [23], reported malignancy ratios of 68.4% and 73.3%, respectively. These differences may be related to regional characteristics as contraceptive use [19] and delay in the search for veterinary assistance. In this study, benign mixed tumor was the most frequent benign neoplasm (56.2%), but it was the second most frequently diagnosed (40%) by Filho *et al.* (2010) [23]. Likewise, carcinoma in mixed tumor represented 47.5% of malignant neoplasms in this study, and 20.5% on the study by Filho *et al.* (2010) [23]. Frequencies reported in this study for each histological type differ from international literature reports [2] [15] [16], probably due to a lack of histological standardization for canine mammary tumors [24].

Surgical technique, performed as proposed by Brodey *et al.* (1983) [16] and Sorenmo *et al.* (2013) [5], was related to patient staging in 40.9% of the population in this study. There was a correlation between staging and patient age in 24.7% of cases, which implied the need for more aggressive surgery on older animals. World Health Organization (WHO) stage III, IV or V in older patients may be related to interval between tumor development and veterinary assistance, leading to the need of more aggressive procedures in these animals [25]. Gilbertson *et al.* (1983) [15] reported that some mammary lesions are associated with a higher risk for the development of invasive malignant neoplasms. Cassali *et al.* (2011) [6], reported alterations on the mammary epithelium molecular expression pattern suggesting intraepithelial and intraductal lesions, as the ones reported in this study, which may represent pre-neoplastic lesions and a premature level of canine breast cancer development, and substantiates premature and simpler surgical procedures.

Unlike the report by Stratmann *et al.* (2008) [2], there was no significant difference in ipsilateral and contralateral tumor development between surgical techniques, probably because, in this study, surgical technique was not randomly chosen, but based on macroscopic disease and clinical features. In addition, there was no correlation between subsequent lesions, probably due to a more detailed histopathological evaluation of each lesion.

Survival and disease free interval estimates were higher for dogs submitted to lumpectomy or mammectomy. This result may be related to early staging of these patients, which has better prognostic factors.

As MacEwen *et al.* (1985) [17] reported for dogs and Fisher (1977) [10] for women, surgical technique must be chosen based on prognostic factors described on literature and there is no benefit on overall survival, disease free interval and new lesion development interval in dogs treated randomly by radical mastectomy [5]. The effectiveness of a surgical treatment depends on the surgeon's overall understanding of the overall health of the patient, type and stage of cancer, adjuvant therapies available and expected prognosis [26].

5. Conclusion

Therefore, we conclude that surgical technique does not influence overall survival, disease free interval and new lesion development interval. Nevertheless, oncological surgery principles and established prognostic factors must be respected; patients must have routine checkups and, any lesion, however small, must be prematurely removed by surgery and; canine mammary tumors must be removed by the simplest procedure, with the goal of removing the entire lesion and the main lymphatic connections.

Funding

This article was developed at the Federal University of Minas Gerais on the year 2012 and was financed by the National Counsel of Technological and Scientific Development.

References

[1]   Johnson, S.D. (1993) Reproductive Systems. In: Slatter, D., Ed., *Textbook of Small Animal Surgery*, 2nd Edition, Saunders Company, Philadelphia, 2177-2192.

[2]   Stratmann, N., Failing, K., Richter, A. and Wehrend, A. (2008) Mammary Tumor Recurrence in Bitches after Regional Mastectomy. *Veterinary Surgery*, **37**, 82-86. http://dx.doi.org/10.1111/j.1532-950X.2007.00351.x

[3]   Mohammed, R.A.A., Martin, S.G., Mahmmod, A.M., Macmillan, R.D., Green, A.R., Paish, E.C. and Ellis, I.O. (2011) Objective Assessment of Lymphatic and Blood Vascular Invasion in Lymph Node-Negative Breast Carcinoma: Findings from a Large Case Series with Long-Term Follow-Up. *Journal of Pathology*, **223**, 358-365. http://dx.doi.org/10.1002/path.2810

[4]   Sorenmo, K. (2003) Canine Mammary Gland Tumors. *Veterinary Clinics of North America*: *Small Animal Practice*, **33**, 573-596. http://dx.doi.org/10.1016/S0195-5616(03)00020-2

[5]   Sorenmo, K.U., Worley, D.R. and Goldschmidt, M.H. (2013) Tumors of the Mammary Gland. In: Withrow, S.J., Vail, D.M. and Page, R.P., Eds., *Withrow and MacEwen's Small Animal Clinical Oncology*, 5th Edition, Saunders Company, Philadelphia, 538-556. http://dx.doi.org/10.1016/B978-1-4377-2362-5.00027-X

[6]　Cassali, G.D., Lavalle, G.E., De Nardi, A.B., Ferreira, E., Bertagnolli, A.C., Estrela-Lima, A., *et al.* (2011) Consensus for the Diagnosis, Prognosis and Treatment of Canine Mammary Tumors. *Brazilian Journal of Veterinary Pathology*, **4**, 153-180.

[7]　Patsikas, M.N. and Dessiris, A. (2006) The Lymph Drainage of the Neoplastic Mammary Glands in the Bitch: A Lymphographic Study. *Anatomy Histology and Embryology*, **35**, 228-234.
http://dx.doi.org/10.1111/j.1439-0264.2005.00664.x

[8]　Pereira, C.T., Rahal, S.C., De Carvalho Balieiro, J.C. and Ribeiro, A.A. (2003) Lymphatic Drainage on Healthy and Neoplastic Mammary Glands in Female Dogs: Can It Be Really Altered? *Anatomy Histology and Embryology*, **32**, 282-290. http://dx.doi.org/10.1046/j.1439-0264.2003.00485.x

[9]　Hedlund, C.S. (2008) Cirurgia dos Sistemas Reprodutivo e Genital. In: Fossum, T.W., Hedlund, C.S., Johnson, A.L., Schulz, K.S., Seim, H.B., Willard, M.D., Bahr, A. and Carrol, G.L., Eds., *Cirurgia de Pequenos Animais*, 3th Edition, Elsevier, Rio de Janeiro, 702-774.

[10]　Fisher, B., Montague, E., Redmond, C., Barton, B., Borland, D., Fisher, E.R., *et al.* (1977) Comparison of Radical Mastectomy with Alternative Treatments for Primary Breast Cancer. A First Report of Results from a Prospective Randomized Clinical Trial. *Cancer*, **39**, 2827-2839.
http://dx.doi.org/10.1002/1097-0142(197706)39:6<2827::AID-CNCR2820390671>3.0.CO;2-I

[11]　Bland, C.S. (1981) The Halsted Mastectomy: Present Illness and Past History. *The Western Journal of Medicine*, **134**, 549-555.

[12]　Fergunson, R.H. (1985) Canine Mammary Gland Tumors. *Veterinary Clinics of North America: Small Animal Practice*, **15**, 501-511.

[13]　Olson J.S. (2005) Bathsheba's Breast: Women, Cancer & History. 1st Edition, John Hopkins University Press, Baltimore, 302 p.

[14]　Cotlar, A.M., Dubose, J.J. and Rose, D.M. (2003) History of Surgery for Breast Cancer: Radical to Sublime. *Current Surgery*, **60**, 329-337. http://dx.doi.org/10.1016/S0149-7944(02)00777-8

[15]　Gilbertson, S.R., Kurzman, I.D., Zachrau, R.E., Hurvitz, A.I. and Black, M.M. (1983) Canine Mammary Epithelial Neoplasms: Biological Implications of Morphologic Characteristics Assessed in 232 Dogs. *Veterinary Patholgy*, **20**, 127-142.

[16]　Brodey, R.S., Goldschmidt, M.H. and Roszel, J.R. (1983) Canine Mammary Gland Neoplasms. *Journal of American Animal Hospital Association*, **19**, 61-90.

[17]　MacEwen, E.G., Harvey, H.J., Patnaik, A.K., Mooney, S., Hayes, A., Kurzman, I. and Hardy Jr., W.D. (1985) Evaluation of the Effect of Levamizole and Surgery on Canine Mammary Cancer. *Journal of Biological Response Modifiers*, **4**, 418-426.

[18]　Daleck, C.R., Franceschini, P.H., Alessi, A.C., Santana, A.E. and Martins, M.I.M. (1998) Aspectos Clínico e Cirúrgicos do Tumor Mamário Canino. *Ciência Rural*, **28**, 95-100. http://dx.doi.org/10.1590/S0103-84781998000100016

[19]　De Nardi, A.B., Rodaski, S., Souza, R.S., Costa, T.A., Macedo, T.R., Rodigheri, S.M., Rios, A. and Piekarz, C.H. (2002) Prevalência de Neoplasias e Modalidades de Tratamentos em Cães Atendidos no Hospital Veterinário da Universidade Federal do Paraná. *Archives of Veterinay Science*, **7**, 15-26.

[20]　Zatloukal, J., Lorenzova, J., Tichy, F., Necas, A., Kecova, H. and Kohout, P. (2005) Breed and Age Risk Factors for Canine Mammary Tumours. *Acta Veterinaria Brno*, **74**, 103-109. http://dx.doi.org/10.2754/avb200574010103

[21]　Fowler, E.H., Wilson, G.P. and Koester, A. (1974) Biologic Behavior of Canine Mammary Neoplasms Based on a Histogenic Classification. *Veterinay Pathology*, **11**, 212-229. http://dx.doi.org/10.1177/030098587401100303

[22]　Benjamin, S.A., Lee, A.C. and Saunders, W.J. (1999) Classification and Behavior of Canine Epithelial Neoplasms Based on Life-Span Observations in Beagles. *Veterinary Pathology*, **36**, 423-436.
http://dx.doi.org/10.1354/vp.36-5-423

[23]　Filho, J.C., Kommers, G.D., Masuda, E.K., Marques, B.M.F.P.P., Fighera, R.A., Irigoyen, L.F. and Barros, C.S.L. (2010) Estudo Retrospectivo de 1647 Tumores Mamários em Cães. *Pesquisa Veterinária Brasileira*, **30**, 177-185.
http://dx.doi.org/10.1590/S0100-736X2010000200014

[24]　Salgado, B.S. and Cassali, G.D. (2012) Perspectives for Improved and More Accurate Classification of Canine Mammary Gland Neoplasms. *Veterinary Pathology Online*, **0**, 1-2.

[25]　Campos, C.B., Horta, R.S., Cobucci, G.C., Botelho, F.P.R., Lavalle, G.E. and Cassali, G.D. (2012) Abordagem Cirúrgica das Neoplasias Mamárias em Pequenos Animais: Perfil do Paciente, Comportamento e Epidemiologia Tumoral. *Veterinária e Zootecnia (Suplemento)*, **18**, 7-1.

[26]　Fisher, B. (2008) Biological Research in the Evolution of Cancer Surgery: A Personal Perspective. *Cancer Research*, **68**, 10007-10020. http://dx.doi.org/10.1158/0008-5472.CAN-08-0186

5

Evaluation of Breast Cancer Awareness among Female University Students in University of Sharjah, UAE

Abduelmula R. Abduelkarem*, Fatima Khalifa Saif, Salma Saif, Talal Ali Alshoaiby

College of Pharmacy, University of Sharjah, Sharjah, UAE
Email: *aabdelkarim@sharjah.ac.ae

Abstract

Objective: The objectives of this study were to assess the knowledge of breast cancer among female students at the College of Pharmacy at the University of Sharjah, UAE, and to evaluate the impact of the intervention program designed by the researchers on the student's knowledge on the disease risk factors, screening methods, and their perception towards its treatment outcomes. Method: A cross-sectional questionnaire survey of a convenience sample of 166 pharmacy students ((n = 110; the 4th year) and (n = 56; the 5th year)) in the University of Sharjah, Sharjah, UAE. The 26-item questionnaire covered the personal information and socio-demographic characteristics, breast cancer general knowledge, knowledge of breast cancer risk factors, knowledge of breast cancer symptoms and screening tests, and perception of management and outcomes of breast cancer. Key Findings: A total of 120 pharmacy students from the 4th year (n = 70) and the 5th year (n = 50) had completed the survey for the pre-intervention phase of the study. For the post intervention phase of the study, only 63 students from the 4th year and 48 students from the 5th year returned their completed questionnaire, giving a response rate of 90% and 96% respectively. Almost one quarter (59 (25.5)) of the students included in the study reported that they had a history of breast cancer in their family respectively. A high proportion (206 (89.2%)) of the students from both levels showed their interest in participating in activities to promote breast awareness, despite the fact that almost three quarters (161 (70%)) of the students reported that they had never been participated in any previous breast awareness programs. The awareness of students under investigation about self-examination was clearly improved at the end of the study period. Eighty (66.7%) of the students from both levels reported that the breast self-examination is recommended for female "once a month". This figure was increased to 103 (92.8%) post the intervention sessions (P value χ^2 < 0.001). Conclusion: The high incidence of breast cancer in the

---

*Corresponding author.

UAE may be attributed to the low level of awareness of the disease among females. Our findings can be used to promote discussion in the profession and with stakeholders about the future role of pharmacists in breast cancer care.

Keywords

Breast Cancer, Awareness, Sharjah, UAE, Knowledge and Perception

1. Introduction

Breast cancer is a malignant growth affecting the breast tissue, which may either affect the milk-producing ducts or the tubules carrying milk. There are two main histological types of breast cancer, namely, tubular and ductal carcinoma, and it may occur in males, though the incidence in females is much higher than in males [1]. Increasing age, family history, genetic factors, obesity, early menstruation, late menopause and nulliparity are all recognized as contributory factors [1].

Signs of breast cancer may include a palpable breast lump, nipple discharge and skin changes. Mammography detecting early signs of the disease is a valuable diagnostic test, while a pathological examination of a biopsy (fine needle aspiration (FNA), core biopsy, ultrasound-guided core biopsy, stereotactic biopsy, open excisional biopsy, and sentinel node biopsy) from a breast lump aids in differentiation of the types of cancer and survival rate. Breast cancer prognosis and treatment depend on tumor-node-metastasis staging, lympho-vascular spread, histological grade, hormone receptor status, comorbidities, and the patient's menopausal status. Generally, treatment includes surgical removal of the breast tissue, chemotherapy, hormone therapy, and radiotherapy [2].

Over the past two decades, female breast cancer has become a major health concern in both poor and rich countries due to its high incidence and associated mortality. It has been demonstrated in one particular study [3] that breast cancer is the most common cause of cancer death among women across the world. In 2008, breast cancer caused 480,000 deaths and about 70% of all cancer deaths occurred in low- and middle-income countries [1]. Based on the current estimate of an average annual increase in incidence ranging from 0.5% to 3% per year, the projected incidence increase in 2010 will be 1.4 - 1.5 million [4]. More recently, it has been reported that breast cancer is the most prevalent cancer affecting women worldwide with 1.7 million new cases diagnosed in 2012, representing 25% of all cancers in women and recording the second leading cause of death among women [5].

Despite the fact that there is scary of data regarding breast cancer in the Arab world and developing countries, one can speculate that the incidence of breast cancer to be very high and is rising at a faster rate [3] [6]. In the United Arab Emirates (UAE), breast cancer is the most commonly diagnosed cancer in females, accounting for about 28% of female deaths [7]. The high incidence of breast cancer in the UAE may be attributed to the low level of awareness of the disease among females and the cultural taboos associated with this disease. Furthermore, it has been concluded in one particular study [8] that in most of the developing countries, patients will seek medical advice and treatment from such problem, when it is in an advanced stage and little or no benefit can be expected from any sorts of therapy.

The recent fall of death from breast cancer in western nations is particularly explained by earlier diagnosis as a result of early presentation. It has been demonstrated that delayed presentation of symptomatic breast cancer for several months ($\geq$3 months) from the first detection to the time of diagnosis and treatment has been associated with increased tumor size [9] and poor long-term survival [9] [10]. The negative sociocultural perception of breast cancer, strong beliefs in traditional medicine and perhaps strong religious beliefs are the main reasons for the delay in presentation in the Arab world and developing countries [11] [12]. It has been demonstrated that the majority of breast cancer cases in the UAE are diagnosed late with involvement of regional lymph nodes or distant metastasis [7].

Emphasis on early screening of breast cancer helps in earlier diagnosis and higher survival rates, and it has been estimated that a 100% survival rate is achievable for stages 0 and 1 of breast cancer cases [13]. Early diagnosis of female breast cancer can be achieved by mass screening, mammography, Clinical Breast Examination

(CBE) and self-breast examination (SBE) or by the combination of three [14]. Even though mammography is the best choice for screening, breast self-examination is also equally important and beneficial for mass awareness, especially in countries with limited recourses or in a country where health care system still needs a lot of reforms and rearrangement, as in the case of many countries in the Arab world. It seems that pursuing a population based mass female screening program in most of developing countries is not a realistic approach. According to stepwise approach of Global Summit Panel 2002, SBE would be the approach for early detection [15]. However, lack of awareness, attitude and knowledge about the early detection of breast cancer and the benefits of screening tests is a real problem among women in developing countries and not very well documented. It has been reported that the public awareness of the importance of screening and early detection of breast cancer in the UAE women remains low [14], although increasing efforts from the Ministry of Health, public and private health sectors in the country, media and healthcare providers increase awareness of the public of this disease. Preventive behavior is essential for reducing cancer mortality. Knowledge is a necessary predisposing factor for behavioral change. Knowledge also plays an important role in improvement of health seeking behavior. Knowledge may not only dramatically improve the attitude, disbelieve and misconception, but also consequently enhance screening practice. That's why, to reduce the number of deaths from breast cancer, there was a shift in emphasis from breast self-examination to breast awareness after 1991 [16]. Besides, several studies also show that knowledgeable women and beliefs about breast cancer and its management may contribute significantly to medical help-seeking behaviors and increase their adherence to recommended breast cancer screening [17]-[19]. Furthermore, understanding the factors that influence patients' delay in seeking breast cancer treatment is therefore necessary to improve its treatment outcomes [20].

It is crucial for healthcare providers to educate the public about the importance of early detection of breast cancer, and engage in health awareness programs for breast cancer prevention, detection and treatment. Pharmacists, as a member of health care team, may play an important role in the improvement of public awareness about breast cancer. Providing information regarding mammography, education about available screening tests for breast cancer and designing pamphlets for women of the available tests and explaining the risk factors of this disease were recognized as an important role of pharmacists in breast cancer community care [14].

Fighting against cancers, specially breast cancer, is in the bottom of the priority list of the policy makers, though breast cancer is the second leading cause of cancer death among women worldwide. Considering the fact that breast cancer has become a global health care concern, several studies have been conducted worldwide to investigate women's knowledge and beliefs, and explore their awareness about breast cancer [17] [21]-[23]. However, none of these studies aimed at elicit awareness, attitude and knowledge of women about breast cancer in UAE. The objectives of this study were to assess the knowledge of breast cancer among female students at the College of Pharmacy at the University of Sharjah, UAE, and to evaluate the impact of the intervention program designed by the researchers on the student's knowledge on the disease risk factors, screening methods, and their perception towards its treatment outcomes.

2. Method

A cross-sectional study, using a validated questionnaire was used to conduct a face to face interview with each participant and to collect information (pre-intervention and post-intervention) from each student who agreed to take part in the study from the 4th and the 5th year pharmacy students, College of pharmacy, University of Sharjah, UAE. Students with no personal history of breast cancer and those able to understand the questionnaire were recruited for the study. Recruited students were asked to agree on a verbal informed consent before they allowed completing the study survey.

According to the university registration office and the college record system, the total number of the students registered in the 4th year and the 5th year pharmacy during the academic year 2013 was 110 and 56 students respectively. Based on the above database of student's registration, the minimum effective sample size was estimated to be 86 from the 4th year pharmacy students and 49 students of the 5th year using the online sample size calculator [24] with a confidence interval of 95%, 5% margin of error, and 50% for the expected response distribution.

They survey was adapted and modified with permission from authors of one particular study [22]. The questionnaire with 26 items was designed to cover 5 sections: 1) personal information and socio-demographic characteristics (eight items: 1 - 8); 2) general knowledge (eight items: 9 - 16); 3) knowledge of breast cancer risk factors (eleven items: 17 - 27); 4) knowledge of breast cancer symptoms and screening tests (eight items: 28 -

35); 5) perception of management and outcomes of breast cancer (eight items: 36 - 43). For most survey items, the respondents were asked to rate their response using the multiple choice options. A five point Likert type scale (from strongly agree to strongly disagree) was used to elicit the perception of the students towards management and treatment outcomes of breast cancer. There are many examples in the literature to support the use of such answer options in breast cancer studies [22] [23]. There was a section inviting comments at the end of questionnaire. (A copy of the questionnaire is available from the author).

There was no requirement to obtain ethical approval for such a study in the UAE. However, the approval was sought from the College of Pharmacy Research Committee. The study was carried out over a period of three months (from February 5th, 2014 to May 7th, 2014).

2.1. Validity and Reliability Testing

The validity of an instrument is the extent to which it actually measures what it is designed to measure. In survey work, this refers to the extent to which the questions collect accurate data relevant to the study's objectives. Evidence of validity may be gained through observation, expert and lay judgment, and empirical inquiry. Despite the fact that the tool used for this particular study was a validated survey and being extensively used in previous study [22] [23], to ensure the face validity of the instrument after being little bit modified to suit our target sample, the questionnaire was sent to two faculty member and one physician with a wide experience in survey design study. Furthermore, the researcher's three students from College of Pharmacy, University of Sharjah, UAE were also asked to read the survey and to give their feedback, if they will have any. All of their views and comments were considered and then incorporated into the final version of the questionnaire.

To assess test-retest reliability, the questionnaire was sent on two separate occasions to 10 students (not included in the final sample) randomly chosen in an area of study interest. The second response was elicited two weeks after the initial test. No problems were highlighted, and test-retest reliability was calculated using Spearman's correlation coefficient (r). The rho value was 0.73, which implies an acceptable level of test re-test reliability. The alpha coefficient was 0.81; indicating that most of the items included make a valid contribution to the overall score.

For baseline purposes (pre-intervention phase of the study), the students under investigation were asked to complete the survey. During the intervention phase of the study, a clear and concise standardized information on different aspects of breast cancer were provided during the "Pharmacy Open Day" of the College to the participant students using different tools such as focus group lectures, distributing brochures that cover brief information on breast cancer such as definition, prevalence, signs and symptoms, stages, diagnosis, risk factors, treatment and prevention. Brief counseling session on how to conduct self-examination was carried out and pictures about breast cancer self-examination were distributed among the participants.

To increase and encourage students to participate in the study, T-shirts and mugs with special statements about breast cancer awareness written on them (Keep calm and support breast cancer, Early detection saves lives) were distributed as a gift to those who took part in the test your knowledge competition that was held near to our stand during the pharmacy open day event of the college. Furthermore, a Face book page with a name "Go pink" was created by the researchers and people, including the 4th and the 5th year pharmacy students of the college were invited to the page posted articles, posters and pictures related to breast cancer awareness. An instagram page was also developed and students under investigation were all invited this page. In this page we uploaded pictures and information regarding breast cancer and how to manage the condition.

2.2. Data Analysis

The participants' responses were encoded and the data were analyzed using Statistical Package for the Social Sciences (SPSS, version 20.0, Chicago, IL, USA). Descriptive analysis was used to calculate the proportion of each group of respondents answer on each statement in the questionnaire. Also, Chi Square test was used to identify any significant difference among the participants' responses regarding certain statements or questions in the questionnaire. Mann Whitney U test was used when it is possible. Furthermore, when analysing the responses data from the five-point scale regarding the perception of the students towards management and treatment outcomes of breast cancer, the responses were reduced to three categories: strongly agree/agree, neutral, and strongly disagree/disagree. This enabled more reader comprehensible confidence intervals for the relative proportions to be calculated. The level of statistical significance was set at P value of <0.05.

3. Results

A total of 120 pharmacy students from the 4th year (70 students) and the 5th year (50 students) had completed the survey for the pre-intervention phase of the study. For the post intervention phase of the study, only 111 pharmacy students from the 4th year (63 students) and the 5th year (48 students) returned their completed questionnaire, giving a response rate of 90% and 96% respectively. The average age of the students under investigation was 22.06 ± 0.84 years (range = 21 - 23 years).

With regard to students' nationality, they were divided into four regions (Eastern Asia, Iraq and GCC countries, Arab countries in Africa, and Arab countries in Middle East). More than half 120 (51.9%) of the students included in the study reported that they were from Arab countries in the Middle East region. The majority of the students from the 4th year (126; 94.7%) and 5th year (92; 93.9%) reported that they were not involved in any type of work during the study period. Almost one quarter 35 (26.3) and 24 (24.5) of the investigated 4th and 5th year students reported that they have had a history of breast cancer in their family respectively. Interestingly, high proportion 206 (89.2%) of the students from both levels showed their interest to participate in activities to promote breast awareness, despite the fact that almost 161 (70%) of them reported that they have never been participated in any of previous breast awareness programs. **Table 1** summarizes participant student's characteristics.

4. General Knowledge of Breast Cancer

When the participants included in the study were questioned if breast cancer only occurs in women, 80 (60.2%) of the 4th and 77 (78.6%) of the 5th year students answered no (P value $\chi^2 = 0.01$). When inquired if breast cancer is the number one type of cancer that occurs in the Arab world, 66 (49.6%) of the 4th and 41 (41.8%) of the 5th year agreed this was the case (P value $\chi^2 = 0.27$).

Before the intervention, close to half of our participants 54 (45%) were aware of the symptoms of breast cancer; after the intervention, close to three quarters of the study population 81 (73%) claimed that they do (P value $\chi^2 < 0.001$).

Table 1. Participant student's characteristics.

Items	The 4th Year Student	The 5th Year Student	Total	P Value χ^2
Study design				
Pre-intervention	70 (52.6)	50 (51.0)	120 (51.9)	0.46[*]
Post-intervention	63 (47.4)	48 (49.0)	111 (48.1)	
Age (years):				
Mean	21.7	22.6	22.06	
SD	0.79	0.63	0.84	<0.001[**]
Range	21 - 23	21 - 23	21 - 23	
Nationality:				
Eastern Asia	21 (15.8)	17 (17.3)	38 (16.5)	
Iraq and GCC countries	22 (16.5)	12 (12.2)	34 (14.7)	0.21[*]
Arab countries in Africa	17 (12.8)	22 (22.4)	39 (16.9)	
Arab countries in Middle East	73 (54.9)	47 (48.0)	120 (51.9)	
Employment status				
Unemployed	126 (94.7)	92 (93.9)	218 (94.4)	0.49[*]
Employed	7 (5.3)	6 (6.1)	13 (5.6)	
History of breast cancer				
Yes	35 (26.3)	24 (24.5)	59 (25.5)	0.44[*]
no	98 (73.7)	74 (75.5)	172 (74.5)	
Previously participation in breast awareness				
Yes	45 (33.8)	25 (25.5)	70 (30.3)	0.11[*]
no	88 (66.2)	73 (74.5)	161 (69.7)	
Interested in activities to promote breast awareness				
Yes	124 (93.2)	82 (83.7)	206 (89.2)	0.02[*#]
no	9 (6.8)	16 (16.3)	25 (10.8)	

[*]One sample Chi-Square test (χ^2); [**]Mann-Whitney U test; [#]The significant of 0.02 is due to the 5th year students responses (Std Residual = 1.7).

Students from the 5th year were more confident in their ability to check their beast for any symptoms related to breast cancer. Seventy six (57.1%) students from the 4th year and 59 (60.2%) from the 5th year reported that they have enough confidence in checking their breast (P value $\chi^2 = 0.21$).

As regard, the age in which breast cancer occurs more, close to three quarters of the study population before and after the intervention, 78 (65%) and 84 (75.7%) respectively, answered that breast cancer occurs more in the 31 - 49 years age group (P value $\chi^2 = 031$). Interestingly, there was significant difference (P value $\chi^2 < 0.001$) in students under investigation answers when they were asked if only females are affected by breast cancer. The majority 90 (81.1%) of the participants answered "no" after the intervention compared with only 67 (55.8%) before the intervention. **Table 2** summarizes the general knowledge of breast cancer among participants and according to their educational levels.

Table 2. General knowledge of breast cancer according to the educational levels and study design.

Item	Education Levels			Study Design		
	The 4th Year n (%)	The 5th Year n (%)	P Value χ^2	Pre-Intervention n (%)	Post-Intervention n (%)	P Value χ^2
Only females are affected by breast cancer						
Yes	34 (25.6%)	15 (15.3%)		38 (31.7%)	11 (9.9%)	
No	80 (60.2%)	77 (78.6%)	0.011	67 (55.8%)	90 (81.1%)	<0.001
Don't know	19 (14.3%)	6 (6.1%)		15 (12.5%)	10 (9%)	
Breast cancer can be transmitted						
Yes	2 (1.5%)	4 (4.1%)		2 (1.7%)	4 (3.6%)	
No	125 (94%)	91 (92.9%)	0.42	112 (93.3%)	104 (93.7%)	0.45
Don't know	6 (4.5%)	3 (3.1%)		6 (5%)	3 (2.7%)	
Breast cancer is number 1 in most of Arab countries						
Yes	66 (49.6%)	41 (41.8%)		30 (25%)	77 (69.4%)	
No	16 (12%)	9 (9.2%)	0.27	15 (12.5%)	10 (9%)	<0.001
Don't know	51 (38.3%)	48 (49%)		75 (62.5%)	24 (21.6%)	
Awareness about symptoms						
Yes	74 (55.6%)	61 (62.2%)		54 (45%)	81 (73%)	
No	17 (12.8%)	11 (11.2%)	0.60	27 (22.5%)	1 (0.9%)	<0.001
Don't know	42 (31.6%)	26 (26.5%)		39 (32.5%)	29 (26.1%)	
Are you confident that you know how to check your breasts?						
Yes	76 (57.1%)	59 (60.2%)		43 (35.8%)	92 (82.9%)	
No	57 (42.9%)	37 (37.8%)	0.21	77 (64.2%)	17 (15.3%)	<0.001
Don't know	0.0 (0.0%)	2 (2%)		0 (0.0%)	2 (1.8%)	
Breast cancer occurs more at the age of						
Under 30 years	2 (1.5%)	5 (5.1%)		3 (2.5%)	4 (3.6%)	
31 - 49 years	97 (72.9%)	65 (66.3%)	0.23	78 (65%)	84 (75.7%)	0.13
Over 50 years	34 (25.6%)	28 (28.6%)		39 (32.5%)	23 (20.7%)	
How often do you check your breasts?						
At least once a month	22 (16.5%)	23 (23.5%)		26 (21.7%)	19 (17.1%)	
Once a month to once a year	31 (23.3%)	19 (19.4%)	0.40	16 (13.3%)	34 (30.6%)	0.006
Never	80 (60.2%)	56 (56.1%)		78 (65%)	58 (52.3%)	
Which of the following is not a treatment used of breast cancer						
Surgery	4 (3%)	2 (2%)		4 (3.3%)	2 (1.8%)	
Chemotherapy	4 (3%)	1 (1%)		4 (3.3%)	1 (0.9%)	
Radiation Therapy	2 (1.5%)	4 (4.1%)	0.05	6 (5%)	0.0 (0.0%)	<0.001
Hormone Therapy	23 (17.3%)	6 (6.1%)		28 (23.3%)	1 (0.9%)	
Ultraviolet light therapy	100 (75.2%)	85 (86.7%)		78 (65%)	107 (96.4%)	

5. Knowledge of Breast Cancer Symptoms and Screening Test

There was a clear significant difference (P value $\chi^2 < 0.001$) in the students under investigation responses between the pre-intervention (63; 52.5%) and post-intervention (99; 89.2%) phase of the study regarding their knowledge of painless breast lump as a symptom of breast cancer.

The awareness of students under investigation about self-examination was clearly improved at the end of the study period. Eighty (66.7%) of the students from both levels reported that the breast self-examination is recommended for female "Once a month". This figure was increased to 103 (92.8%) post the intervention sessions (P value $\chi^2 < 0.001$). Interestingly, more than three quarter 103 (77.4%) of the 4th year students reported that self-examination of the breast should be conducted once a month compared to 80 (81.6%) students from the 5th year reported that once a year is the recommended plan for breast self-examination (**Table 3**).

More than three quarters of the participants 92 (76.7%) reported that pain in breast region was a sign/symptom of breast cancer during the pre-intervention phase of the study. However, this figure was dramatically increased into almost 100% at the end of the study period (P value $\chi^2 < 0.001$).

Respondent's opinion and views regarding clinical breast examination, Dimpling of breast skin, Change in the shape of breast, Nipple discharge, Lump under armpit according to educational levels and according to pre- and post-intervention design of the study are summarized in **Table 3**.

Table 3. Knowledge of breast cancer symptoms and screening tests according to education levels and study design.

Item	Education Levels			Study Design		
	The 4th Year n (%)	The 5th Year n (%)	P Value χ^2	Pre-Intervention n (%)	Post-Intervention n (%)	P Value χ^2
Painless breast lump						
Yes	94 (70.7)	68 (69.4)		63 (52.5)	99 (89.2)	
No	17 (12.8)	4 (4.1)	0.02	20 (16.7)	1 (0.9)	<0.001
Don't know	22 (16.5)	26 (26.5)		37 (30.8)	11 (9.9)	
Lump under armpit						
Yes	91 (68.4)	73 (74.5)		66 (55)	98 (88.3)	
No	16 (12)	13 (13.3)	0.33	23 (19.2)	6 (5.4)	<0.001
Don't know	26 (19.5)	12 (12.2)		31 (25.8)	7 (6.3)	
Nipple discharge						
Yes	106 (79.7)	86 (87.8)		83 (69.2)	109 (98.2)	
No	12 (9.0)	4 (4.1)	0.22	14 (11.7)	2 (1.8)	<0.001
Don't know	15 (11.3)	8 (8.2)		23 (19.2)	0 (0)	
Change in the shape of breast						
Yes	125 (94)	93 (94.9)		107 (89.2)	111 (100)	
No	2 (1.5)	2 (2)	0.82	4 (3.3)	0 (0)	0.005
Don't know	5 (3.8)	3 (3.1)		9 (7.5)	0 (0)	
Pain in breast region						
Yes	119 (89.5)	84 (85.7)		92 (76.7)	111 (100)	
No	6 (4.5)	9 (9.2)	0.35	15 (12.5)	0 (0)	<0.001
Don't know	8 (6)	5 (5.1)		13 (10.8)	0 (0)	
Dimpling of breast skin						
Yes	116 (87.2)	77 (78.6)		87 (72.5)	106 (95.5)	
No	3 (2.3)	4 (4.1)	0.21	7 (5.8)	0 (0)	<0.001
Don't know	14 (10.5)	17 (17.3)		26 (21.7)	5 (4.5)	
Breast self-examination (BSE) is recommended for females						
Once a month	103 (77.4)	0 (0)		80 (66.7)	103 (92.8)	
Once a year	10 (7.5)	80 (81.6)	0.52	13 (10.8)	6 (5.4)	<0.001
Once in five years	1 (0.8)	9 (9.2)		1 (0.8)	0 (0)	
Don't know	19 (14.3)	9 (9.2)		26 (21.7)	2 (1.8)	
Clinical breast examination (CBE) is recommended for females						
Once a month	5 (3.8)	3 (3.1)		6 (5)	2 (1.8)	
Once a year	92 (69.2)	74 (75.5)	0.13	64 (53.3)	102 (91.9)	<0.001
Once in five years	6 (4.5)	9 (9.2)		15 (12.5)	0 (0)	
Don't know	30 (22.6)	12 (12.2)		35 (29.2)	7 (6.3)	

6. Risk Factors of Breast Cancer

Despite the fact of similar responses on the majority of risk factors of breast cancer items reported by the 4th year and the 5th pharmacy students, there were a clear significant difference (P value $\chi^2 < 0.001$) between their answers reported on of the items related to risk factors of breast cancer in the pre-intervention and after the completion of breast cancer awareness program designed by the study researchers for the study purpose (**Table 4**).

Prior to the intervention, more than half of the examined participants 66 (55%) and 83 (69.2%) reported that they "don't know" as whether early appearance of menses or cigarette smoking increases the risk for developing of breast cancer respectively. However, the majority 97 (87.4%) and 105 (94.6%) of the interviewed students agreed on the statement that early onset of menses (<12 years) and cigarette smoking increases the risk of breast cancer at the end of the study.

Breast feeding decreases the risk of breast cancer was reported by 49 (40.8%) of the interviewed student at the baseline data (pre-intervention). Almost three quarter 83 (74.8%) of the students reported that breast feeding decreases the risk of breast cancer after participation in the different awareness sessions conducted by the research over the study period. Responses of the study involved students on obesity, low fat diet, old age, family history of breast cancer, and hormone replacement therapy are all summarized in **Table 4**.

7. Perception of Management and Outcomes of Breast Cancer

Twenty three (19.2%) of participants were either strongly agreed or agreed on the statement that surgical removal of affected breast is the only treatment available. At the end of the study, the students under investigation either agreed or strongly agreed on the statement declined to 11 (9.9%) (95% CI = 10.17 - 19.26). The majority 105 (87.5%) of the participants (pre-interventions phase) and 110 (99.1) (95% CI = 89.82 - 96.33) were either strongly agreed or agreed that having a mother or sister with breast cancer means you are more likely to get it. Seventy (60.8%) of the students included in the study were either strongly disagreed or disagreed that treatment for breast cancer is embarrassing. Interestingly, the majority 100 (90.1%) of the students either disagreed or strongly disagreed on the statement (P value $\chi^2 < 0.001$; 95% CI = 5.76 - 13.29).

The perception of the interviewed students on early detection of breast cancer leads improved survival rate was not improved at the end of the study despite of the awareness intervention sessions. One hundred and twelve students (93.3%) either strongly agreed or agreed on the above statement at the beginning of the study. This figure decreased into 99 (89.2%) at the end of the study period (P value $\chi^2 = 0.5$; 95% CI = 87.73 - 94.95). The perception of participants on the statements "a woman after receiving treatment for breast cancer can enjoy a good quality of life", "the treatment for breast cancer is a long and painful process", "treatments for breast cancer are more helpful to young people", and "treatment of breast cancer results in loss of physical beauty" are summarized in **Table 5**.

8. Discussion

In the Arab world, including the Gulf region, the incidence of female breast cancer is alarming and affecting a younger population compared to the West side of the world. In the Arab world countries, there are very few breast cancer awareness programs [14] [25]. Lack of knowledge about the breast cancer common risk factors and the understanding of the importance of breast self-examination were the recognized as the most findings in different studies conducted in Saudi Arabia different regions [25]-[27]. Several more studies assessed the awareness of breast cancer and the practice of breast self-examination among females of western [28] population, as well as Arab women in the Middle East [29] and in the Gulf region [25] [30]-[32]. However, few studies were conducted to address breast cancer among UAE females and none of the previous studies were designed to elicit the problem among university female students in Sharjah, UAE. Therefore the objective of this study is to investigate the level of breast cancer awareness among the pharmacy female students from fourth and fifth year of the college's five years study plan.

As regards general knowledge of breast cancer, the breast cancer cannot be transmitted was the most frequent knowledge identified by fourth and fifth year students, (94%) and (92.9%) respectively. This finding is consistent with what was reported by Hadi *et al.* [22] and reported that 91.5% of the students included in the study answered this question correctly.

Students from the 5th year were more confident in their ability to check their beast for any symptoms related to

Table 4. Risk factors of breast cancer according to the educational level of the study group.

Item	Education Levels			Study Design		
	The 4th Year n (%)	The 5th Year n (%)	P Value χ^2	Pre-Intervention n (%)	Post-Intervention n (%)	P Value χ^2
Old age						
Increases risk	111 (83.5)	91 (92.9)		93 (77.5)	109 (98.2)	
Decreases risk	1 (0.8)	0 (0)	0.017	1 (0.8)	0 (0)	<0.001
No effect	6 (4.5)	6 (6.1)		10 (8.3)	2 (1.8)	
Don't know	15 (11.3)	1 (1)		16 (13.3)	0 (0)	
Family history of breast cancer						
Increases risk	129 (97)	96 (98)		114 (95)	111 (100)	
Decreases risk	0 (0)	0 (0)	0.455	0 (0)	0 (0)	0.058
No effect	2 (1.5)	2 (2)		4 (3.3)	0 (0)	
Don't know	2 (1.5)	0 (0)		2 (1.7)	0 (0)	
Cigarette smoking						
Increases risk	107 (80.5)	81 (82.7)		83 (69.2)	105 (94.6)	
Decreases risk	2 (1.5)	3 (3.1)	0.75	3 (2.5)	2 (1.8)	<0.001
No effect	13 (9.8)	7 (7.1)		17 (14.2)	3 (2.7)	
Don't know	11 (8.3)	7 (7.1)		17 (14.2)	1 (0.9)	
Low fat diet						
Increases risk	15 (11.3)	8 (8.2)		15 (12.5)	8 (7.2)	
Decreases risk	63 (47.4)	56 (57.1)		39 (32.5)	80 (72.1)	
No effect	6 (4.5)	6 (6.1)	0.38	12 (10)	0 (0)	<0.001
Don't know	49 (36.8)	28 (28.6)		54 (45)	23 (20.7)	
First child at late age (≥30 years)						
Increases risk	71 (53.4)	68 (69.4)		40 (33.3)	99 (89.2)	
Decreases risk	1 (0.8)	2 (2)	0.04	1 (0.8)	2 (1.8)	<0.001
No effect	13 (9.8)	8 (8.2)		19 (15.8)	2 (1.8)	
Don't know	48 (36.1)	20 (20.4)		60 (50)	8 (7.2)	
Early onset of menses (<12 years)						
Increases risk	68 (51.1)	54 (55.1)		25 (20.8)	97 (87.4)	
Decreases risk	5 (3.8)	1 (1)	0.58	6 (5)	0 (0)	<0.001
No effect	15 (11.3)	12 (12.2)		23 (19.2)	4 (3.6)	
Don't know	45 (33.8)	31 (31.6)		66 (55)	10 (9)	
Late menopause (>55 years)						
Increases risk	78 (58.6)	58 (59.2)		43 (35.8)	93 (83.8)	
Decreases risk	6 (4.5)	6 (6.1)	0.79	12 (10)	0 (0)	<0.001
No effect	14 (10.5)	7 (7.1)		17 (14.2)	4 (3.6)	
Don't know	35 (26.3)	27 (27.6)		48 (40)	14 (12.6)	
Use of oral contraceptives						
Increases risk	97 (72.9)	83 (84.7)		70 (58.3)	110 (99.1)	
Decreases risk	2 (1.5)	1 (1)	0.21	3 (2.5)	0 (0)	<0.001
No effect	7 (5.3)	3 (3.1)		9 (7.5)	1 (0.9)	
Don't know	27 (20.3)	11 (11.2)		38 (31.7)	0 (0)	
Obesity						
Increases risk	113 (85)	86 (87.8)		92 (76.7)	107 (96.4)	
Decreases risk	0 (0)	2 (2)	0.28	1 (0.8)	1 (0.9)	<0.001
No effect	2 (1.5)	1 (1)		2 (1.7)	1 (0.9)	
Don't know	18 (13.5)	9 (9.2)		25 (20.8)	2 (1.8)	
Hormone replacement therapy						
Increases risk	97 (72.9)	77 (78.6)		71 (59.2)	103 (92.8)	
Decreases risk	1 (0.8)	4 (4.1)	0.16	3 (2.5)	2 (1.8)	<0.001
No effect	2 (1.5)	1 (1)		3 (2.5)	0 (0)	
Don't know	33 (24.8)	16 (16.3)		43 (35.8)	6 (5.4)	
Breast feeding						
Increases risk	16 (12)	7 (7.1)		19 (15.8)	4 (3.6)	
Decreases risk	73 (54.9)	59 (60.2)	0.63	49 (40.8)	83 (74.8)	<0.001
No effect	14 (10.5)	11 (11.2)		18 (15)	7 (6.3)	
Don't know	30 (22.6)	21 (21.4)		34 (28.3)	17 (15.3)	

Table 5. Perception of management and outcomes of breast cancer.

Items	Pre-Intervention (120) n (%)	Post-Intervention (111) n (%)	Total (n = 231) n (%)	P Value χ^2	95% CI for Single Proportion for Strongly Agree/Agree Responses
Surgical removal of affected breast is the only treatment available					
Strongly agree/agree	23 (19.2)	11 (9.9)	34 (14.7)		
Neutral	7 (5.8%)	13 (11.7%)	20 (8.7%)	0.05	10.17 - 19.26
Strongly disagree/disagree	90 (75%)	87 (78.4%)	177 (76.6%)		
Early detection of breast cancer leads improved survival rate					
Strongly agree/agree	112 (93.3)	99 (89.2)	211 (91.3)		
Neutral	4 (3.3%)	10 (9.0%)	14 (6.1%)	0.15	87.73 - 94.95
Strongly disagree/disagree	4 (3.3%)	2 (1.8%)	6 (2.6%)		
Having a mother or sister with breast cancer means you are more likely to get it					
Strongly agree/agree	105 (87.5)	110 (99.1)	215 (93.1)		
Neutral	10 (8.3%)	0 (0.0%)	10 (4.3%)	0.002	89.82 - 96.33
Strongly disagree/disagree	5 (4.2%)	1 (0.9%)	6 (2.6%)		
A woman after receiving treatment for breast cancer can enjoy a good quality of life					
Strongly agree/agree	76 (63.3)	109 (98.2)	185 (80.1)		
Neutral	32 (26.7%)	2 (1.8%)	34 (14.7%)	<0.001	74.96 - 85.21
Strongly disagree/disagree	12 (10.0%)	0 (0.0%)	12 (5.2%)		
The treatment for breast cancer is a long and painful process					
Strongly agree/agree	80 (66.7)	110 (99.1)	190 (82.3)		
Neutral	36 (30.0%)	1 (0.9%)	37 (16.0%)	<0.001	77.35-87.15
Strongly disagree/disagree	4 (3.3%)	0 (0.0%)	4 (1.7%)		
Treatments for breast cancer are more helpful to young people					
Strongly agree/agree	70 (58.3)	105 (94.6%)	175 (15.8%)		
Neutral	40 (33.3%)	2 (1.8%)	42 (18.2%)	<0.001	70.26 - 81.26
Strongly disagree/disagree	10 (8.3%)	4 (3.6%)	14 (6.1%)		
Treatment for breast cancer is embarrassing					
Strongly agree/agree	22 (18.3)	0 (0.0%)	22 (9.5%)		
Neutral	25 (20.8%)	11 (9.9%)	36 (15.6%)	<0.001	5.76 - 13.29
Strongly disagree/disagree	73 (60.8%)	100 (90.1%)	173 (74.9%)		
Treatment of breast cancer results in loss of physical beauty					
Strongly agree/agree	68 (56.7)	71 (64.0%)	139 (60.2)		
Neutral	31 (25.8%)	34 (30.6%)	65 (28.1%)	0.017	53.89 - 66.45
Strongly disagree/disagree	21 (17.5%)	6 (5.4%)	27 (11.7%)		

breast cancer. Seventy six (57.1%) students from the 4th year and 59 (60.2%) from the 5th year reported that they have enough confidence in checking their breast.

Despite the fact of non-significant difference (P value χ^2 = 0.21) in the responses of the students from the 4th year (57; 57.1%) and the 5th year (59; 60.2%) when they were asked about their confident to check their breast for any sign of cancer, fifth year students were more positive regarding their ability to check their breasts, this could be attributed to the fact of prior exposure to material dealing with breast cancer as part of their curriculum. The importance of exposure to breast cancer educational material and awareness interventions about breast cancer were also demonstrated by the findings of this study. Only 43 (35.8%) of the participants reported that they have enough confident to check their breasts at the beginning of the study, compared to 92 (82.9%) after the completion of awareness program (brochures and the illustrating pictures about breast cancer self-examination) that was distributed by the researchers over the study period.

Regarding awareness of breast cancer warning signs, breast lump was the most frequently symptom identified by almost half of participants (50.5%) in the study conducted on Saudi females in Jeddah [33]. The result of Saudi females in Jeddah is in disagreement with that was reported by Malaysia study [22] and the results the present study. The most identified symptom by the students in Malaysia and this study was the change in shape of the breast, 81% and 89.2% respectively. Interestingly, in the present study the awareness materials about the breast cancer were effective in improving the knowledge of breast cancer signs and symptoms among participants. Almost 100% of the students under investigation were able to identify that change in the shape of the breast and pain in breast as the most important sign/symptom for the breast cancer problem.

In the present study, it was found that although the majority of participants were aware of the breast self-examination for breasts in females, the majority of participants are neither aware of the frequency of performing breast self-examination. More than three quarter 103 (77.4%) of 4th year pharmacy students reported that it should be recommended for once a month. On the other hand, 80 (81.6%) from the 5th year reported that it should be recommended for once a year. These findings are congruent with previous studies investigating awareness and knowledge of breast cancer and practices of breast self-examination among women and university students in Saudi Arabia [26] [32]-[34].

Regarding awareness of breast cancer risk factors, the majority of participants (97%) fourth year and (98%) fifth year reported that having family history with breast cancer is considered a risk factor that might lead to developing breast cancer among the family members. This result is similar to those results presented in Saudi Arabia study [33] and Malaysia study. (91%) [22], which revealed that more than half (57.5%) of females Saudi and the majority (91%) of Malaysia females included in the study knew about family history and having a close relative with breast cancer as established risk factors for the disease. More than half 71 (59.2%) and 70 (58.3) of the students under investigation were aware of hormone replacement therapy and uses of oral contraceptives as other risk factors of breast cancer respectively. However, knowledge of other risk factors of breast cancer was limited as only few females knew that early onset of menses (<12 years) (25; 20.8%), first child at late age (≥30 years) (40, 33.3%), late menopause (>55 years) (43; 35.8%), and cigarette smoking (83; 69.2%) are risk factors of breast cancer. Intervention awareness program was effective in improving participants awareness of the risk factors associated with breast cancer. Almost three quarter (80, 72.1%) and the majority (105; 94.6%) of the interviewed students were able to identify low fat diet and cigarette smoking as important factor to decrease and increase the risk of developing breast cancer respectively, which is a contrast to the results obtained prior to the intervention, where only 39 (32.5%) and 83 (69.2%) of the students included in the study were able to identify the impact of low fat diet and cigarette smoking on developing of breast cancer (P value $\chi^2 < 0.001$).

The vast majority of our study participants had correct beliefs and positive perception about breast cancer management and its outcomes. At the beginning of our study, most of the studied students (93.3%) reported that early detection of breast cancer leads to improve survival rate. However, 76 (63.3%), 80 (66.7%), and 70 (58.3%) were either strongly agreed or agreed that a woman after receiving treatment for breast cancer can enjoy a good quality of life, the treatment for breast cancer is a long and painful process, and treatments for breast cancer are more helpful to young people respectively. Intervention awareness programs has a dramatic effect on the participants perception regarding a woman after receiving treatment for breast cancer can enjoy a good quality of life, the treatment for breast cancer is a long and painful process, and treatments for breast cancer are more helpful to young people. The majority of participants reported that either agreed or strongly agreed with the statements such as intervention awareness programs has a dramatic effect on the participants perception regarding a woman after receiving treatment for breast cancer can enjoy a good quality of life (109; 98.2%), the treatment for breast cancer is a long and painful process (110; 99.1%), and treatments for breast cancer are more helpful to young people (105; 94.6%). One can contemplate that such observable changes may be attributed to the contents of the brochures that were distributed during the intervention awareness program, which contained detail explanation about how to manage and what are the outcomes of breast cancer. Overall, the intervention helped improve the participant's response to the survey questions; this could indicate that breast cancer campaign can improve the prognosis and survivability.

Study findings directed the light on the importance of raising the level of public awareness about breast cancer to overcome an ever-increasing burden of this disease and reduce the number of new cases that put the UAE at the top of the scale among the other countries with a high rate of breast cancer sufferers. Proper counseling should be routinely given by healthcare providers within hospitals and clinics to improve breast cancer knowledge. The primary goal is to improve the survival rate by promoting early detection and medical help-seeking behaviors among females. The study was conducted among the pharmacy students of University of Sharjah only and therefore might not be a representative of all universities across the UAE.

9. Conclusion

Despite the limitations of this cross sectional survey study (time constrain, reluctant of some students to repeat felling the form, and lack of research attitude among university female students), the findings of the present study provide some insights into changes in students' perception at the baseline and at the end of the study period. Findings indicated that levels of awareness of breast cancer of studied female students, *i.e.* knowledge of breast cancer warning signs, risk factors, screening program and breast self-examination, were very inadequate at the beginning of the study. Surprisingly, most of the findings after the awareness program designed for the purpose of the research study had a dramatic change which indicated that the breast cancer awareness were more likely to be effective and have a larger impact. Indeed, the focus of primary health care providers should be to raise awareness about breast care, not only for females in communities, but also for future health care providers, especially the newly graduates from the health and medical related schools.

Acknowledgements

First of all, we would like to thank our supervisor Prof. Abdulmawla Abdulkarem, whose help, advice and supervision was invaluable. He inspired us greatly to work in this project and we appreciate his valuable guidance and support till the end of our study. Also we would like to thank all of the students who helped us to accomplish our study and who answered our questionnaires. Our thanks go to our college administration for their allowance to participate in the open day to do our study intervention phase. Finally, we would like to thanks our parents for their great help and encouragement through the entire period of the study.

References

[1] World Health Organization (WHO) (2006) Cancer Fact Sheet No. 297.
     http://www.who.int/mediacentre/factsheets/fs297/en/index.html

[2] Maughan, K.L., Lutterbie, M.A. and Ham, P.S. (2010) Treatment of Breast Cancer. *American Family Physician*, **81**, 1339-1346.

[3] Bray, F., MacCarron, P. and Maxwell Parkin, D. (2004) The Changing Global Patterns of Female Breast Cancer Incidence and Mortality. *Breast cancer Research*, **6**, 229-239. http://dx.doi.org/10.1186/bcr932

[4] Smith, R.A., Caleffi, M., Albert, U.-S., Chen, T.H.H., duffy, S.W., *et al.* (2006) Breast Cancer in Limited Resource Countries: Early Detection and Access to Care. *The Breast Journal*, **12**, S16-S26.

[5] Cancer Research UK (2014) Breast Cancer Incidence Statistics.
     http://info.cancerresearchuk.org/cancerstats/types/breast/incidence/

[6] Parkin, D.M., Whelan, S.L., Ferlay, J., Raymond, L. and Young, J. (1997) Cancer Incidence in Five Continents. Vol. 8, IARC Press, Lyon.

[7] Al-Sharbatti, S.S., Shaikh, R.B., Mathew, E. and Al-Biate, M.A.S. (2013) Breast Self-Examination Practice and Breast Cancer Risk Perception among Female University Students in Ajman. *Asian Pacific Journal of Cancer Prevention*, **14**, 4919-4923. http://dx.doi.org/10.7314/APJCP.2013.14.8.4919

[8] Ibrahim, O. and Ibrahim, R. (2013) Community Pharmacists' Involvement in Breast Cancer Health Promotion in United Arab Emirates (UAE). *American Journal of Pharmacology and Toxicology*, **8**, 155-163.
     http://dx.doi.org/10.3844/ajptsp.2013.155.163

[9] Richards, M.A., Westcombe, A.M., Love, S.B., Littlejohns, P. and Ramirez, A.J. (1999) Influence of Delay on Survival in Patients with Breast Cancer: A Systematic Review of the Literature. *The Lancet*, **353**, 1119-1126.
     http://dx.doi.org/10.1016/S0140-6736(99)02143-1

[10] Rossi, S., Cinini, C., Di Pietro, C., Lombardi, C.P., Crucitti, A., Bellantone, R. and Crucitti, F. (1990) Diagnostic Delay in Breast Cancer: Correlation with Disease Stage and Prognosis. *Tumori*, **76**, 559-562.

[11] Rashidi, A. and Rajaram, S.S. (2000) Middle Eastern Asian Islamic Women and Breast Self-Examination: Needs Assessment. *Cancer Nursing*, **23**, 64-70. http://dx.doi.org/10.1097/00002820-200002000-00010

[12] Rajaram, S.S. and Rashidi, A. (1999) Asian-Islamic Women and Breast Cancer Screening: A Socio-Cultural Analysis. *Women & Health*, **28**, 45-58. http://dx.doi.org/10.1300/J013v28n03_04

[13] Venkatramana, M., Sreedharan, J., Muttappallymyalil, J. and Thomas, M. (2011) Opinion of Nurses Regarding Breast Cancer Screening Programs. *Indian Journal of Cancer*, **48**, 423-427. http://dx.doi.org/10.4103/0019-509X.92262

[14] Bener, A., Honein, G., Carter, A., Da'ar, Z., Miller, C. and Dunn, E. (2002) The Determinants of Breast Cancer Screening Behavior: A Focus Group Study of Women in the United Arab Emirates. *Oncology Nursing Forum*, **29**, E91-E98. http://dx.doi.org/10.1188/02.ONF.E91-E98

[15] Anderson, B.O., Braun, S., Lim, S., Smith, R.A., Taplin, S. and Thomas, D.B. (2003) Early Detection of Breast Cancer in Countries with Limited Resources. *The Breast Journal*, **9**, S51-S59. http://dx.doi.org/10.1046/j.1524-4741.9.s2.4.x

[16] English, J. (2003) Importance of Breast Awareness in Identification of Breast Cancer. *Nursing Times*, **99**, 18-19.

[17] Odusanya, O.O. and Tayo, O.O. (2001) Breast Cancer Knowledge, Attitudes and Practice among Nurses in Lagos, Nigeria. *Acta Oncologica*, **40**, 844-848. http://dx.doi.org/10.1080/02841860152703472

[18] Sadler, G.R., Ko, C.M., Cohn, J.A., White, M., Weldon, R. and Wu, P. (2007) Breast Cancer Knowledge, Attitudes, and Screening Behaviors among African American Women: The Black Cosmetologists Promoting Health Program. *BMC Public Health*, **7**, 57. http://dx.doi.org/10.1186/1471-2458-7-57

[19] Grunfeld, E.A., Ramirez, A.J., Hunter, M.S. and Richards, M.A. (2002) Women's Knowledge and Beliefs Regarding Breast Cancer. *British Journal of Cancer*, **86**, 1373-1378. http://dx.doi.org/10.1038/sj.bjc.6600260

[20] Luquis, R.R. and Villanueva Cruz, I.J. (2006) Knowledge, Attitude and Perceptions about Breast Cancer and Breast Cancer Screening among Hispanic Women Residing in South Central Pennsylvania. *Journal of Community Health*, **31**, 25-42. http://dx.doi.org/10.1007/s10900-005-8187-x

[21] Okobia, M.N., Bunker, C.H., Okonofua, F.E. and Osime, U. (2006) Knowledge, Attitude and Practice of Nigerian Women towards Breast Cancer: A Cross-Sectional Study. *World Journal of Surgical Oncology*, **4**, 11. http://dx.doi.org/10.1186/1477-7819-4-11

[22] Hadi, M.A., Hassali, M.A., Shafie, A.A. and Awaisu, A. (2010) Evaluation of Breast Cancer Awareness among Female University Students in Malaysia. *Pharmacy Practice* (Internet), **8**, 29-34.

[23] Hadi, M.A., Hassali, M.A., Shafie, A.A. and Awaisu, A. (2010) Knowledge and Perception of Breast Cancer among Women of Various Ethnic Groups in the State of Penang: A Cross-Sectional Survey. *Medical Principles and Practice*, **19**, 61-67. http://dx.doi.org/10.1159/000252837

[24] Raosoft. An Online Sample Size Calculator. http://www.ezsurvey.com/samplesize

[25] Abdel Hadi, M. (2000) Breast Cancer Awareness among Health Professionals. *Annals of Saudi Medicine*, **20**, 135-136.

[26] Alam, A. (2006) Knowledge of Breast Cancer and Its Risk and Protective Factors among Women in Riyadh. *Annals of Saudi Medicine*, **26**, 272-277.

[27] Dandash, K. and Al-Mohaimeed, A. (2007) Knowledge, Attitudes, and Practices Surrounding Breast Cancer and Screening in Female Teachers of Buraidah, Saudi Arabia. *International Journal of Health Sciences*, **1**, 61-71.

[28] Linsell, L., Burgess, C. and Ramirez, A.J. (2008) Breast Cancer Awareness among Older Women. *British Journal of Cancer*, **99**, 1221-1225. http://dx.doi.org/10.1038/sj.bjc.6604668

[29] Montazeri, A., Vahdaninia, M., Harirchi, I., Harirchi, A.M., Sajadian, A., Khaleghi, F., *et al.* (2008) Breast Cancer in Iran: Need for Greater Women Awareness of Warning Signs and Effective Screening Methods. *Asia Pacific Family Medicine*, **7**, 6. http://dx.doi.org/10.1186/1447-056X-7-6

[30] Alharbi, N., Alshammari, M., Almutairi, B., Makboul, G. and El-Shazly, M. (2012) Knowledge, Awareness, and Practices Concerning Breast Cancer among Kuwaiti Female School Teachers. *Alexandria Journal of Medicine*, **48**, 75-82.

[31] Bener, A., El Ayoubi, H., Moore, M., Basha, B., Joseph, S. and Chouchane, L. (2009) Do We Need to Maximize the Breast Cancer Screening Awareness? Experience with an Endogamous Society with High Fertility. *Asian Pacific Journal of Cancer Prevention*, **10**, 599-604.

[32] Jahan, S., Al-Saigul, M. and Abdelgadir, M.H. (2006) Breast Cancer: Knowledge, Attitudes and Practices of Breast Self-Examination among Women in Qassim Region of Saudi Arabia. *Saudi Medical Journal*, **27**, 1737-1741.

[33] Radi, S.M. (2013) Breast Cancer Awareness among Saudi Females in Jeddah. *Asian Pacific Journal of Cancer Prevention*, **14**, 4307-4312. http://dx.doi.org/10.7314/APJCP.2013.14.7.4307

[34] Habib, F., Salman, S., Safwat, M. and Shalaby, S. (2010) Awareness and Knowledge of Breast Cancer among University Students in Al Madina Al Munawara Region. *Middle East Journal of Cancer*, **1**, 159-166.

6

Non-Axillary Sentinel Node in Breast Cancer. Are we Staging Correctly? A Multicenter Study

Javier Encinas Méndez[1], Joan Francesc Julián Ibáñez[2], Manel Cremades Pérez[2*], Jordi Navinés[2], Josep Verge Schulte-Eversum[1], Manel Fraile López-Amor[2], Manel Armengol Carrasco[3]

[1]Consorci Sanitari Garraf. H. Sant Camil, Sant Pere de Ribes, Spain
[2]Hospital Germans Trias i Pujol, Badalona, Spain
[3]H. U. Vall d' Hebron, Barcelona, Spain
Email: *Mcremades@outlook.com

Abstract

Purpose: The study of the sentinel lymph node is the best technique to stage, have a prognosis and decide the adequate treatment in breast cancer. The usual technique implies studding the axillary lymph node. Our work tries to identify affected nodes in other regions apart from the axilla and its possible impact in staging and treatment. Methods: The sentinel lymph node technique was performed on 1660 patients included in an observational and multicentric study designed to observe the presence of metastatic cells in axillary and non-axillary lymph nodes. Results: In 19% of the patients the sentinel lymph node was detected in non-axillary regions. In these cases metastatic cells were more frequent which could suppose a change in the stage and/or treatment. As protective factor against non-axillary nodes involvement we found the localization of the cancer in external quadrants while youth and injecting the tracer inside the tumor were found to be risk factors. Conclusions: Detecting and studding non-axillary lymph nodes in breast cancer leads to a more precise staging of the disease which could imply a change in the optimal treatment.

Keywords

Breast Neoplasms, Sentinel Lymph Node Biopsy, Neoplasm Staging

1. Introduction

Sentinel lymph node (SLN) assessment is the gold standard method to achieve a correct breast cancer staging [1]

---
*Corresponding author.

and, subsequently, decide its optimal treatment. Moreover, it is known to be one of the main prognostic factors in this disease [2].

It is remarkable that its use has usually been focused on the axillary lymph nodes, undervaluing hypothetic positive nodes in other areas and its possible consequences [3].

Nevertheless, traditional interpretation of SLN biopsy (SLNB) results is recently being questioned. As almost 70% of positive axillary SLN patients do not have metastasis performing an axillary lymph node dissection (ALND) seems to be overtreatment [4]. Selected patients with specific tumor characteristic, even with a positive axillary SLN, may benefit from a conservative attitude, thus eliminating complications of axillary surgery with no adverse effect on survival [5] [6].

Currently not many trials have been done to confirm this hypothesis so more research in this field is needed.

However, despite the decisions taken after this possible new interpretation, the SLN technique remains the main staging test in breast cancer.

That is why it is relevant to identify and examine sentinel lymph nodes located in other areas than the axilla to reach a more precise staging [7] [8] of the disease, changing its treatment if necessary.

2. Material and Methods

A prospective, multicenter cohort study was undertaken in 9 different hospitals in Catalonia (Spain) from January 2000 to February 2008.

All patients diagnosed of breast cancer who underwent a sentinel lymph node assessment and accomplished the selection criteria (**Table 1**, **Table 2**) were enrolled.

The sample size was calculated using the ENE program and fixed to 1660 patients. As reference we took an estimated prevalence of 20% of positive non-axillary nodes (CI 95% and accuracy +/−2%).

We focused our study on nodal identification, whether axillary or non-axillary.

As secondary variables, and related to the breast cancer, we assessed the patients age, preoperative diagnostic, radiological diagnostic, margin status, palpable nodes, presence of micrometastasis, single or multiple nodal involvement, location, histological type, vascular or lymphatic infiltration, tumor size, positive hormone receptors and/or Erb2 and type of treatment.

Related to the SLN biopsy we studied the injection method, the number of nodes identified in the lymphoscintigraphy, the number of nodes identified in the dissection and the number of nodal metastasis.

To carry out the study all the institutions followed the same protocol.

Table 1. Inclusion criteria.

Inclusion Criteria
Infiltrative carcinomas, less than 3 cm wide, with clinically negative axillary nodes
Multifocal tumor in the same breast quadrant
Large intraductal *in situ* carcinoma (>3 cm, high grade and/or comedo)
Male patients with breast cancer and the same characteristics

Table 2. Exclusion criteria.

Exclusion Criteria
Patients with no nodal involvement after SLNB
Pregnancy
Multicentric tumors
Patients with advanced disease who require preoperative chemotherapy or those who present metastatic axillary nodes after FNA
Inflammatory breast carcinoma
Previous axillary radiotherapy
Previous axillary surgery

The day before surgery patients were visited and, after and axillary sonography to rule out suspicious unpalpable lymph nodes, 0.3 ml of tracer (99 m-Tc labeled human albumin) was injected either inside of the tumor, peritumorally, subdermally or subareorarly. No colorant was used.

In case of positive sonography fine needle aspiration (FNA) cytology was performed.

Sentinel nodes (SNs) were initially identified with lymphoscintigraphy to ease surgical location and dissection. Surgery took place the day after the lymphoscintigraphic study and a hand-held γ-probe was used to identify SNs following the 10% rule.

Cytology was carried out perioperatively when axillary SNs were located, proceeding to perform an axillary lymph node dissection (ALND) if positive. On the other hand, when internal mammary SNs were located its study was completed postoperatively as results would not modify the surgical procedure.

Next, all SNs were studied with immunohistochemical analysis to detect unseen metastasis in the cytology.

In case of positive results our therapeutic approach varied depending on the size and location:

- More than 2 mm: We performed a complete ALND;
- Between 0.2 and 2 mm (micrometastasis): Patients joined a clinical trial where ALND and routine controls were compared [9];
- Less than 0.2 mm: Were considered as isolated tumor cells (ITC) so no ALND was carried out;
- If located in the internal mammary radiotherapy was indicated.

Once all data was collected we carried out descriptive, bivariate and multivariate analysis with the statistical softwares SPSS and G-Stat with a P value < 0.05.

3. Results

A middle age woman, with a single palpable tumor located in the upper outer quadrants was the most common presentation. Infiltrative ductal carcinoma with hormone receptor expression represented the typical histology. The most frequent nodal location was axillary followed by simultaneous axillary and non-axillary drainage.

Lymph node metastasis varied depending on its location. Thus, patients with drainage to axillary and non-axillary nodes, without involvement of internal mammary ones, were the group of patients who presented a higher rate of metastasis. Afterwards, we found those who had involvement of non-axillary nodes with exception of internal mammary ones, followed by those who presented simultaneous axillary and internal mammary nodes. It is not until the fourth group that we found patients with only axillary drainage and, finally, patients with only involvement of internal mammary nodes.

Patients, tumor and drainage characteristics are presented in **Table 3**.

4. Bivariate Statistical Analysis

Patients that presented non-axillary drainage were statistically younger, with an average age of 52 yo, in comparison with those who had axillary drainage (p < 0.001) (**Table 4**). Similarly, younger patients presented a greater proportion of non-axillary drainage.

Regarding the injection technique, intratumoral and peritumoral injection also showed a greater tendency towards non-axillary nodes [10] [11] than subdermal or subareolar injection (p = 0.009) (**Table 5**).

It's also remarkable that the number of sentinel nodes detected was statistically larger when non-axillary drainage was present (p < 0.001) and the incidence of metastatic nodes was higher too in this scenario (p < 0.001).

Tumor location, as described in the literature, is clearly related to lymph drainage. Accordingly, in our study, tumors in outer quadrants tended to have a lymphatic drain towards axillary nodes (53% vs 39%; p < 0.001) while those in inner quadrants presented opposite results (47% vs 61%; p < 0.001).

Patients with non-axillary nodes affected had more aggressive tumors. Mastectomies were more frequent in these cases than tumorectomies (18 vs 13%; p = 0.014) and vascular and lymphatic infiltration were more prevalent (33% vs 18%) although the difference was not statistically significant (p = 0.064).

There were no apparent differences in tumor size, presence of free margins after surgery, micrometastasis, hormone receptors, HER 2 expression, histologic type and grade of cancer.

5. Multivariate Statistical Analysis

A logistic regression was carried out to identify important dependent variables related with axillary and non-axillary lymph draining.

As dependent variables we included the tumor location, the number of nodes dissected, the number of metastatic nodes, the age and the tracer injection method. The model was statistically significant with p < 0.001.

Results showed that being less than 50 yo (OR = 2.21) and intratumoral and peritumoral tracer injection (OR = 1.52) were risk factors to present non-axillary lymph nodes involvement (**Table 6**).

Table 3. Patient, tumor and drainage characteristics.

Number of Patients	1660 Women
Mean Age	57 years old
Major Incidence Range	50 to 63 years old
Palpable Tumor	53% of cases
Single Tumor	89% of cases
Location	34.96% upper outer quadrant
	16.20% upper quadrant union
	11.44% upper inner quadrant
	10.38% outer quadrant union
	9.19% inner quadrant union
	8.38% areolar
	5.13% lower outer quadrant
	4.32% lower inner quadrant
Histology	70.4% infiltrative ducal carcinoma
	11.87% intraductal *in situ* carcinoma
	5.86% infiltrative intraductal carcinoma
	5.73% lobulillar carcinoma
	8.14% others
Size	1.82 cm (SD 0.98; range 0.2 - 8.1 cm)
Vascular or Linfatic Infiltration	28% of cases
Positive Hormone Receptors	83% of cases
Positive Erb2	30% of cases
Tracer Injection	59.81% intratumoral
	31.57% intratumoral + subdermal
	6.44% peritumoral
	2.19% subareolar
Number of Nodes Biopsied	1.44 (SD 0.69)
Number of Metastatic Sentinel Nodes	0.3 (SD 0.56)
Nodal Location	1.364 axillary (82.2%)
	267 axillary and non-axillary (16.1%)
	29 extra-axillary (1.7%)
Surgical Treatment	86.45% tumorectomy
	13.55% mastectomy
Axillary Lymph Node Dissection	24% of cases
Metastatic Nodes	0.87 (SD 2.15; range 0 - 21)

Table 4. Quantitative variables comparing axillary vs non-axillary drainage.

	Non-Axillary (mean)	Axillary (mean)	p-Value
Age	52	58	<0.001
Nodes Identified	2.05	1.29	<0.001
Mestatatic Nodes	0.46	0.26	<0.001
Tumoral Size (cm)	1.87	1.81	0.299

Table 5. Qualitative variables comparing axillary vs non-axillary drainage.

	Non-Axillary N (%)	Axillary N (%)	p-Value
Age			<0.001
<50 yo	155 (49.4)	379 (28.6)	
>50 yo	159 (50.6)	945 (71.4)	
Injection Method			0.009
Intratumoral	204 (65.2)	781 (58.5)	
Peritumoral	24 (7.7)	82 (6.1)	
Subdermal	84 (26.8)	436 (31.6)	
Subareolar	1 (0.3)	35 (2.6)	
Treatment			0.014
Tumorectomy	261 (82.1)	1162 (87.5)	
Mastectomy	57 (17.9)	166 (12.5)	
Tumor Location			<0.001
Outer Quadrants	122 (39.2)	685 (53.2)	
Inner Quadrants	189 (60.8)	603 (46.8)	
Vascular/Lymphatic Infiltration			
Yes	54 (33.5)	375 (26.3)	0.064
No	107 (66.5)	522 (73.7)	
Number of Nodes			
1 or more	101 (31.8)	328 (24.4)	0.007
0	217 (68.2)	1014 (75.6)	
Free Margins			0.501
Cytology			0.169
Micrometastasis			0.843
Single/Multiple			0.346
Histology			0.130
Hormone Receptors			0.222
Erb2			0.184

Table 6. Multivariate analysis.

	p-Value	OR	CI 95%
Age	<0.001	2.21	1.64 - 2.98
Number of nodes	<0.001	0.22	0.18 - 0.28
Metastasic nodes	0.579		
Location	<0.001	0.49	0.36 - 0.67
Injection method	<0.001	1.52	1.10 - 2.10

On the contrary, outer quadrants location of the tumor seemed to be a protective factor (OR = 0.49).

The number of nodes detected remained higher when non-axillary drainage was detected but the number of metastatic nodes was not statistically different when analyzed simultaneously with the number of nodes detected (p = 0.579).

6. Discussion

Breast cancer is a very prevalent illness and implies important clinical and aesthetic consequences, mainly in women. Nevertheless, thanks to the evolution of diagnostics and treatments, almost 80% of patients get cured.

But not only rates of cure must be taken into account. To avoid consequences of surgical treatment the SLNB technique was developed, saving lots of unnecessary axillary dissections.

Nowadays this question is more up-to-date than ever given that, even with a positive axillary SLN, the necessity of performing an ALND is being questioned in the literature [4]-[6] [12]. Essentially, this implies that to improve our treatments and adapt them to each patient needs, an accurate staging must previously be carried out.

Consequently, although axillary draining is the most common and its implications have been well studied, non-axillary drainage is often underestimated. Current research shows draining towards internal mammary nodes in a range between 2.4% and 23.3% [7] [13] [14]. Obviously, this proportion gets higher when Rotter, intramammary or intercostal nodes are also included. This fact may lead to suppose that an incorrect staging is sometimes performed, meaning that a suboptimal treatment could be given.

It is important to highlight that almost 20% of breast neoplasm present lymphatic draining to non-axillary nodes, the vast majority with concomitant draining to axillary ones, being more frequently metastatic.

The presence of metastatic nodes in non-axillary regions would imply a change in the illness stage in case of negative axillary ones. Moreover, those patients presenting both axillary and non-axillary metastatic nodes would remain in the same illness stage but optimal treatment would require addition of radiotherapy, at least in internal mammary nodal chain [14].

Another interesting consequence is that, traditionally, it has been proposed that the presence of nodal metastasis could imply a lymphatic block that could lead to alternative drainage pathways. This may be the reason why there seems to be more metastatic nodes when simultaneous drainage to axillary and non-axillary regions is present [10]. However, more studies need to be done to confirm this hypothesis.

If that was the case, the attitude in patients with positive preoperative axillary nodes should be reconsidered as, currently, the SLNB is dismissed and an ALND is directly performed. Consequently, we fail to know if there is simultaneous draining towards non-axillary nodes which would be an indication of postoperative radiotherapy.

Unfortunately, given the usual difficulty to reach non-axillary nodes, its dissection is hardly ever performed.

In conclusion, we consider that doing a biopsy of non-axillary nodes is an important factor to carry out an accurate staging of the disease, and therefore, decide the optimal treatment in each patient [8]. Moreover, traditional staging should also be reconsidered given that atypical nodal location is not considered.

References

[1] Moncayo, V.M., Aarsvold, J.N., Grant, S.F., Bartley, S.C. and Alazraki, N.P. (2013) Status of Sentinel Lymph Node for Breast Cancer. *Seminars in Nuclear Medicine*, **43**, 281-293. http://dx.doi.org/10.1053/j.semnuclmed.2013.02.004

[2] García Fernández, A., Chabrera, C., García Font, M., Fraile, M., Lain, J.M., Barco, I., González, C., Gónzalez, S., Reñe, A., Veloso, E., Cassadó, J., Pessarrodona, A. and Giménez, N. (2013) Positive versus Negative Sentinel Nodes in Early Breast Cancer Patients: Axillary or Loco-Regional Relapse and Survival. A Study Spanning 2000-2012. *Breast*, **22**, 902-907. http://dx.doi.org/10.1016/j.breast.2013.04.015

[3] Kim, H., Shin, M.J., Kim, S.J., Kim, I.J. and Park, I. (2014) The Relation of Visualization of Internal Mammary Lymph Nodes on Lymphoscintigraphy to Axillary Lymph Node Metastases in Breast Cancer. *Lymphatic Research and Biology*, **21**.

[4] Grabau, D., Dihge, L., Fernö, M., Ingvar, C. and Rydén, L. (2013) Completion Axillary Dissection Can Safely Be Omitted in Screen Detected Breast Cancer Patients with Micrometastases. A Decade's Experience from a Single Institution. *European Journal of Surgical Oncology (EJSO)*, **39**, 601-607. http://dx.doi.org/10.1016/j.ejso.2013.03.012

[5] Krishnan, MS, Recht, A., Bellon, J.R. and Punglia, R.S. (2013) Trade-Offs Associated with Axillary Lymph Node Dissection with Breast Irradiation versus Breast Irradiation Alone in patients with a Positive Sentinel Node in Relation to the Risk of Non-Sentinel Node Involvement: Implications of ACOSOG Z0011. *Breast Cancer Research and Treatment*, **138**, 205-213.

[6]   Suyoi, A., Bains, S.K., Kothari, A., Douek, M., Agbaje, O., Hamed, H., Fentiman, I., Pinder, S. and Purushotham, A.D. (2014) When Is a Completion Axillary Lymph Node Dissection Necessary in the Presence of a Positive Sentinel Lymph Node? *European Journal of Cancer*, **50**, 690-697. http://dx.doi.org/10.1016/j.ejca.2013.11.024

[7]   Gnerlich, J.L., Barreto-Andrade, J.C., Czechura, T., John, J.R., Turk, M.A., Kennedy, T.J. and Winchester, D.J. (2014) Accurate Staging with Internal Mammary Chain Sentinel Node Biopsy for Breast Cancer. *Annals of Surgical Oncology*, **21**, 368-374. http://dx.doi.org/10.1245/s10434-013-3263-4

[8]   Caudle, A.S., Yi, M., Hoffman, K.E., Mittendorf, E.A., Babiera, G.V., Hwang, R.F., Meric-Bernstam, F., Sahin, A.A. and Hunt, K.K. (2014) Impact of Identification of Internal Mammary Sentinel Lymph Node Metastasis in Breast Cancer Patients. *Annals of Surgical Oncology*, **21**, 60-65. http://dx.doi.org/10.1245/s10434-013-3276-z

[9]   Solá, M., Alberro, J.A., Fraile, M., Santesteban, P., Ramos, M., Fabregas, R., Moral, A., Ballester, B. and Vidal, S. (2013) Complete Axillary Lymph Node Dissection versus Clinical Follow-Up in Breast Cancer Patients with Sentinel Node Micrometastasis: Final Results from the Multicenter Clinical Trial AATRM 048/13/2000. *Annals of Surgical Oncology*, **20**, 120-127. http://dx.doi.org/10.1245/s10434-012-2569-y

[10] Garcia-Manero, M., Olartecoechea, B. and Royo, P. (2010) Different Injection Sites of Radionuclide for Sentinel Lymph Node Detection in Breast Cancer: Single Institution Experience. *European Journal of Obstetrics & Gynecology and Reproductive Biology*, **153**, 185-187. http://dx.doi.org/10.1016/j.ejogrb.2010.06.024

[11] Noushi, F., Spillane, A.J., Uren, R.F., Cooper, R., Allwright, S., Snook, K.L., Gillet, D., Pearce, A.M. and Gebski, V. (2013) High Discordance Rates between Sub-Areolar and Peri-Tumoural Breast Lymphoscintigraphy. *European Journal of Surgical Oncology* (*EJSO*), **39**, 1053-1060. http://dx.doi.org/10.1016/j.ejso.2013.06.006

[12] Gatzemeier, W. and Mann, G.B. (2013) Which Sentinel Lymph-Node (SLN) Positive Breast Cancer Patient Needs an Axillary Lymph-Node Dissection (ALND)—ACOSOG Z0011 Results and beyond. *Breast*, **22**, 211-216.

[13] Van der Ploeg, I.M., Tanis, P.J., Valdés Olmos, R.A., Kroon, B.B., Rutgers, E.J. and Nieweg, O.E. (2008) Breast Cancer Patients with Extra-Axillary Sentinel Nodes Only May Be Spared Axillary Lymph Node Dissection. *Annals of Surgical Oncology*, **15**, 3239-3243. http://dx.doi.org/10.1245/s10434-008-0120-y

[14] Cong, B.B., Qiu, P.F. and Wang, Y.S. (2014) Internal Mammary Sentinel Lymph Node Biopsy: Minimally Invasive Staging and Tailored Internal Mammary Radiotherapy. *Annals of Surgical Oncology*, **21**, 2119-2121. http://dx.doi.org/10.1245/s10434-014-3650-5

7

Adenoma of the Nipple, Mimicking Paget's Disease of the Breast: Report of a Case

Ahmed Abbas*, Ali Al-Zaher, Ali El Arini, Ikram Chaudhry

Department of Surgery, King Fahad Specialist Hospital, Dammam, KSA
Email: *ahmednci@gmail.com

Abstract

Nipple adenoma is a rare benign condition that simulates malignancy. A 37-year-old woman presented with unilateral bloody nipple discharge for 1-year duration followed by severe nipple erosion. As biopsy revealed nipple adenoma and therefore, complete local excision was done. The final histopathology showed florid papillomatosis which was adequately excised. Nipple adenoma although rare entity this should be included in the differential diagnosis of any nipple erosion such as carcinoma and Paget's disease of the breast specially when associated with bloody discharge in premenopausal women.

Keywords

Nipple Adenoma, Benign Breast Lesion, Florid Papillomatosis of the Nipple

1. Introduction

Nipple adenoma is a rare benign neoplasm which originates from the nipple of the breast. In 1955 Jones described this first time as florid papillomatosis. Also this condition is known as erosive adenomatosis or superficial papillary adenomatosis. Although this is a benign tumor clinically it is very difficult to differentiate between malignant conditions like carcinoma and Paget's disease of the breast [1]. Patient usually presents with subareolar nodule, pain, nipple discharge, erythema and ulceration

Proper pre-operative diagnosis is essential because any misinterpretation of histopathological report can lead to undue mastectomy as reported by Carter *et al.* [2].

2. Case Presentation

A 36-year-old woman presented with a history of a left sided bloody nipple discharge for one year duration.

---

*Corresponding author.

Subsequently she developed severe nipple ulceration. The patient was seen by a dermatologist and was given systemic antibiotics and local corticosteroids with no response. On physical examination, the left nipple was completely eroded with extensive skin ulceration. Otherwise, both breasts and axillae were clinically free with no palpable lymphadenopathy.

Clinical differential diagnoses included: Paget's disease of the nipple and skin malignancy. However, nipple adenoma was not clinically suspected. Bilateral breast ultrasound and mammogram did not show any abnormality. Small incisional biopsy showed nipple adenoma. A complete excision of the eroded left nipple and part of the surrounded areola was achieved in addition to part of the retro-areolar breast tissue (**Figure 1**). Microscopically, the nipple showed lesion featuring complex ducts composed of bland oval cells with variable degree of hyperplasia which were focally continuous with squamous epithelium of the skin. The epithelial cells did not display any significant pleomorphism, mitotic activity or necrosis. Focal nipple ulceration is also noted (**Figure 2** and **Figure 3**), without evidence of malignancy. The picture was consistent with nipple adenoma. Nipple reconstruction was planned at a later stage.

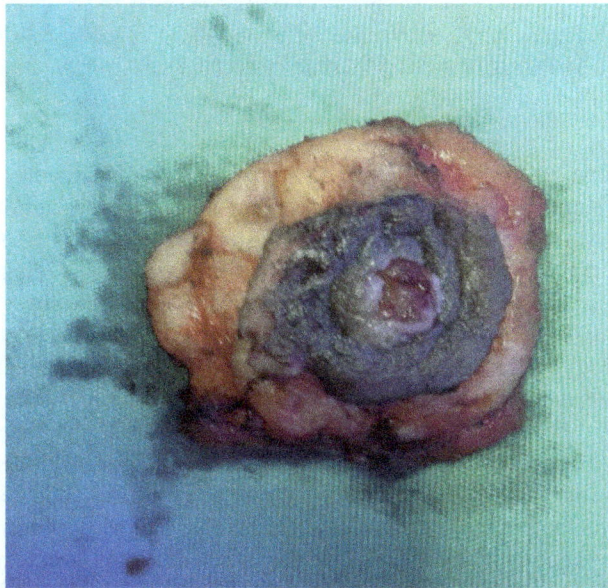

Figure 1. gross picture of the resected specimen including the eroded nipple, part of the areola and underlying breast tissue.

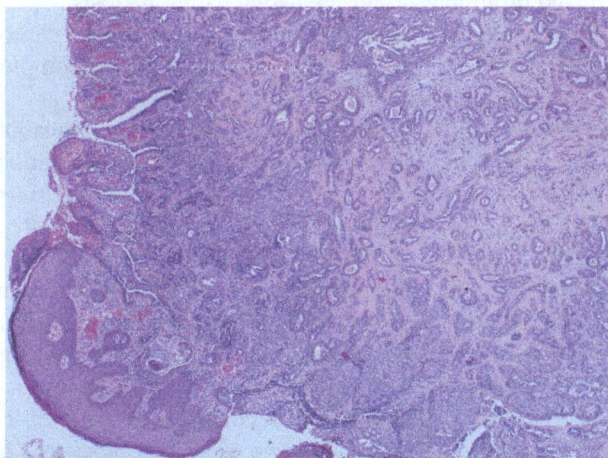

Figure 2. Complex ductal architecture underlying the surface epithelium with focal ulceration. (4× Low-power photomicrograph).

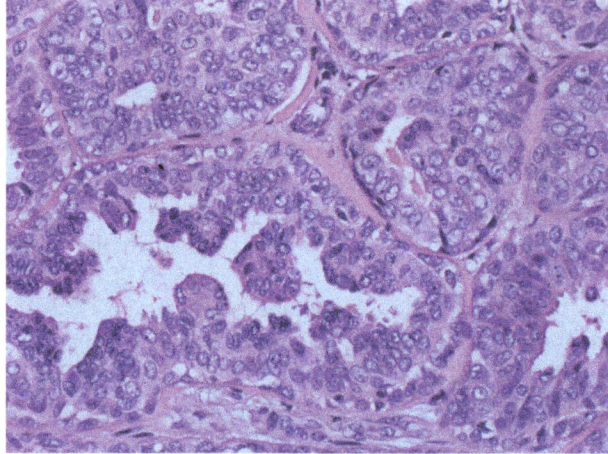

Figure 3. Ducts comprised of bland-looking epithelial cells with variable hyperplasia. (20× High-Power photomicrograph).

3. Discussion

Nipple adenoma, also known as florid papillomatosis, erosive adenomatosis or superficial papillary adenomatosis is a benign condition simulating malignancy such as breast carcinoma and/or Paget's disease clinically [1]. Women in their 4th and 5th decades commonly affected and usually they presents with unilateral, serous or bloody nipple discharge in the presence of crusting. The main differential diagnosis is Paget's disease of the nipple based on similar clinical features like soreness, ulceration and swelling of the nipple, sometimes with discharge [3] [4]. However, Paget's disease is more common in older women and Paget's cells can be detected by aspiration biopsy cytology. Whereas adenoma of the nipple tends to occur in premenopausal women.

The pathological characteristics of adenoma of the nipple are the maintenance of a double layer composed of epithelial and myoepithelial cells, no accompanying epithelial necrosis, and a definite direction of the duct cell arrangement in a pattern of pseudo invasion. It can be difficult to distinguish adenoma of the nipple from ductal carcinoma when the adenoma shows a marked proliferation of epithelial cells accompanied by pseudo invasion [5]. The coexistence of carcinoma and nipple adenoma has been noticed before by many investigators, and the reported incidence of this phenomenon varies in different studies. Fisher *et al.*, found that, in a group of 967 patients with carcinoma, 1.2% had associated nipple adenoma [6].

Nipple adenomas are papillary or solid adenomas developing within the nipple where proliferation of papillary epithelium is remarkable [2] [7]. The histological patterns of nipple adenoma are described by Rosen as adenosis, papillomatosis, mixed proliferative and sclerosing papillomatosis [8].

There is no evidence of metastasis in this disease but local recurrences can occur when the neoplasm is incompletely excised. Hence, nipple reconstruction is usually planned after completeness of excision is confirmed histologically.

Bloody or serous nipple discharge is the most common presenting complaint in 65% - 70% of the patients, followed by enlargement and induration of the nipple associated with ulceration, which have been reported in medical literature [9]-[11]. However, histopathological evidence is medatory for the diagnosis of this rare condition. Afetab *et al.*, described 19 cases of nipple adenoma over a period of 14 years; all patients were females with age ranging from 23 to 63 years. Most of the cases presented clinically with induration and ulceration. The diagnosis was clinically suspected in only 3 cases and the final diagnosis was confirmed by histology alone [12].

Similarly, our patient presented with bloody nipple discharge associated with extensive erosion raising the clinical suspicion of Paget's disease. Incisional biopsy was performed and histopathology report revealed a diagnosis, adenoma of nipple. Since complete excision is curative, local recurrence has been reported in 30% of incompletely excised lesions [13], our patient underwent complete excision of the eroded nipple and part of the areola together with part of the retro-areolar breast tissue to achieve adequate excision and minimize local recurrence. The final histopathologic diagnosis showed adequately excised nipple adenoma.

In conclusion we report a rare case of nipple adenoma mimicking Paget's disease of breast which is a diagnostic challenge. Nipple adenoma should be considered as a part of differential diagnosis when there is severe nipple erosion. Complete excision is the treatment of choice to avoid local reccurence.

Acknowledgments

We thank Dr. Abdul-Wahed Meshikhes, Consultant surgeon at Department of Surgery, King Fahad Specialist Hospital, Dammam 31444, Saudi Arabia, for revising the manuscript.

References

[1]   Kijima, Y., Matsukita, S., Yoshinaka, H., Owaki, T. and Aikou, T. (2006) Adenoma of the Nipple: Report of a Case. *Breast Cancer*, **13**, 95-99. http://dx.doi.org/10.2325/jbcs.13.95

[2]   Carter, E. and Dyess, D.L. (2004) Infiltrating Syringomatous Adenoma of the Nipple: A Case Report and 20-Year Retrospective Review. *The Breast Journal*, **10**, 443-447. http://dx.doi.org/10.1111/j.1075-122X.2004.21518.x

[3]   Tavassoli, F.A. and Devillee, P. Editors (2003) World Health Organisation Classification of Tumours: Pathology and Genetics of Tumours of the Breast and Female Genital Organs. IARC Press, Lyon.

[4]   Healy, C.E., Dijikstra, B., Walsh, M., Hill, A.D. and Murphy, J. (2003) Nipple Adenoma: A Differential Diagnosis for Paget's Disease. *The Breast Journal*, **9**, 325-326. http://dx.doi.org/10.1046/j.1524-4741.2003.09417.x

[5]   Sato. T., Muto, I., Hasegawa, M., Aono, T., Okada, T., Tamura, T., *et al.* (2007) A Rare Case of Invasive Ductal Carcinoma with Hyperprolactinemia. *Breast Cancer*, **14**, 302-306. http://dx.doi.org/10.2325/jbcs.14.302

[6]   Jones, M.W. and Tavassoli, F.A. (1995) Co-Existance of Nipple Duct Adenoma and Breast Carcinoma: A Clinicopathologic Study of 5 Cases and Review of Literature. *Modern Pathology*, **8**, 633-636. http://dx.doi.org/10.1097/00000478-198307080-00003

[7]   Rosen, P.P. (1983) Syringomatous Adenoma of the Nipple. *The American Journal of Surgical Pathology*, **7**, 739-745.

[8]   Rosen, P.P. (2009) Rosen's Breast Pathology. 3rd Edition, Lippincott William & Wilkins, Philadelphia.

[9]   Da Costa, D., Taddese, A., Cure, M.L., Gerson, G., Poppiti Jr., R. and Esserman, L. (2007) Common and Unusual Diseases of the Nipple-Areolar Complex. *Radiographics*, **27**, S65-S77. http://dx.doi.org/10.1148/rg.27si075512

[10] Montemarano, A.D., Sau, P. and James, W.D. (1995) Superficial Papillary Adenomatosis of the Nipple: A Case Report and Review of the Literature. *Journal of the American Academy of Dermatology*, **33**, 871-875. http://dx.doi.org/10.1016/0190-9622(95)90425-5

[11] Tavassoli, F.A. (1999) Pathology of the Breast. 2nd Edition, Appleton & Lange, Stamford.

[12] Afetab, K., Indrees, R., Rauf, F. and Kayani, N. (2010) Nipple Adenoma of Breast: A Masquerader of Malignancy. *Journal of the College of Physicians and Surgeons Pakistan*, **20**, 472-474.

[13] Chang, C.K., Jacobs, I.A., Calilao, G. and Salti, G.I. (2003) Metastatic Infiltrating Syringomatous Adenoma of the Breast. *Archives of Pathology Laboratory Medicine*, **127**, E155-E156.

8

Ultrasound Alongside with Mammogram in Women with Physically Dense Breast

Fadak S. Alshayookh, Howayda M. Ahmed, Ibrahim A. Awad, Saddig D. Jastaniah*

Department of Diagnostic Radiology, Faculty of Applied Medical Sciences, King Abdulaziz University, Jeddah, KSA

Email: *sjastaniah@kau.edu.sa

Abstract

We report usefulness of ultrasound used as an adjunct diagnostic tool to mammogram in routine annual checkup for women breasts of certain ages and breast mass. The purpose of breast imaging is to detect areas of tissue distortion and breast cancers. A mammogram is the common diagnostic imaging modality used to find breast diseases but sometimes the mammogram might not give the doctor enough information especially in women with dense breasts. As a result, the patient may be asked to undergo ultrasound or magnetic resonance imaging as a better mean of judgment to the case. Because ultrasound is widely used, simple and safe to patients we were encouraged to emphasis on exploring its role adjunct to mammogram. A retrospective observation study was done at the diagnostic radiology department at King Abdulaziz University Hospital (KAUH) in the period from January 2012 to June 2012; we covered all women with dense breasts in mammography and ultrasound units. The study group was 40 patients. All patients were imaged with both mammography and ultrasound. The statistical measures of accuracy, sensitivity and specificity were calculated using the SPSS program. The results we obtained suggest that age and the physical density of breast potentially affect mammogram images of women with 41 years or smaller with sensitivity 66% and specificity 68%. Therefore, we recommend using ultrasound alongside the mammogram in women with dense breast for better diagnosis of small cancers that were not identified on mammography or clinical breast examination alone.

Keywords

Ultrasound, Mammogram, Dense Breasts, Women Breasts

1. Introduction

Regular, systematic imaging of breast tissue is fundamental to the detection of altered breast architecture, al-

*Corresponding author.

lowing for sampling, analysis and identification of benign or malignant potential. Breast imaging can be achieved with magnetic resonance imaging, mammography and ultrasound alone or in combination, although, performance of obtaining information from mammography is reduced due to overlying of tissues in dense breast [1].

Breast density refers to the relative amount of fibrous and glandular tissue which attenuates x-rays on a mammogram. The breast density impacts breast cancer detection. While there are limitations of breast density measures, multiple studies demonstrate that breast cancer risk is increased for women with dense breasts. The decreased sensitivity of mammography in dense breasts is a major limitation of mammography [2].

Dense breasts do not indicate abnormality, but may increase risk of breast cancer. However, experts do not agree which modality should be used in such cases in addition to mammograms [3].

It has been reported [4] that the density of dense structures such as the milk ducts is similar to the tumor making it difficult to interpret. Increased breast density is known to cause a parallel decrease in mammographic sensitivity suggesting there is a need for additional imaging if adequate interrogation of breast tissue is to occur [5].

Recent research documents that increased breast density can be acknowledged as an independent risk factor for breast cancer, with imaging of both mammography and bilateral whole breast ultrasound now considered to be the best practice. Patients with dense breast tissue may additionally have other risk factors and even though a mammographic examination may have a negative result, it is appropriate to provide additional imaging [6].

Mammographic images are assessing for the presence of mass/es, asymmetric focal density, architectural distortion and the presence of micro-calcifications. The clinical findings should be document including comment on palpable lumps, tissue thickening, and skin puckering or nipple retractions. The size, shape, density and margins of all masses are noted. The distribution and morphology of micro-calcifications, multi-focal and multi-centric lesions, architectural distortion of the breast tissue and skin thickening are all reported [7].

Ultrasound is widely used, simple and safe to patients [8]. It images tissues of the breast to the chest wall via a technique known as cross-sectional technique in order to display the tissue with no overlap [5] [9].

Breast ultrasound as is it known today, had its roots in military technology, with initial developments occurring more than 50 years ago. In the past it was noted that ultrasound was "not seen as a breast screening tool" but was commonly used to evaluate breast abnormalities found at mammography [10]. In the current clinical setting, breast ultrasound is often seen as an integral part of breast imaging programs. The ultrasound has revolutionized the evaluation of breast abnormalities with providing a rapid, cost effective, and accurate guidance method for a wide range of interventional techniques [11]. Targeted breast ultrasound is used to interrogate a specific area of breast tissue, and is widely accepted as a diagnostic tool for the evaluation of palpable and non-palpable breast abnormalities in conjunction with mammography [12].

The ultrasound is not a screening tool and cannot replace mammography. This study aims at demonstrating the importance of using ultrasound as together with mammography to each annual screen for women with dense breasts.

2. Materials and Methods

2.1. Patients and Methods

Our observation study was done at the diagnostic radiology department at KAUH after obtaining research ethical approval. The study was done during the academic year 2012. Within about the first six months of 2012; we covered all women with dense breasts in mammography and ultrasound department. After exclusion unwanted cases, the group study was 40 patients. Patients imaged both using mammography and ultrasound (**Figure 1** and **Figure 2**). The statistical measures of accuracy, sensitivity and specificity were calculated using the SPSS program.

2.2. Patients

The study was a retrospective, nonrandomized, observational clinical case series. We retrospectively analyzed the records of patients diagnosed they have problem related with dense breast and registered in the clinic between January 2012 and Jun 2012. The total number of patients who presented for breast imaging during this time was 356 patients. The exclusion criteria were patients who either had previous breast diseases (113 pa-

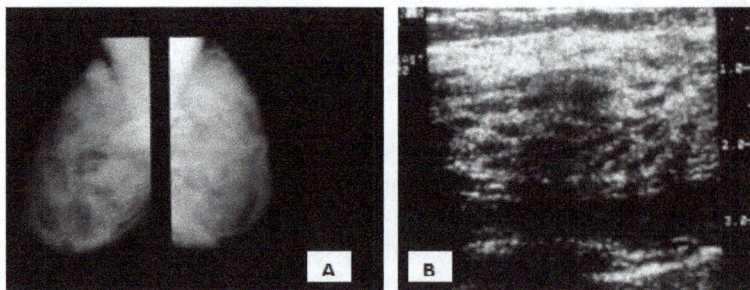

Figure 1. Normal mammographic (A) and ultrasound (B) images of dense breast.

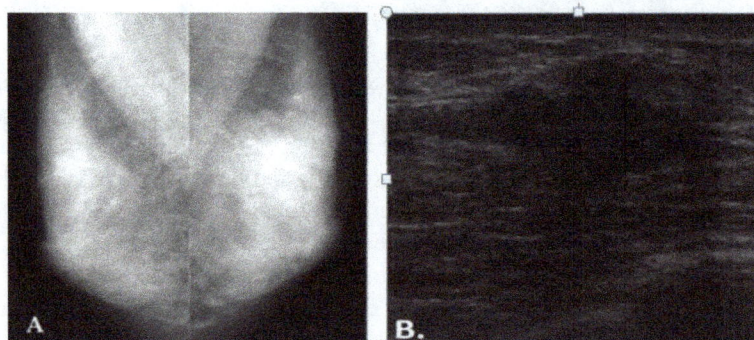

Figure 2. Palpable left dense breast lump. (A) Whole-breast mediolateral mammographic image reveals no abnormality; (B) Ultrasound image shows solid mass with irregular shape, indistinct and angular margins. Histopathology revealed invasive ductal carcinoma.

tients), or who has fatty breast parenchyma—not a dense breast—(93 patients), or only mammography examination was done (75 patients), or only ultrasound examination was done (35 patients). So, our sample is 40 patients with dense breast parenchyma. The patients' ages range from 34 to 61 years. All the patients within the study group had both mammogram and ultrasound examinations in the standard technique which is mentioned in the previous chapter. The images then sent to PACS.

2.3. Image Interpretation

The images produced were autonomously evaluated using PACS workstations with the help of qualified radiologist with good experience in breast mammogram and ultrasound .The images of each patient were reviewed with computer aided analysis in the plans which are performed. The radiologist also makes comments on the presence of anatomical variations of breast including flat nipple, inverted nipple, large breast and large nipple, etc.

2.4. Statistical Analysis

Demographic data of participants together with mammogram and ultrasound findings were collected and statistically analyzed using the SPSS program to find and show the relationship between both findings and which is stronger modality in case of dense breast by the sensitivity and specificity test.

3. Results

The total of 40 patients was collecting from KAU hospital within about the first six months of 2012, their age ranged from 34 to 61. According to the World Health Organization for the division of ages (WHO), the category of young adult patient will be aged from 20 to 40 years old and the category of middle adult patient will be aged from 40 to 65 years old. The mean in this sample is 45.5 years and standard deviation is 6.82 years indicate to variation and skewness is 0.355 indicate to most of age distribution less than mean. This means the average of age is 45.5 years which is located within interval +6.820, −6.820 and most of age less than 35 years. As we see (**Table 1**) represented basic statistics of age as mean, standard deviation and skewness. **Figure 3** also shows distribution of age by category: Young adult (20 - 40) and Middle adult (40 - 65). In **Figure 4** below we can see the method of diagnosis which is used. The Mammogram was detect perfectly as Ultrasound (same result) in 37.5%, 4 of patient was in young adult category and 11 was in middle adult category. While the Ultrasound was superiority in diagnosis and detects 62.5% of cases, 7 patients was in young adult category and 18 were in middle adult category. Cross tabulation shows the methods used in each age category (**Table 2**) and graph it that in (**Figure 5**).

When the sensitivity and Specificity test was done, the area under the curve was 0.511 with standard error for them was 0.096 and 95% confidant interval from 0.322 to 0.699 as shown in (**Table 3**). But we can see the area under the curve was not a significant which means that may diagnosed by Mammogram and Ultrasound doesn't have any sense different if patient age equal or greater than 41.5 years old. In the patient age less than 41.5 years old, the sensitivity of mammogram is decreased and the differences between mammogram and ultrasound results will appear.

As a result, the best cut-off that maximize (sensitivity + specificity) was 41.5 years old. At this duration, the sensitivity was 0.667 and specificity was 0.680 (1 − Specificity = 0.320). The ROC Curve obtained by different cut-offs shows Curve of Sensitivity & Specificity (**Figure 6**).

For diagnostic method, the odds ratio was 1.069. So, we can say the odds of diagnosed by Ultrasound among age ranged are 1.069 times the odds of diagnosed by Mammogram among age ranged (**Table 4**). The risk ratio of US was 1.025. That means the ultrasound diagnosed 1.025 times as more useful to Mammogram diagnosed specially for young adult age. While the limits for odds ratio and risk ratio of mammogram and ultrasound. Risk ratio of both mammogram for middle adult age and ultrasound was 0.959 times as less useful to ultrasound diagnosed alone specially (**Table 4**) shows all the previous with lower and upper.

Table 1. The basic statistics of age as mean, standard deviation and skewness.

Descriptive Statistic			
Variables	Mean	Standard Deviation	Skewness
Age	45.50	6.820	0.355

Table 2. Cross tabulation.

Variables		Diagnosis Method	
		Ultrasound	Mammo. & US
Age	Young Adult	7	4
	Middle Adult	18	11

Table 3. ROC Curve variables.

Receiver Operator Characteristic (ROC) Curve				95% CI	
Variables	Area	Std. Error	P-Value	Lower	Upper
Age	0.511	0.096	0.911	0.322	0.699

Table 4. The odds and risk ratio.

Risk & Odds			
Ratio	Estimate	95% CI	
		Lower	Upper
Odds	1.069	0.254	4.511
Risk for US	1.025	0.604	1.741
Risk for US & MG	0.959	0.386	2.381

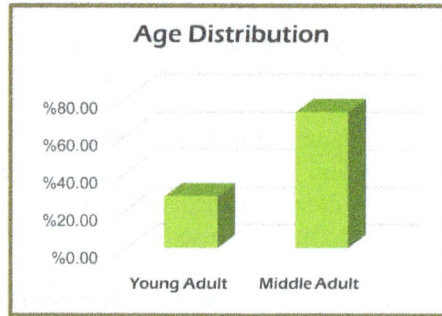

Figure 3. The distribution of age by category: Young adult (20 - 40 Y) & Middle adult (40 - 65 Y).

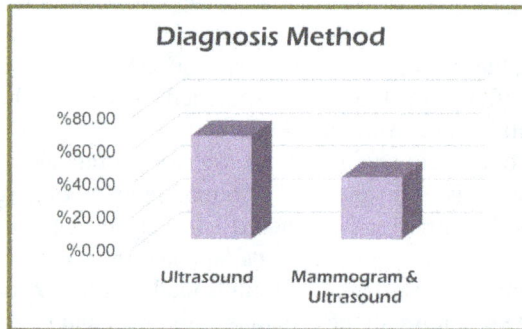

Figure 4. The method of diagnosis (Ultrasound & Mammogram).

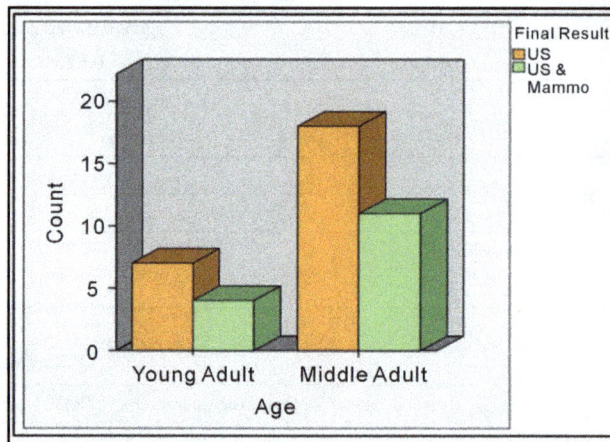

Figure 5. The imaging modality and age category.

4. Discussion

Mammographic sensitivity is proven to be significantly compromised when imaging dense breast tissue and research now documents dense tissue as an independent risk factor. Imaging with both mammography and ultrasound is now suggested by several authors as best practice for these patients, with mammography no longer viewed as the gold standard of imaging. Many authors comment on the comparative sensitivity of mammography and ultrasound and several studies have attempted to quantify the differences in sensitivity and detection rates relative to patient ages and breast density. Several authors agree that the use of ultrasound and mammography may have a combined sensitivity as high as 96% - 100%.

Lumps, both benign and cancerous, appear white on a mammogram; similarly, dense tissue also appears white.

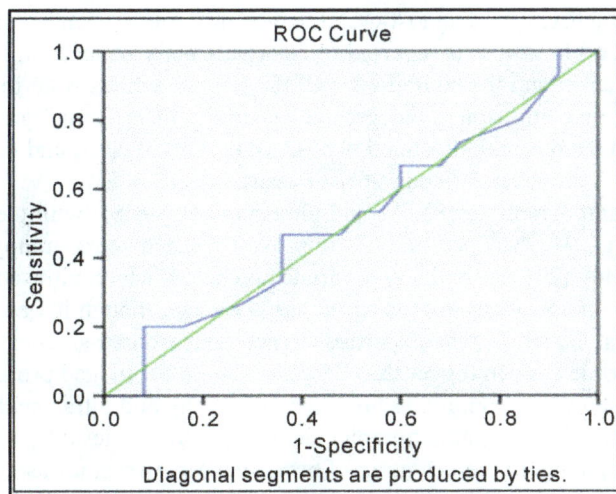

Figure 6. Diagnosed curve of sensitivity & specificity.

Therefore, mammograms is not helpful in women with dense breasts [2] [13].

Breast density is not fixed but may change over time. Paradoxically, breast density tends to gradually decreases with age although overall risk increases with age showing survival benefit of screening women with dense breasts with supplemental whole breast ultrasound screening (WB-US) in addition to mammography. Screening WB-US has been investigated in high-risk women and in women with dense breasts. WB-US in addition to screening mammography has increased cancer detection compared to mammography alone. At prevalent screening, the cancer detection rate increased from 7.6/1000 by mammography alone to 11.8/1000 with mammography and WB-US [14].

Other research has shown that dense breast tissue provides additional risk factor for breast cancer, and the level of that risk has been quantified at 4 - 6 times the normal risk or radiographic density reduces the sensitivity of mammography in women whose tissue density is to <60% [15] [16]. Overall, given a normally distributed mammography screening population, mammography is considered to be 80% - 90% effective in detecting cancers in women without symptom [17].

The dense glandular tissue appears white on the mammogram, while fatty breast tissue appears black. Unfortunately, cancers also typically appear white, allowing the dense tissue to mask cancers and other lesions. This is particularly true of small cancers that may be hidden "behind" even a small area of density [18].

On the other hand, ultrasound should not be used alone for screening women with dense breast tissue because there are certain tissue characteristics, like micro calcifications, that are imaged very well by mammography, but poorly or not at all by ultrasound. Micro-calcifications are commonly associated with DCIS, and also with one particularly aggressive form of breast cancer. Ultrasound does not image calcifications as well as mammography [19]. Ultrasound and mammogram together found 82% of the breast cancers. Mammogram alone found only 53% of the cancers [20] [21].

We believe that ultrasound is of great value as a first line of imaging in the assessment of young or pregnant symptomatic women, followed by mammography if deemed necessary this is in agreement with previous studies [22]. The ultrasound has a greater ability than mammography to demonstrate lesion characteristics as the transducer can be maneuvered through multiple planes [7]. The main goal of ultrasound has been preventing unnecessary biopsies of benign lesions and finding carcinomas that are missed by clinical and/or mammographic evaluation. Ultrasound is seen as attractive for supplemental screening as it is widely available, well tolerated by patients, and relatively inexpensive, involving no radiation [12]. With the development of improved technology and higher-frequency transducers, ultrasound has been indicated as a tool to help differentiate benign from malignant solid breast masses [23]. High resolution real-time ultrasound allows detailed visualization of many abnormal breast masses, with further stating in a 2002 study that ultrasound was vital in the diagnosis of breast cysts and has "shown promise in the differentiation of benign from malignant solid masses [22].

When combined using mammography and ultrasound, [24] stated that the sensitivity is higher than from using mammogram alone. Ultrasound deems superior to mammography for the "vast proportion of patients and worthy of consideration as a first-line diagnostic and screening tool, to stand alongside mammography in equal partnership". And further, ultrasound is reported to be significantly better than mammography in case of detection of invasive breast cancer and the combination of the two modalities is an improvement, [25] agree with the previous authors stating that "ultrasound has greater sensitivity than mammography in the detection of soft tissue abnormalities within the breast. Ultrasound is positive in 93% of cases and mammography 87%, whereas the combination of modalities proved positive in 96% of cases.

The sensitivity of mammography as 83.7% and ultrasound as 89.1%, with the combined sensitivity of mammography and ultrasound, 94.6%. Specificity is improved when mammography and ultrasound are combined (92%) [26]. In a later study [27] assess the appropriate age below which ultrasound would be the more accurate breast imaging test. The choice of imaging is based partly on age, though it was not based on clear evidence for specific imaging choices. Generally, the expertise suggest that women smaller than 35 years in age should be imaged by ultrasound, while women bigger than 35 years should be imaged primary with mammography.

Results of this study show that combining both mammography and ultrasound has a greater sensitivity (96%) than either sonography (81.7%) or mammography alone (75.8%). Reviews by [28] assess the role of ultrasound as an adjunct to mammography in the detection of breast cancer. Breast ultrasound can lower the number of indeterminate findings of mammography, by defining them as benign or malignant. An additional 0.35% breast cancer detection rate when ultrasound is used in conjunction with mammography for screening women with non-fatty breasts heterogeneously dense or extremely dense breast parenchyma [29].

5. Conclusion

The physical density of breast and the patient age potentially affect the accuracy of mammography. Our results showed that age and the physical density of breast potentially affect mammogram images of women with 41 years or younger with sensitivity 66% and specificity 68%. Sensitivity improved with mammography in women older than 41 years. As a result, the diagnosis by using ultrasound alongside the mammogram are preferable imaging combination in such cases of women and considered that mammography and ultrasound the new gold standard in breast screening.

References

[1]   Birdwell, R.L., Ikeda, D.M., O'Shaughnessy, K.F. and Sickles, E.A. (2001) Mammographic Characteristics of 115 Missed Cancers Later Detected with Screening Mammography and the Potential Utility of Computer-Aided Detection. *Radiology*, **219**, 192-202. http://dx.doi.org/10.1148/radiology.219.1.r01ap16192

[2]   Pinsky, R.W. and Helvie, M.A. (2010) Mammographic Breast Density: Effect on Imaging and Breast Cancer Risk. *Journal of the National Comprehensive Cancer Network*, **8**, 1157-1164.

[3]   Wirth, W., Nikitenko, D. and Lyon, J. (2005) Segmentation of Breast Region in Mammograms Using a Rule-Based Fuzzy Reasoning Algorithm. *ICGST Graphics, Vision and Image Processing Journal*, **5**, 45-54.

[4]   Asselin-Labat, M.L., Vaillant, F., Sheridan, J.M., Pal, B., Wu, D., Simpson, E.R., Yasuda, H., Smyth, G.K., Martin, T.J., Lindeman, G.J. and Visvader, J.E. (2010) Control of Mammary Stem Cell Function by Steroid Hormone Signalling. *Nature*, **465**, 798-802. http://dx.doi.org/10.1038/nature09027

[5]   Baker, S., Wall, M. and Bloomfield, A. (2005) Breast Cancer Screening for Women Aged 40-49 Years—What Does the Evidence Mean for New Zealand? *The New Zealand Medical Journal*, **118**, 1-8.

[6]   Carney, P.A., Miglioretti, D.L., Yankaskas, B.C., Kerlikowske, K., Rosenberg, R., Rutter, C.M., Geller, B.M., Abraham, L.A., Dignan, M., Cutter, G. and Ballard-Barbash, R. (2003) Individual and Combined Effects of Age, Breast Density, and Hormone Replacement Therapy Use on the Accuracy of Screening Mammography. *Annals of Intern Medicine*, **138**, 168-175. http://dx.doi.org/10.7326/0003-4819-138-3-200302040-00008

[7]   Dummin, L.J., Cox, M. and Plant, L. (2007) Prediction of Breast Tumor Size by Mammography and Sonography—A Breast Screen Experience. *The Breast Journal*, **16**, 38-46. http://dx.doi.org/10.1016/j.breast.2006.04.003

[8]   David, N., Jackie, S., Butler, L. and Lewis, R. (2006) Hole's Human Anatomy and Physiology. 11th Edition, McGraw Hill Higher Education, 880-881.

[9]   Liberman, L., Feng, T.L., Dershaw, D.D., Morris, E.A. and Abramson, A.F. (1998) US-Guided Core Breast Biopsy: Use and Cost-Effectiveness. *Radiology*, **208**, 717-723.

[10] Warner, E., Plewes, D.B., Hill, K.A., Causer, P.A., Zubovits, J.T., Jong, R.A., Cutara, M.R., DeBoer, G., Yaffe, M.J, Messner, S.J., Meschino, W.S., Piron, C.A. and Narod, S.A. (2004) Surveillance of BRCA1 and BRCA2 Mutation

Carriers with Magnetic Resonance Imaging, Ultrasound, Mammography, and Clinical Breast Examination. *Journal of the American Medical Association*, **292**, 1317-1325. http://dx.doi.org/10.1001/jama.292.11.1317

[11] Dempsey, P.J. (2004) The History of Breast Ultrasound. *Journal of Ultrasound in Medicine*, **23**, 887-894.

[12] Berg, W.A., Gutierrez, L., NessAiver, M.S., Carter, B., Bhargavan, M., Lewis, R.S. and Ioffe, O.B. (2004) Diagnostic Accuracy of Mammography, Clinical Examination, US, and MR Imaging in Preoperative Assessment of Breast Cancer. *Radiology*, **233**, 830-849. http://dx.doi.org/10.1148/radiol.2333031484

[13] Kopans, D.B. (2008) Basic Physics and Doubts about Relationship between Mammographically Determined Tissue Density and Breast Cancer Risk. *Radiology*, **246**, 348-353

[14] American College of Radiology (2003) Breast Imaging Reporting and Data System (BI-RADS). 4th Edition, American College of Radiology, Reston.

[15] Vacek, P.M. and Geller, B.M. (2004) A Prospective Study of Breast Cancer Risk Using Routine Mammographic Breast Density Measurements. *Cancer Epidemiology, Biomarkers Prevention*, **13**, 715-722.

[16] Barlow, W.E., White, E., Ballard-Barbash, R., Vacek, P.M., Titus-Ernstoff, L., Carney, P.A., Tice, J.A., Buist, D.S.M., Geller, B.M., Rosenberg, R., Yankaskas, B.C. and Kerlikowske, K. (2006) Prospective Breast Cancer Risk Prediction Model for Women Undergoing Screening Mammography. *Journal of the National Cancer Institute*, **98**, 1204-1214. http://dx.doi.org/10.1093/jnci/djj331

[17] American Cancer Society (2009-2010) Breast Cancer Facts & Figures. American Cancer Society, Inc., Atlanta.

[18] Pisano, E.D., Hendrick, R.E., Yaffe, M.J., Baum, J.K., Acharyya, S., Cormack, J.B., *et al.* (2008) Diagnostic Accuracy of Digital Mammography versus Film Mammography: Exploratory Analysis of Selected Population Subgroups in DMIST. *Radiology*, **246**, 376-383. http://dx.doi.org/10.1148/radiol.2461070200

[19] Tabar, L., Chen, H.H.T., Yan, M.F.A., Tot, T., Tung, T.H., Chen, L.S., Chiu, Y.H., Duffy, S.W. and Smith, R.A. (2004) Mammographic Tumor Features Can Predict Long-Term Outcomes Reliably in Women with 1-14-mm Invasive Breast Carcinoma. *Cancer*, **101**, 1745-1759. http://dx.doi.org/10.1002/cncr.20582

[20] Berg, W.A. (2007) Beyond Standard Mammographic Screening: Mammography at Age Extremes, Ultrasound, and MR Imaging. *Radiologic Clinics of North America*, **45**, 895-906. http://dx.doi.org/10.1016/j.rcl.2007.06.001

[21] Berg, W.A., Blume, J.D., Cormack, J.B., Mendelson, E.B., Lehrer, D., Böhm-Vélez, M., Pisano, E.D., Jong, R.A., *et al.* (2008) Combined Screening with Ultrasound and Mammography vs Mammography Alone in Women at Elevated Risk of Breast Cancer. *JAMA*, **299**, 2151-2163. http://dx.doi.org/10.1001/jama.299.18.2151

[22] Baker, J.A. and Soo, M.S. (2002) Breast Ultrasound: Assessment of Technical Quality and Image Interpretation. *Radiology*, **23**, 229-238.

[23] Stavros, A.T., Thickman, D., Rapp, C.L., Dennis, M.A., Parker, S.H. and Sisney, G.A. (1995) Solid Breast Nodules: Use of Sonography to Distinguish between Benign and Malignant Lesions. *Radiology*, **196**, 123-134.

[24] Benson, S.R., Blue, J., Judd, K. and Harman, J.E. (2004) Ultrasound Is Now Better than Mammography for the Detection of Invasive Breast Cancer. *American Journal of Surgery*, **188**, 381-385. http://dx.doi.org/10.1016/j.amjsurg.2004.06.032

[25] Boonjunwetwat, D., Chyutipraiwan, U., Sampatanukul, P. and Chatamra, K. (2007) Sensitivity of Mammography and Ultrasonography on Detecting Abnormal findIngs of Ductal Carcinoma *in Situ*. *Journal of the Medical Association of Thailand*, **90**, 539-545.

[26] Malur, S., Wurdinger, S., Moritz, A., Michels, W. and Schneider, A. (2001) Comparison of Written Reports of Mammography, Sonography and Magnetic Resonance Mammography for Preoperative Evaluation of Breast Lesions, with Special Emphasis on Magnetic Resonance Mammography. *Breast Cancer Research*, **3**, 55-60. http://dx.doi.org/10.1186/bcr271

[27] Houssami, N., Irwig, L., Simpson, J.M., McKessar, M., Blome, S. and Noakes, J. (2003) Sydney Breast Imaging Accuracy Study: Comparative Sensitivity and Specificity of Mammography and Sonography in Young Women with Symptoms. *American Journal of Roentgenology*, **180**, 935-940.

[28] Flobbe, K., Nelemans, P.J., Kessels, A.G., Beets, G.L., von Mevenfeldt, M.F. and van Engelshoven, J.M. (2002) The Role of Ultrasonography as an Adjunct to Mammography in the Detection of Breast Cancer: A Systematic Review. *European Journal of Cancer*, **38**, 1044-1050. http://dx.doi.org/10.1016/S0959-8049(01)00388-4

[29] Robinson, M. and Offit, K. (2007) Management of an Inherited Predisposition to Breast Cancer. *New England Journal of Medicine*, **357**, 154-162. http://dx.doi.org/10.1056/NEJMcp071286

9

An Autoantibody Based Protein Microarray Blood Test to Enhance the Specificity of a Negative Screening Mammogram

T. M. Allweis[1*], L. Strauss[2], Z. Malyutin[2], A. Bassein Kapov-Kagan[2], I. Novikov[2],
T. B. Bevers[3], S. Iacobelli[4], M. T. Sandri[5], A. Bitterman[6], P. Engelman[7],
B. Piura[2], M. Rosenberg[8], G. Yahalom[1*#]

[1]Kaplan Medical Center, Rehovot, Israel
[2]Eventus Diagnostics (Israel) LTD, Ora, Israel
[3]University of Texas, MD Anderson Cancer Center, Houston, USA
[4]Media Pharma Srl, Chieti, Italy
[5]Laboratory Medicine Division, Istituto Europeo di Oncologia, Milan, Italy
[6]Carmel Medical Center, Surgery A, Haifa, Israel
[7]Zvulun Breast Center, Clalit Organization, Kiryat Bialik, Israel
[8]Eventus Diagnostics Inc., Miami, USA
Email: [#]galit@eventusdx.com

Abstract

Background: Current screening mammography for breast cancer is associated with misdiagnosis in as many as 30% of cases. Objectives: To develop and clinically evaluate a unique autoantibody based protein microarray blood test to improve the accuracy of breast cancer screening. Materials and Methods: A microarray was constructed from commercial antigens and antigens selected from screened cDNA libraries of breast cancer tissue samples. A training set containing 439 healthy controls and 276 biopsy proven breast cancer cases was used to establish a set of separating models between the two groups. These models were used to assign a diagnosis to 285 blind samples from 120 breast cancer patients and 165 healthy controls. Results: The test identified 82 of the 120 breast cancer patients and 160 of the 165 healthy controls. These results can be translated into a sensitivity of 68.3% [CI: 59% - 77%] and a specificity of 97% [CI: 93% - 99%], with a PPV for this validation set of 94.3% (CI: 87.10% - 98.11%), NPV of 80.81% [CI: 74.62% - 86.05%] and an AUC of

---

[*]Equally contributed.
[#]Corresponding author.

89.2% [CI: 78% - 87%]. Conclusions: The protein microarray can be utilized to reduce the false negative rate of routine screening mammography. Women with a negative mammography and a negative blood test can be reassured and encouraged to continue routine breast cancer screening. A positive test should alert the physician about the possible presence of a breast cancer not detected by routine screening mammography and drive to perform additional investigation, such as breast ultrasound and MRI.

Keywords

Autoantibodies, Breast Cancer, Diagnostic, Screening

1. Introduction

Worldwide, breast cancer is the most common cancer and the most common cause of death from cancers among women. Lifetime incidence of breast cancer is reported by the American Cancer Society to be between 12% and 13% in the US, with similar rates in the western world [1]. Imaging modalities for breast cancer detection include mammography, ultrasound (US) and magnetic resonance imaging (MRI). However, the mainstay of screening for breast cancer is mammography which is currently the only recommended screening modality for women over 40 - 50 years of age in much of the developed world [2]. The issue of recommended mammography is specifically challenged in the subpopulation of women with dense breast tissue. While mammography has an overall sensitivity of 50% - 70% [3], in younger women and in women with dense breast tissue the sensitivity is greatly reduced [4]. Approximately 50% of women have dense breasts (50% or more of breast volume occupied by fibroglandular tissue on mammography) on initial screening mammography. It has been demonstrated that women with dense breast are at higher risk of developing breast cancer, as well as at greater risk of missing a tumor on mammography due to masking by fibroglandular tissue [5] [6]. Thus, it has been suggested that women with dense breasts and a negative screening mammography undergo further supplemental imaging such as breast ultrasound and/or breast MRI.

An American College of Radiology Imaging Network (ACRIN) study comparing mammography alone to mammography with the addition of ultrasound in women with dense breast showed a breast cancer detection rate of 7.6 cancers per 1000 women screened with mammography alone versus 11.8 cancers detected per 1000 women screened with the combination of mammography and ultrasound [4] [7]. Other studies showed an improved cancer detection rate for women with dense breast from 0.25% to 0.46% [6] or by 20% [8]. The majority of cancers detected solely by supplemental ultrasound were node-negative invasive carcinomas, corresponding to a lower stage and allowing the possibility of earlier treatment and improved survival. However, a decrease in specificity by 7% with the combination of mammography and ultrasound versus mammography alone was reported as well. Although the increase in cancer detection rate of mammography combined with ultrasound may be beneficial, the increased biopsy rate, especially of unnecessary biopsies, results in increased morbidity [4] [7]. MRI is another imaging method proposed to improve screening. The lack of ionizing radiation and the fact that it is not affected by breast tissue density makes it a promising option. Many studies have shown increased breast cancer detection rates with MRI after a negative mammography in women with an elevated risk for breast cancer [9]-[11]. The ACRIN 6666 investigators demonstrated that an additional 14.7 cancers were detected per 1000 women screened using MRI after mammography [2] [4] [7]. Nevertheless, MRI also showed a high false-positive rate: 7% of women in the ACRIN 6666 study underwent biopsy on the basis of MRI findings alone, but only 18.6% of them were found to have breast cancer [4]. High false-positive rates ultimately increase patient morbidity without improving mortality. Furthermore, MRI is generally less well tolerated by patients than ultrasound. The high cost and need for injection of contrast material also make MRI a less attractive technique for widespread screening except in very high risk patients such a BRCA mutation carriers [5].

The drawbacks of current breast cancer screening modalities support the general consensus among breast cancer surgeons and the public where there is an urgent and unmet need to develop more accurate, non-invasive, simple and low risk additions or alternatives for screening and early diagnosis of breast cancer [12]. The immune system as a potential tool to help in diagnosis of cancer has been challenged many times for many different cancers. Thus far, only a small number of circulating autoantibodies specific to breast carcinoma antigens have been identified and investigated [13]. The best known are Her2 [14] and Muc1 [15], both of which can be over expressed in breast tumors, and are involved in the production of specific autoantibodies. So far, current efforts to predict or diagnose breast cancer based on autoimmunity have not resulted in clinically applicable serologic biomarkers with accurate and definitive predictive and diagnostic capabilities. There are several explanations for this phenomenon. First, most of the autoantibodies against cancer cells are present in high enough levels (3SD above background) in only a small proportion of cancer patients, as well as in a similar proportion of healthy individuals [16]-[19]. Second, some antibodies tend to appear in several types of cancer, and thus lack the sensitivity needed [17] [19]. Lastly, some antibodies appear in disease states other than cancers [16] [20] [21]. These facts led to the hypothesis that a panel of autoantibodies, rather than a single antibody, would be much more helpful in the diagnosis of cancer by this method [19] [22]-[25].

We have recently reported that an autoantibody panel has the potential to serve as an additional tool for breast cancer diagnosis [26]. In this previous report, a panel of 15 antigens was used to develop a highly sensitive blood test. This tool can be especially helpful for the sub-population of women with dense breast, in whom mammography loses much of its sensitivity. In order to utilize such a blood test for women after negative mammography, a test with high specificity is needed. High specificity will assure a low rate of false positive results, which are the major cause for unnecessary procedures. In this report, we described the development and performance of a microarray based on antigens that were derived from cDNA libraries. The unique microarray was developed using a set of 715 known plasma samples, and tuned to achieve high specificity. After establishing algorithms based on these known plasma samples, the microarray was tested on a set of 285 blind plasma samples in order to estimate its sensitivity and specificity.

2. Materials and Methods

Study design All participants were female subjects over the age of 18 with a breast abnormality detected by clinical breast examination, mammogram, ultrasound, or breast MRI, and women presenting for routine screening with a negative mammography (BIRADS 1, 2). All women who had an indeterminate/suspicious abnormality underwent a pathological diagnosis by core needle or surgical biopsy of the lesion. Those with pathologically proven breast cancer (invasive ductal, invasive lobular and ductal carcinoma in situ) were considered as "cases", and those with negative mammography and/or benign biopsy result (fibroademoas, fibrocystic changes including ADH, ALH and LCIS) were "controls". Although both DCIS and ADH are similar entities with the diagnosis being a quantitative difference in the atypical cells present on the biopsy, biologically, there may not be significant differences between the two, which should be further explored in future studies, the reason for this difference lies within the different treatment given to each group. In situations where there was a discrepancy between the results of the needle biopsy and surgery, the pathologic findings at surgery overruled the needle biopsy results. Patients with biopsy samples with no pathological report, or with no final diagnosis, were excluded from the study. Women were not eligible to participate if they had a previous or concurrent malignancy including hematologic malignancies, were receiving chemotherapy, or had chemotherapy or steroid-based therapy in the past 6 months. Women undergoing immunosuppressive treatments or women with an autoimmune disorder were also excluded. The study in the different centers was conducted under local Institutional Review Board (IRB) approvals (trial registration ID: NCT01343849), and subjected to signing informed consent by each participant. Data forms were completed by each site to obtain clinical information and final pathological diagnosis.

Blood samples collection Plasma was collected from whole blood using heparin tubes (Greiner Cat. No. 455084) centrifuged at 4000 RPM for 10 min at room temperature and aliquots were stored frozen at $-80°C$ until microarray analysis.

cDNA libraries construction Four breast cancer tissues were used to construct a cDNA library. All tissues were originated from invasive ductal carcinoma. Two were triple positive (ER, PR, Her2), one was ER positive and the forth was Her2 positive. In short, RNA was extracted using NucleoSpin® RNA (Macherey-Nagel Cat. No. 740955.10) extraction kit according to manufacturer instructions. Using In-Fusion® SMARTer Directional cDNA Library Construction Kit (Clonetech Cat. No. 634933) a library of at least 1E6 different clones was constructed from each tissue.

Screening for reactive antigens Clones from 4 different cDNA libraries were produced using auto-induction protocol and purified using Hispur Ni-ANT resin (Pierce, Cat. No. 88221). Individual clones were picked, and arrayed on NEXTERION® Slide E (Schott Cat. No. 1066643) using a Micro Grid II microarrayer (Digilab) with split pins. Protein microarrays were blocked using Blockit plus (Arrayit, Cat. No. BKTPL) for 1 hour at room temperature followed by 1 hour incubation with human plasma samples diluted 1:100 in blocking buffer. After 1 hour incubation at 37°C with gentle agitation, microarrays were washed 3 times with 0.1% PBST followed by 3 washes with PBS. 1:500 Goat-anti-Human-Cy3 conjugated (Jackson Immuno Research, Cat. No. 109-165-003) was added for 30 min at 37°C with gentle agitation, followed by same washing procedures.

Data acquisition and analysis Microarrays were scanned with Innoscan710 scanner (Innopsys) at 532 nm, and quantified using Mapix software. In the first round of selection, each antigen was screened against 70 plasma samples (35 breast cancer cases and 35 controls) and evaluated by their t-test. In addition, each clone was used individually to derive a receiver operating characteristic (ROC) curve that was ranked according to the area under curve produced for each antigen. Antigens with t-test statistic t > 2 or area under curve (AUC) above 0.6 were chosen for the second round of selection—screening against plasma from 150 breast cancer cases and 150 controls. The same acceptance criteria were applied to the antigens in the second round. The second round of selection resulted with the 39 antigens that were printed on the protein microarray slides in order to evaluate their performance on blind samples.

Protein microarray printing All antigens were diluted to a printing concentration of (0.1 - 1 mg/ml) in a 384 well plates (Arrayit Cat. No. MMP384), and arrayed on NEXTERION® Slide E (Schott cat. No. 1066643) using a Micro Grid II microarrayer (Digilab) with split pins. The slides were blocked using Blockit plus (Arrayit, Cat. No. BKTPL) for 1 hour at room temperature, and stored at 4°C under vacuum until use.

Protein microarray slide development Samples were defrosted and loaded on an MF membrane (GE healthcare Cat. No. MF1 8122-2250) for a period of 24 hours at room temperature followed by extraction with reaction buffer (Arrayit, Cat. No. PMRB), and loaded on the protein microarrays in dilutions of 1:10 - 1:20. After 1 hour incubation at 37°C with gentle agitation, microarrays were washed 3 times with 0.1% PBST followed by 3 washes with PBS. 1:500 Goat-anti-Human-Cy3 conjugated (Jackson Immuno Research, Cat. No. 109165003) was added for 30 minutes at 37°C with gentle agitation, followed by same washing procedures. Microarrays were scanned with Innoscan710 scanner (Innopsys) at 532 nm, and quantified using Mapix software.

Protein microarray data analysis The samples were randomly divided into two groups, 715 samples were designated as the training set, and the remaining 285 samples as blind samples. The results obtained from the 57 antigens were log transformed and normalized to the median of each sample. The results of the samples in the training set were applied to the IBM SPSS modeler that produced separating models based on machine learning algorithms (Neural Network, Chaid, CRT and C5). These models were applied to the blind set sample data, and resulted with a score of "0" or "1" for each sample. The score was compared to the clinical status that was obtained for each sample to calculate sensitivity, specificity, NPV and PPV.

3. Results

Study participants A total of 1000 plasma samples were obtained from five centers. The samples tested in this study were randomly divided into two groups (training set and blind validation set), with similar average age distribution of breast cancer cases and controls between the two groups (see **Table 1**).

Of the 1000 samples collected, 604 were controls (either with negative mammography or negative/benign biopsy results) and 396 were cases (327 invasive ductal breast cancer, 25 had invasive lobular breast cancer and 44 had ductal carcinoma in situ) (see **Figure 1**).

Library construction Four different cDNA libraries were constructed from 4 different invasive ductal breast cancer tissue samples (two triple positive IDC, one Her2 positive ER/PR negative and one ER positive). Each library contained at least 1E6 clones. The cDNA libraries were pooled and screened for reactive antigens.

High throughput protein microarray screening for selection of reactive antigens A total of 119,808 clones were randomly selected from the pool libraries. These clones were printed on microarrays and screened in two rounds of selection. The first round consisted of 70 plasma samples (35 breast cancer cases and 35 controls), and the second round of selection consisted of 150 breast cancer cases and 150 controls. Each antigen received a score based upon t-test and AUC (see materials and methods). In order to pass a selection round, a potential antigen had to have either t-test > 2 or AUC > 0.6. The average t-test was 2.7 for antigens being selected at the first round and 3.4 for those being selected at the second round. The average AUC was 0.7 for the first selection round and 0.64 for the second round. A total of 39 antigens passed at least one of the criteria in the second selection round (see supplementary data in **Table S1**).

Table 1. Age information of subjects participating in the study divided to controls and breast cancer cases in the training set and the blind validation set.

		Controls	Breast cancer cases
Training set	mean (age) ± sd.	48.8 ± 14.5	58.8 ± 12.9
	range	18 - 81	32 - 91
	% above 50	51%	74%
Blind validation set	mean (age) ± sd.	49.0 ± 14.0	60.5 ± 13.3
	range	20 - 82	31 - 93
	% above 50	53%	81%

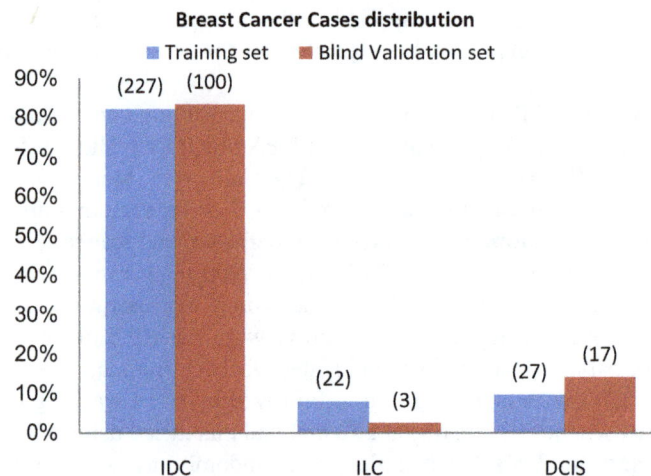

Figure 1. Percentage distribution of breast cancer cases (according to diagnosis) in the training and blind validation sets.

Microarray construction A total of 39 antigens derived from the cDNA libraries which showed the best separation probability together with 17 commercial antigens, all reported to be associated with a humoral response in breast cancer, were printed on epoxy slides (a total of 56 antigens examined). Of the 17 commercial antigens used, 15 were previously reported as highly sensitive in predicting the presence of breast cancer as a part of a panel of antigens [26]. The commercial antigens used are summarized in **Table 2**.

Protein microarray performances In order to evaluate the performance of the protein microarray, a total of 1000 plasma samples were used (one sample per a participant). All samples were tested on the protein microarray using the same protocol (see materials and methods). The samples were divided into two groups—a total of 715 were a part of the training set that was used to develop a set of prediction models, upon which the remaining 285 blinded samples (blind validation set) were tested and given a predicted clinical status.

Prediction using the Protein microarray The training set containing serum from 439 controls (negative mammography or benign lesions) and 276 breast cancer cases was used to establish the mathematical algorithms. After processing the samples, each sample, with a known clinical status, received a set of values, one per each antigen, which corresponded to the relative amount of each autoantibody (see materials and methods). These values were used to establish the separating algorithm between the breast cancer patients and the healthy controls. The algorithm was tuned to achieve at least 95% specificity and at least 50% sensitivity.

The remaining 285 blinded samples were then tested, and received a score of either "0" (control) or "1" (case) based on the algorithm (see supplementary **Table S2**). The results were compared to the clinical data in order to evaluate the sensitivity and specificity of the test. A total of 82 (out of the 120) breast cancer cases were diagnosed correctly translating to a sensitivity of 68.3% (CI: 59.2% - 76.5%). A total of 160 (out of 165) controls were diagnosed correctly translating to a specificity of 96.97% (CI: 93.1% - 99.0%), see **Table 3**. The NPV for this validation set was 80.8% (CI: 74.6% - 86.1%) and PPV for this validation set was 94.3% (CI: 87.1% - 98.1%). The overall AUC obtained for this set was 89.2% (CI: 78% - 87%), as seen in the ROC analysis in **Figure 2**.

Table 2. List of commercial antigens used on the microarray construction.

No.	Sequence	Origin	reference
Ag1	QRASPLTSIISAVVGI	ErbB-2	[14]
Ag2	TAPLQPEQLQVFETLEEI	ErbB-2	[14]
Ag3	NGTSFDIHYGSGSLSGYLS	Cathepsin D	[29]
Ag4	HSP27	HSP27	[38]
Ag5	EPPLSQETFSDLWKLLPENNVLSPL	p53	[30]
Ag6	DDLMLSPDDIEQWFTEDPGP	p53	[30]
Ag7	NHEPSVTQVILDRPY	Phage display	[31]
Ag8	HoxB7	HoxB7	[32]
Ag9	LGALS3BP	LGALS3BP	[33]
Ag10	GIPC	GIPC	[34]
Ag11	VFETLEEITGYLYISAWPD	her2	[14]
Ag12	TPO	TPO	[35]
Ag13	Cathepsin D	Cathepsin D	[29]
Ag14	p53	p53	[36]
Ag15	Biotin-KAAELIPLHKLAAK	chd1	[29]
Ag16	ErbB-2	ErbB-2	[14]
Ag17	CEA	CEA	[37]

Table 3. Prediction on a blind set of 285 samples using mathematical algorithm based on protein microarrays results.

Clinical status	Controls	Cases
Protein microarray results		
negative	160	38
positive	5	82
	Specificity	Sensitivity
	97%	68%
	NPV	PPV
	81%	94%

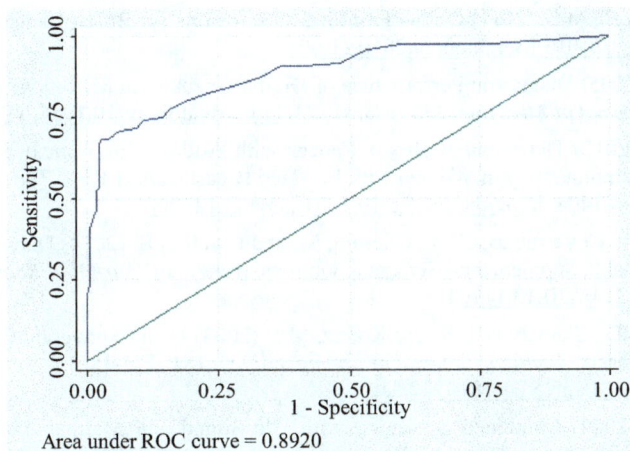

Area under ROC curve = 0.8920

Figure 2. ROC for the prediction set of 285 blind samples. An AUC of 89.2% was achieved, representing 97% specificity and 68% sensitivity.

4. Discussion

Screening mammography as a standalone modality for the early detection of breast cancer has several limitations, especially in women with dense breasts. Here, we demonstrated that this newly developed blood test based on a panel of antigen selectively chosen to recognize breast cancer autoantibodies has a high specificity (97%) with a moderate sensitivity (68%), and an AUC of 89% for breast cancer detection. These results compare favorably with screening mammography as a standard standalone test whose sensitivity is 70% - 80% (range: 29% - 97%) [27] and specificity 35% - 98% [28].

Because of these characteristics (high specificity and moderate sensitivity), the new test can be used as a second line screening for women with negative mammography. Particularly, in this sub-population, 68% of the undiagnosed women can be detected with the autoantibody-based blood test at the cost of 3% false positive results. Patients displaying positive results should be referred to additional and more sensitive imaging modalities (such as US or MRI). The benefit of utilizing this blood test prior to other imaging modalities lies in the possibility to reduce many false positive results of the other modalities that will occur if the test is not performed prior to MRI.

Some patients' sub-populations, specifically women with dense breast tissue, in whom mammography is highly inaccurate, may benefit more from using a blood test. After receiving a negative mammography result, these women can undergo a blood test that will refer them to additional and more sensitive imaging techniques. To this end, additional clinical studies should be performed in order to evaluate the sensitivity and specificity of the autoantibody based blood test, specifically for the dense breast sub-population.

Breast imaging, either anatomical or functional, is limited by many factors. Tumor antigenicity as a tool for breast cancer detection is only beginning to be explored, but shows a promise in taking cancer screening to a biological era.

Acknowledgements

The authors greatly appreciate the cooperation and efforts of M.D. Anderson Cancer Center, University G. D'Annunzio, Division of Senology, European Institute of Oncology, Carmel Medical Center Zvulun Breast Center and Kaplan Medical Center, who have generously provided all the specimens for this study. We also thank M.D. Anderson's research personnel Diane M Weber (RN, BSN) and Valerie O Sepeda (RN, BSN), for help in obtaining the breast cancer samples used in this study. In addition we would like to thank Sarah (Luna) Cohen (CRA), Svetlana Rothe (CRA), Ortal Karazi and Eva Yadin for their extensive labor. The authors would like to acknowledge the huge contribution of the late Prof. Donny Strosberg for his scientific involvement in this project.

References

[1]   IARC (2012) IARC [Online]. http://globocan.iarc.fr/Pages/fact_sheets_population.aspx

[2]   D'Orsi, C.J. and Newell, M.S. (2011) On the Frontline of Screening for Breast Cancer. *Seminars in Oncology*, **38**, 119-127. http://dx.doi.org/10.1053/j.seminoncol.2010.11.004

[3]   Pisano, E.D., *et al.* (2005) Diagnostic Performance of Digital versus Film Mammography for Breast-Cancer Screening. *The New England Journal of Medicine*, **353**, 1773-1783. http://dx.doi.org/10.1056/NEJMoa052911

[4]   Berg, W.A., *et al.* (2012) Detection of Breast Cancer with Addition of Annual Screening Ultrasound or a Single Screening MRI to Mammography in Women with Elevated Breast Cancer Risk. *The Journal of the American Medicine Association*, **307**, 1394-1404. http://dx.doi.org/10.1001/jama.2012.388.

[5]   Ho, J.M., Jafferjee, N., Covarrubias, G.M., Ghesani, M. and Handler, B. (2014) Dense Breasts: A Review of Reporting Legislation and Available Supplemental Screening Options. *American Journal of Roentgenology*, **203**, 449-456. http://dx.doi.org/10.2214/AJR.13.11969.

[6]   Crystal, P., Strano, S.D., Shcharynski, S. and Koretz, M.J. (2003) Using Sonography to Screen Women with Mammographically Dense Breasts. *American Journal of Roentgenology*, **181**, 177-182. http://dx.doi.org/10.2214/ajr.181.1.1810177.

[7]   Berg, W.A., *et al.* (2008) Combined Screening with Ultrasound and Mammography vs. Mammography Alone in Women at Elevated Risk of Breast Cancer. *The Journal of the American Medicine Association*, **299**, 2151-2163. http://dx.doi.org/10.2214/ajr.181.1.1810177.

[8]   Kolb, T.M., Lichy, J. and Newhouse, J.H. (2002) Comparison of the Performance of Screening Mammography, Physical Examination, and Breast US and Evaluation of Factors that Influence Them: An Analysis of 27,825 Patient Evalua-

tion. *Radiology*, **225**, 165-175. http://dx.doi.org/10.1148/radiol.2251011667.

[9]   Kuhl, C.K., *et al.* (2005) Mammography, Breast Ultrasound, and Magnetic Resonance Imaging for Surveillance of Women at High Familial Risk for Breast Cancer. *Journal of Clinical Oncology*, **23**, 8469-8476. http://dx.doi.org/10.1200/JCO.2004.00.4960.

[10]   Lehman, C.D., *et al.* (2007) Cancer Yield of Mammography, MR, and US in High-Risk Women. *Radiology*, **244**, 381-388. http://dx.doi.org/10.1148/radiol.2442060461.

[11]   Warner, E., Plewes, D.B., Shumak, R.S., Catzavelos, G.C., Di Prospero, L.S., Yaffe, M.J., *et al.* (2001) Comparison of Breast Magnetic Resonance Imaging, Mammography, and Ultrasound for Surveillance of Women at High Risk for Hereditary Breast Cancer. *Journal of Clinical Oncology*, **19**, 3524-3531.

[12]   Weigelt, B., Geyer, F.C. and Reis-Filho, J.S. (2010) Histological Types of Breast Cancer: How Special Are They? *Molecular Oncology*, **4**, 192-208. http://dx.doi.org/10.1016/j.molonc.2010.04.004

[13]   Piura, E. and Piura, B. (2010) Autoantibodies to Tummor-Associated Antigens in Breast Carcinoma. *Journal of Oncology*, **2010**, Article ID: 264926.

[14]   Baselga, J., Seidman, A.D., Norton, L. and Rosen, P.P. (1997) HER2 Overexpression and Paclitaxel Sensitivity in Breast Cancer: Therapeutic Implications. *Oncology*, **11**, 43-48.

[15]   Yang, E., Hu, X.F. and Xing, P.X. (2007) Advances of MUC1 as a Target for Breast Cancer Immunotherapy. *Histology and Histopathology*, **22**, 905-922.

[16]   Daniels, T., Zhang, J.Y., Gutierrez, I., Elliot, M.L., Yamada, B., Jo Heeb, M., *et al.* (2005) Antinuclear Autoantibodies in Prostate Cancer: Immunity to LEDGF/p75, a Survival Protein Highly Expressed in Prostate Tumors and Cleaved during Apoptosis. *The Prostate*, **62**, 14-26. http://dx.doi.org/10.1002/pros.20112

[17]   Soussi, T. (2000) p53 Antibodies in the Sera of Patients with Various Types of Cancer: A Review. *Cancer Research*, **60**, 1777-1788.

[18]   Rohayem, J., Diestelkoetter, P., Weigle, B., Oehmichen, A., Schmitz, M., Mehlhorn, J., Conrad, K., Rieber, E.P., *et al.* (2000) Antibody Response to the Tumor-Associated Inhibitor of Apoptosis Protein Survivin in Cancer Patients. *Cancer Research*, **60**, 1815-1817.

[19]   Zhang, J.Y., Casiano, C.A., Peng, X.X., Koziol, J.A., Chan, E.K. and Tan, E.M. (2003) Enhancement of Antibody Detection in Cancer Using Panel of Recombinant Tumor-Associated Antigens. *Cancer Epidemiology, Biomarkers & Prevention*, **12**, 136-143.

[20]   Ganapathy, V., Daniels, T. and Casiano, C.A. (2003) LEDGF/p75: A Novel Nuclear Autoantigen at the Crossroads of Cell Survival and Apoptosis. *Autoimmunity Reviews*, **2**, 290-297. http://dx.doi.org/10.1016/S1568-9972(03)00063-6

[21]   Ganapathy, V. and Casiano, C.A. (2004) Autoimmunity to the Nuclear Autoantigen DFS70 (LEDGF): What Exactly Are the Autoantibodies Trying to Tell Us? *Arthritis & Rheumatism*, **50**, 684-688. http://dx.doi.org/10.1002/art.20095

[22]   Ludwig, N., Keller, A., Comtesse, N., Rheinheimer, S., Pallasch, C., Fischer, U., *et al.* (2008) Pattern of Serum Autoantibodies Allows Accurate Distinction between a Tumor and Pathologies of the Same Organ. *Clinical Cancer Research*, **14**, 4767-4774. http://dx.doi.org/10.1158/1078-0432.CCR-07-4715

[23]   Leidinger, P., Keller, A., Ludwig, N., Rheinheimer, S., Hamacher, J., Huwer, H., *et al.* (2008) Towards an Early Diagnosis of Lung Cancer: An Autoantibody Signature for Squamous Cell Lung Carcinoma. *International Journal of Cancer*, **123**, 1631-1636. http://dx.doi.org/10.1002/ijc.23680

[24]   Lin, H.S., Talwar, H.S., Tarca, A.L., Ionan, A., Chatterjee, M., Ye, B., *et al.* (2007) Autoantibody Approach for Serum Based Detection of Head and Neck Cancer. *Cancer Epidemiology, Biomarkers & Prevention*, **16**, 2396-2405. http://dx.doi.org/10.1158/1055-9965.EPI-07-0318

[25]   Piura, E. and Piura, B. (2011) Autoantibodies to Tailor-Made Panels of Tumor Associated Antigens in Breast Carcinoma. *Journal of Oncology*, **2011**, Article ID: 982425.

[26]   Yahalom, G., Weiss, D., Novikov, I., Bevers, T.B., Radvanyi, L.G., Liu, M., *et al.* (2013) An Antibody-Based Blood Test Utilizing a Panel of Biomarkers as a New Method for Improved Breast Cancer Diagnosis. *Biomarkers in Cancer*, **5**, 71-80. http://dx.doi.org/10.4137/BIC.S13236

[27]   Smith-Bindman, R., Chu, P., Miglioretti, D.L., Quale, C., Rosenberg, R.D., Cutter, G., *et al.* (2005) Physician Predictors of Mammographic Accuracy. *Journal of the National Cancer Institute*, **97**, 358-367. http://dx.doi.org/10.1093/jnci/dji060

[28]   Beam, C.A., Conant, E.F., Sickles, E.A. and Weinstein, S.P. (2003) Evaluation of Proscriptive Health Care Policy Implementation in Screening Mammography. *Radiology*, **229**, 534-540. http://dx.doi.org/10.1148/radiol.2292021585

[29]   Chinni, S.R., Falchetto, R., Gercel-Taylor, C., Shabanowitz, J., Hunt, D.F. and Taylor, D.D. (1997) Humoral Immune Response to Cathepsin D and Glucose Regulated Protein 78 in Ovarian Cancer Patients. *Clinical Cancer Research*, **3**, 1557-1564.

[30] Lubin, R., Schlichtholz, B., Bengoufa, D., Zalcman, G., Trédaniel, J., Hirsch, A., *et al.* (1993) Analysis of p53 Antibodies in Patients with Various Cancers Define B-Cell Epitopes of Human p53: Distribution on Primary Structure and Exposure on Protein Surface. *Cancer Research*, **53**, 5872-5876.

[31] Hansen, M.H., Nielsen, H. and Ditzel, H.J. (2001) The Tumor-Infiltrating B Cell Response in Medullary Breast Cancer Is Oligoclonal and Directed against the Autoantigen Actin Exposed on the Surface of Apoptotic Cancer Cells. *Proceedings of the National Academy of Sciences of the United States of America*, **98**, 12659-12664. http://dx.doi.org/10.1073/pnas.171460798

[32] Erkanli, A.I., Taylor, D.D., Dean, D., Eksir, F., Egger, D., Geyer, J., *et al.* (2006) Application of Bayesian Modeling of Autologous Antibody Responses against Ovarian Tumor-Associated Antigens to Cancer Detection. *Cancer Research*, **66**, 1792-1798. http://dx.doi.org/10.1158/0008-5472.CAN-05-0669

[33] Natoli, C., Iacobelli, S. and Kohn, L. (1996) The Immune Stimulatory Protein 90K Increases Major Histocompatibility Complex Class I Expression in a Human Breast Cancer Cell Line. *Biochemical and Biophysical Research Communications*, **225**, 617-620. http://dx.doi.org/10.1006/bbrc.1996.1219

[34] Yavelsky, V., Rohkin, S., Shaco-Levy, R., Tzikinovsky, A., Amir, T., Kohn, H., *et al.* (2008) Native Human Autoantibodies Targeting GIPC1 Identify Differential Expression in Malignant Tumors of the Breast and Ovary. *BMC Cancer*, **8**, 247-258. http://dx.doi.org/10.1186/1471-2407-8-247

[35] Smyth, P.P., Shering, S.G., Kilbane, M.T., Murray, M.J., McDermott, E.W., Smith, D.F., O'Higgins, N.J., *et al.* (1998) Serum Thyroid Peroxidase Autoantibodies, Thyroid Volume, and Outcome in Breast Carcinoma. *Journal of Clinical Endocrinology and Metabolism*, **83**, 2711-2716.

[36] Nicolini, A., Capri, A. and Tarro, G. (2006) Biomolecular Markers of Breast Cancer. *Frontiers in Bioscience*, **11**, 1818-1843. http://dx.doi.org/10.2741/1926

[37] Gold, P. and Freeman, S.O. (1965) Specific Carcino Embryonic Antigens of the Human Digestive System. *Journal of Experimental Medicine*, **122**, 467-481. http://dx.doi.org/10.1084/jem.122.3.467

[38] Korneeva, I., Bongiovanni, A.M., Girotra, M., Caputo, T.A. and Witkin, S.S. (1999) Serum Antibodies to the 27-kd Heat Shock Protein in Women with Gynecologic Cancers. *American Journal of Obstetrics and Gynecology*, **183**, 18-21. http://dx.doi.org/10.1016/S0002-9378(00)72431-8

Supplement

Table S1. T test auc of self antigens.

Ag1	t test (1)	Auc (1)	t test (2)	Auc (2)
EBC01	2.19	0.61	2.47	
EBC02	2.58	0.64	2.96	0.61
EBC03	2.03	0.66	2.19	
EBC04	2.21	0.76	4.44	0.63
EBC05	2.33	0.61	2.63	
EBC06	2.93	0.7	3.91	
EBC07	2	0.67	3.28	
EBC08	2.8	0.77	4.32	0.62
EBC09	2.09	0.64	2.75	
EBC10		0.69	3.6	
EBC11	3.54	0.79	3.24	0.61
EBC12	2.23	0.67	2.9	0.64
EBC13	2.41	0.64	2.51	
EBC14	3.27	0.67	3.8	0.64
EBC15	2	0.7	2.3	
EBC16	3.61	0.74	4	0.66
EBC17	2.35	0.81	2.43	0.73
EBC18	3.08	0.7	2.74	0.6
EBC19	3.61	0.62	3.72	0.61
EBC20	2.45	0.77	4.27	
EBC21	2.52	0.73	3.43	0.73
EBC22	2.58	0.8	3.4	0.62
EBC23	2.37	0.71	3.25	0.67
EBC24	3.07	0.64	3.96	0.61
EBC25	2.8	0.73	3.87	
EBC26	2.35	0.67	2.69	
EBC27	3.6	0.72	3.97	0.65
EBC28	3.3	0.8	3.6	0.68
EBC29	2.8	0.73	3.72	0.64
EBC30	3.1	0.68	2.82	0.64
EBC31	3.6	0.73	3.57	0.67
EBC32	3.42	0.73	4.04	0.69
EBC33	3.1	0.65	2.73	0.63
EBC34	3.2	0.72	4.39	0.63
EBC35	2.94	0.7	3.26	
EBC36	2.9	0.71	4.12	0.63
EBC37	2.43	0.69	3.29	
EBC38	2.39	0.75	2.39	0.61
EBC39		0.68	5.89	0.62

Table S2. Summary of blind set prediction results.

id	Real	Pred
UK1	0	0
UK2	0	1
UK3	0	0
UK4	0	1
UK5	0	0
UK6	0	0
UK7	0	0
UK8	0	0
UK9	0	0
UK10	0	0
UK11	0	0
UK12	0	0
UK13	0	0
UK14	0	0
UK15	0	0
UK16	0	0
UK17	0	0
UK18	0	0
UK19	0	0
UK20	0	0
UK21	0	0
UK22	0	0
UK23	0	0
UK24	0	0
UK25	0	0
UK26	0	0
UK27	0	0
UK28	0	0
UK29	0	0
UK30	0	0
UK31	0	0
UK32	0	0
UK33	0	0
UK34	0	0
UK35	0	0
UK36	0	0
UK37	0	0
UK38	0	0
UK39	0	0
UK40	0	0
UK41	0	0
UK42	0	0

Continued

UK43	0	0
UK44	0	0
UK45	0	0
UK46	0	0
UK47	0	0
UK48	0	0
UK49	0	0
UK50	0	0
UK51	0	0
UK52	0	0
UK53	0	0
UK54	0	0
UK55	0	0
UK56	0	1
UK57	0	0
UK58	0	0
UK59	0	0
UK60	0	0
UK61	0	0
UK62	0	0
UK63	0	0
UK64	0	0
UK65	0	0
UK66	0	0
UK67	0	0
UK68	0	0
UK69	0	0
UK70	0	0
UK71	0	0
UK72	0	0
UK73	0	0
UK74	0	0
UK75	0	0
UK76	0	0
UK77	0	0
UK78	0	0
UK79	0	0
UK80	0	0
UK81	0	0
UK82	0	0
UK83	0	0
UK84	0	0
UK85	0	0

Continued

UK86	0	0
UK87	0	0
UK88	0	1
UK89	0	0
UK90	0	0
UK91	0	0
UK92	0	0
UK93	0	0
UK94	0	0
UK95	0	0
UK96	0	0
UK97	0	1
UK98	0	0
UK99	0	0
UK100	0	0
UK101	0	0
UK102	0	0
UK103	0	0
UK104	0	0
UK105	0	0
UK106	0	0
UK107	0	0
UK108	0	0
UK109	0	0
UK110	0	0
UK111	0	0
UK112	0	0
UK113	0	0
UK114	0	0
UK115	0	0
UK116	0	0
UK117	0	0
UK118	0	0
UK119	0	0
UK120	0	0
UK121	0	0
UK122	0	0
UK123	0	0
UK124	0	0
UK125	0	0
UK126	0	0
UK127	0	0
UK128	0	0

Continued

UK129	0	0
UK130	0	0
UK131	0	0
UK132	0	0
UK133	0	0
UK134	0	0
UK135	0	0
UK136	0	0
UK137	0	0
UK138	0	0
UK139	0	0
UK140	0	0
UK141	0	0
UK142	0	0
UK143	0	0
UK144	0	0
UK145	0	0
UK146	0	0
UK147	0	0
UK148	0	0
UK149	0	0
UK150	0	0
UK151	0	0
UK152	0	0
UK153	0	0
UK154	0	0
UK155	0	0
UK156	0	0
UK157	0	0
UK158	0	0
UK159	0	0
UK160	0	0
UK161	0	0
UK162	0	0
UK163	0	0
UK164	0	0
UK165	0	0
UK166	1	1
UK167	1	1
UK168	1	0
UK169	1	1
UK170	1	0
UK171	1	1

Continued

UK172	1	0
UK173	1	1
UK174	1	1
UK175	1	1
UK176	1	1
UK177	1	1
UK178	1	1
UK179	1	1
UK180	1	1
UK181	1	0
UK182	1	1
UK183	1	1
UK184	1	1
UK185	1	1
UK186	1	1
UK187	1	0
UK188	1	0
UK189	1	1
UK190	1	1
UK191	1	0
UK192	1	1
UK193	1	0
UK194	1	1
UK195	1	1
UK196	1	1
UK197	1	1
UK198	1	1
UK199	1	0
UK200	1	1
UK201	1	0
UK202	1	0
UK203	1	0
UK204	1	1
UK205	1	1
UK206	1	1
UK207	1	1
UK208	1	0
UK209	1	1
UK210	1	1
UK211	1	0
UK212	1	0
UK213	1	0
UK214	1	0

Continued

UK215	1	1
UK216	1	1
UK217	1	0
UK218	1	1
UK219	1	0
UK220	1	0
UK221	1	1
UK222	1	0
UK223	1	1
UK224	1	1
UK225	1	1
UK226	1	1
UK227	1	1
UK228	1	0
UK229	1	1
UK230	1	0
UK231	1	1
UK232	1	1
UK233	1	1
UK234	1	1
UK235	1	1
UK236	1	1
UK237	1	1
UK238	1	1
UK239	1	1
UK240	1	1
UK241	1	1
UK242	1	1
UK243	1	1
UK244	1	0
UK245	1	1
UK246	1	1
UK247	1	1
UK248	1	0
UK249	1	0
UK250	1	1
UK251	1	1
UK252	1	1
UK253	1	0
UK254	1	0
UK255	1	1
UK256	1	0
UK257	1	1

Continued

UK258	1	1
UK259	1	1
UK260	1	1
UK261	1	1
UK262	1	1
UK263	1	1
UK264	1	1
UK265	1	0
UK266	1	1
UK267	1	1
UK268	1	1
UK269	1	0
UK270	1	1
UK271	1	1
UK272	1	1
UK273	1	1
UK274	1	1
UK275	1	0
UK276	1	1
UK277	1	0
UK278	1	0
UK279	1	0
UK280	1	0
UK281	1	1
UK282	1	1
UK283	1	0
UK284	1	0
UK285	1	1

	True	False
type 0	160	5
type 1	32	82

10

Observer Variability in BI-RADS Ultrasound Features and Its Influence on Computer-Aided Diagnosis of Breast Masses

Laith R. Sultan[1*], Ghizlane Bouzghar[1], Benjamin J. Levenback[1], Nauroze A. Faizi[1], Santosh S. Venkatesh[2], Emily F. Conant[1], Chandra M. Sehgal[1]

[1]Department of Radiology, University of Pennsylvania, Philadelphia, USA
[2]Department of Electrical Engineering, University of Pennsylvania, Philadelphia, USA
Email: *lsultan@mail.med.upenn.edu

Abstract

Objective: Computer classification of sonographic BI-RADS features can aid differentiation of the malignant and benign masses. However, the variability in the diagnosis due to the differences in the observed features between the observations is not known. The goal of this study is to measure the variation in sonographic features between multiple observations and determine the effect of features variation on computer-aided diagnosis of the breast masses. Materials and Methods: Ultrasound images of biopsy proven solid breast masses were analyzed in three independent observations for BI-RADS sonographic features. The BI-RADS features from each observation were used with Bayes classifier to determine probability of malignancy. The observer agreement in the sonographic features was measured by kappa coefficient and the difference in the diagnostic performances between observations was determined by the area under the ROC curve, A_z, and interclass correlation coefficient. Results: While some features were repeatedly observed, $\kappa = 0.95$, other showed a significant variation, $\kappa = 0.16$. For all features, combined intra-observer agreement was substantial, $\kappa = 0.77$. The agreement, however, decreased steadily to 0.66 and 0.56 as time between the observations increased from 1 to 2 and 3 months, respectively. Despite the variation in features between observations the probabilities of malignancy estimates from Bayes classifier were robust and consistently yielded same level of diagnostic performance, A_z was 0.772 - 0.817 for sonographic features alone and 0.828 - 0.849 for sonographic features and age combined. The difference in the performance, ΔA_z, between the observations for the two groups was small (0.003 - 0.044) and was not statistically significant (p < 0.05). Interclass correlation coefficient for the observations was 0.822 (CI: 0.787 - 0.853) for BI-RADS sonographic features alone and for those combined with age was 0.833 (CI: 0.800 - 0.862). Conclusion: Despite the differences in the BI- RADS sonographic features between different observations, the diagnostic performance of computer-aided analysis for differentiating breast masses did not change. Through continual retraining, the computer-aided analysis provides consistent diagnostic performance independent of the variations in the observed sonographic features.

Keywords

Breast Imaging, Breast Cancer, Observer Variability, Computer-Aided Diagnosis

1. Introduction

Despite major advances in diagnostic breast cancer imaging, the yield for biopsying a breast lesion is still low and up to 85% of biopsies are found to be benign [1]. There continues to be a need for further innovations to improve confidence and reliability of breast imaging. In this context, several studies have proposed the use of computer algorithms and machine learning methods to improve the diagnostic value of breast ultrasound [2]-[7]. These computer based systems can serve as a second reader to decrease false positive rates of breast images [2]. In our earlier study, we introduced an approach that combines individual sonographic features quantitatively by machine learning to determine the probability of malignancy of solid breast masses [7]. The results show that the Bayesian method of weighting provides a systematic approach for combining ultrasound BI-RADS features yielding a high level of diagnostic performance, with an A_z of approximately 0.884. While the results are encouraging, variability in the diagnostic performance on repeated assessments is not known. The goal of this study was to determine the extent of variation in the computer-aided diagnosis between repeated interpretations of the breast ultrasound images. In brief, the variability in the diagnosis can result from two factors: 1) differences in feature selection and 2) differences in weighting of the individual features contributing to overall estimate of the probability of malignancy. In this study we investigate the role of both the factors. First, the observer variability in feature selection from three observations of the ultrasound images was measured by inter-rater kappa statistics. Second, the sonographic features from each observation were combined using Bayes model to determine the probability of malignancy. The diagnostic performances of the probability estimates of three observations were compared to determine diagnostic variability. Since the predictive values of the sonographic features are influenced by the age of the patients [7], we also evaluated the diagnostic performance of the sonographic features in conjunction with the patient age.

2. Materials and Methods

2.1. Image Acquisition and Analysis

This retrospective study was approved by institutional Review Board. 264 masses were obtained from 248 female patients with biopsy-proven solid masses and known mammographic BI-RADS. Sonographic images were acquired using broadband 12 - 5 MHz transducer and a Philips ATL 5000 scanner. 5 to 7 B-Scan ultrasound images including color Doppler were acquired per patient in radial and anti-radial planes.

Images were analyzed using the ACR BI-RADS ultrasound lexicon [8]. According to this lexicon, sonographic features of a solid breast mass [9] are grouped into shape, orientation, margin, lesion boundary, echo pattern, and posterior acoustic features. The observer with three-years prior training in general radiology underwent a self study session of the BI-RADS lexicon descriptors and of the training cases of breast images with known BI-RADS and pathology. The observer was blinded to patient age, race, physical examination, family history, mammographic report, and histological diagnosis during analysis.

The BI-RADS features assessment was repeated two more times after the initial assessment. The second observation (observation 2) was one month from the initial observation (observation 1) and the third observation (observation 3) was three months later. In all three observations the same image data was analyzed where the cases were presented to the observer in a random order.

Agreement in the BI-RADS features was determined by kappa statistics which assesses the inter-rater agreement beyond that is expected by chance [10]. According to this approach, $\kappa = 1$ corresponds to complete agreement whereas $\kappa = 0$ represents an agreement comparable to chance. The intermediate values between 0 and 1 represent the degree of agreement. On a five scale system described by Landis and Koch [11], kappa values 0.01 - 0.20, 0.21 - 0.40, 0.41 - 0.60, 0.61 - 0.80 and 0.81 - 1.00 were designated to indicate slight, fair, moderate, substantial, and almost perfect agreement, respectively. Both individual features agreement values and all features combined (overall) agreement values were calculated.

2.2. Computer-Aided Analysis

The sonographic BI-RADS features were used with machine learning algorithm to determine probability of malignancy. This involved training the algorithm using cases with known features and diagnosis. Following the training the algorithm was tested on the unknown cases to predict the probability of malignancy. The predicted values were compared with the biopsy results. The training and testing were performed by using leave-one-sample out cross validation. This involved training the algorithm on all cases of the database except one and predicting the outcome of the remaining last case. The process of training and testing was repeated recursively until the entire dataset has been analyzed. Training and testing was performed by using Bayes model in which the probability of an event (malignancy) is revised based on the accumulation of new evidence (detection of sonographic features). Bayes probability of malignancy in the presence of sonographic features $P(M|F)$ was determined by the approach described earlier [12]. In short, it was determined by multiplying initial estimate of probability $P(M)$ with the probabilities that feature F_i is present in the malignant mass $P(F_i|M)$. $P(F_i|M)$ was determined by dividing the ratio of number of malignant cases with feature F_i over the total number of malignant cases. $P(M)$ was determined by the ratio of number of malignant cases to the total number of cases studied. The diagnostic performance of the Bayes probabilities $P(M|F)$ was measured by calculating the area under the ROC curve (A_z), the standard error, and the 95% confidence intervals [MedCalc Software, Ostend, Belgium].

The statistical difference between the diagnostic performances of the three observations was determined based on p-values [13]. A p-value less than 0.05 was considered to be statistical significant. Additionally, interclass correlation coefficients of the probability estimates were calculated as a measure of the consistency of the diagnostic performance in the three observations.

3. Results

3.1. General Characteristics

Of the 264 lesions, 85 (32%) were malignant and 179 (68%) were benign. Among the malignant lesions, invasive ductal carcinoma was the most common 65 (76%). Other diagnoses included invasive lobular carcinoma 7 (8%), ductal carcinoma in situ 7 (8%) including one papillary carcinoma in situ case, adenocarcinoma 3 (3%), two poorly differentiated carcinomas and one remaining case which was diagnosed as mucinous mammary carcinoma (a rare form of invasive ductal carcinoma). Of the benign masses, 44% were found to be fibroadenomas, 33% were identified as miscellaneous fibrocystic changes, 6% were sclerosing adenosis, and the remaining 17% were identified as benign lesions without atypia in the histopathology report. The mean (±standard deviation) age of all the patient population was 51.5 ± 14.7 years. The mean age of patients with malignant masses was 58.8 ± 12.1 years compared to 48.0 ± 14.5 years for benign cases. The difference in the mean age of the two groups was statistically significant (p = 0.0001).

3.2. Agreement in BI-RADS Feature Selection

Figure 1 shows examples of two breast lesions with high and low agreement in feature selection between three observations. Features like oval shape, microlobulation and hypoechogencity were consistently observed in all three readings in the image shown in **Figure 1(a)**. On the other hand, considerable variation in lesion orientation and margin features was observed between observations in the image shown in **Figure 1(b)**. The results on agreement for each BI-RADS feature for all the cases are summarized in **Table 1**. κ for the individual features ranged from 0.16 to 0.95. The highest intra-observer agreement was found to be on the lesion echo pattern with κ between 0.69 and 0.98 for the three observations. The feature which showed the lowest agreement value was lesion boundary with κ between 0.15 and 0.53.

When all the features were investigated collectively, the overall intra-observer agreement between observa-

(a)

(b)

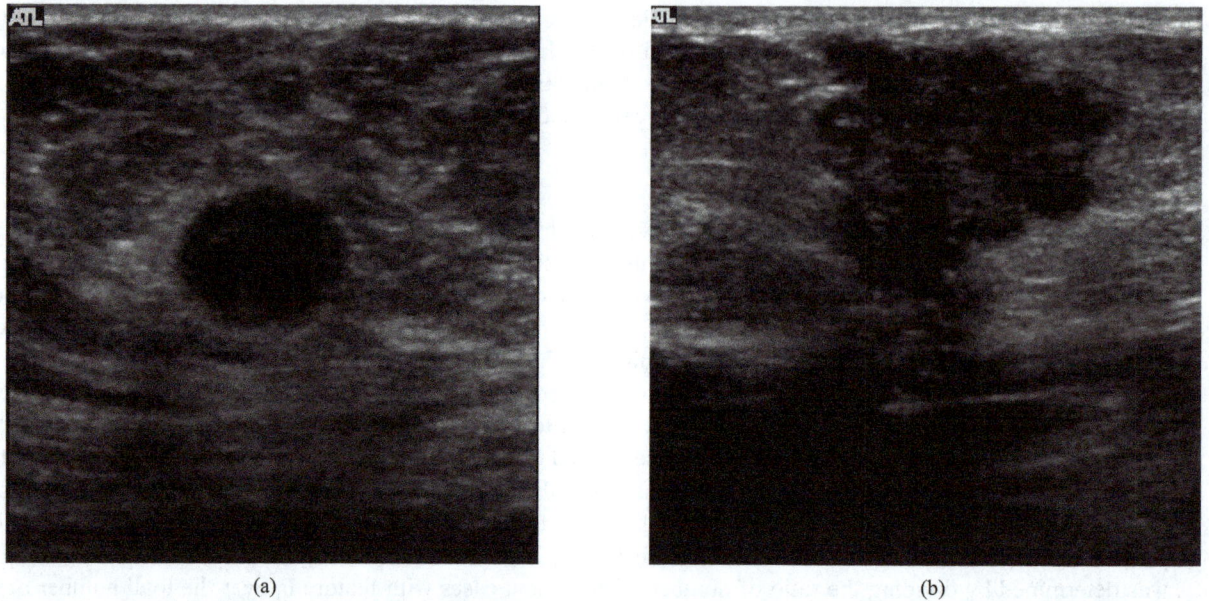

Figure 1. (a) Example of a breast mass that showed high agreement in sonographic features selected between the three observations; (b) Example of a breast lesion that showed lowest agreement in features selected over the three observations.

Table 1. Intra-observer agreement values for BI-RADS US descriptors. The term "overall" represents agreement in all the features together. O1, O2, and O3 refer to first, second and third observations respectively.

Feature	O1 vs. O2 (1 month interval) (κ)	O2 vs. O3 (2 months interval) (κ)	O3 vs. O1 (3 months interval) (κ)	Intra-observer (κ) [15]	Intra-observer (κ) [16]
Shape	0.51	0.75	0.46	0.71	0.7 3
Orientation	0.65	0.71	0.56	0.83	0.68
Boundary	0.16	0.53	0.15	0.85	0.68
Echo pattern	0.98	0.70	0.69	0.67	0.65
Posterior acoustic features	0.98	0.69	0.67	0.82	0.64
Margin	0.95	0.56	0.56	0.59	0.64
Overall	**0.77** (Substantial)	**0.66** (Substantial)	**0.56** (Moderate)	**0.77** (Substantial)	**0.74** (Substantial)

tions 1 and 2 made at an interval of 1 month was 0.77. κ for the agreement between observations 2 and 3 made at a time interval of 2 months was 0.66. For the time interval of 3 months between observations (observation 1 and observation 3) the agreement reduced to 0.56. Thus there was a progressive decrease in agreement (κ) as the time interval between the observations increased from 1 month to 3 months (**Table 1**).

3.3. Diagnostic Performance Analysis

The area under the ROC curve for the ultrasound features alone ranged from 0.772 to 0.817 for the three observations (**Table 2** and **Figure 2**). The difference in the performance (ΔA_z) between the observations was small (0.013 to 0.044) and not statistically significant (p > 0.05, **Table 2**). The diagnostic performance increased markedly (range: 0.828 - 0.849, **Table 3** and **Figure 3**) when the age was included as a risk factor in estimating probability of malignancy. Similar to sonographic features alone, ΔA_z for sonographic features plus age was small (0.003 - 0.021, **Table 3**) and not statistically significant. Inter class correlation coefficient for the three observations was 0.822 (95% CI 0.787 - 0.853) for features alone and 0.833 (95% CI 0.800 - 0.862) for BI-RADS features combined with age.

Table 2. Area under the ROC curve (A_z), the standard error (SE), 95% confidence interval (95% CI) and the p-value for Baysian estimated probabilities in the three observations. Observation 1 represents the initial observation. Observations 2 and 3 were made 1 and 2 months after observation 1.

	$A_z \pm$ SE	95% CI	ΔA_z and p-value		
Observation 1	0.772 ± 0.35	0.717 - 0.822	p = 0.49 $\Delta A_z = 0.013$		
Observation 2	0.786 ± 0.32	0.731 - 0.834		p = 0.08 $\Delta A_z = 0.044$	p = 0 .09 $\Delta A_z = 0.031$
Observation 3	0.817 ± 0.029	0.765 - 0.862			

Table 3. Area under the ROC curve (A_z), the standard error (SE), 95% confidence interval (95% CI) and the p-value for Baysian estimated probabilities combined with patient age in the three observations. Observation 1 represents the initial observation. Observations 2 and 3 were made 1 and 2 months after Observation 1.

	$A_z \pm$ SE	95% CI	ΔA_z and p-value		
Observation 1	0.828 ± 0.0258	0.777 - 0.872	p = 0.87 $\Delta A_z = 0.003$		
Observation 2	0.831 ± 0.027	0.780 - 0.874		p = 0.39 $\Delta A_z = 0.012$	p = 0.17 $\Delta A_z = 0.021$
Observation 3	0.849 ± 0.0248	0.800 - 0.890			

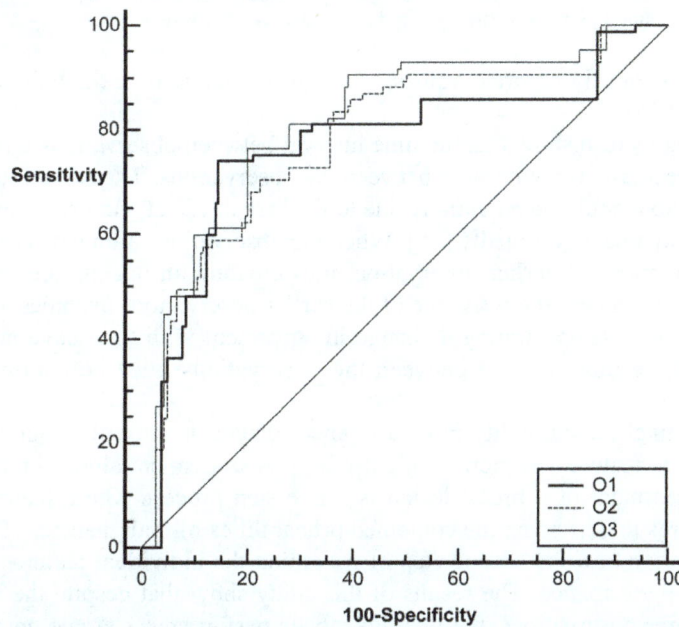

Figure 2. The diagnostic performances of Bayes probabilities estimates from three observations. O1, O2 and O3 refer to first, second and third observations, respectively.

4. Discussion

Previous studies evaluating the observer variability in the interpretation of BI-RADS sonographic features have shown that the agreement between observers can be fair to substantial [14]-[17]. Abdulla *et al.* [14], for instance, demonstrated that inter-observer variability as measured by kappa statistics (κ) for individual features ranged from fair ($\kappa = 0.36$) to substantial ($\kappa = 0.70$). Similarly, Calasa *et al.* [15] demonstrated that intra-observer variability for individual features ranged from moderate ($\kappa = 0.59$) to substantial ($\kappa = 0.85$) with an overall substantial agreement with kappa values ranging from 0.72 to 0.79. In general, variation in features observed in this study

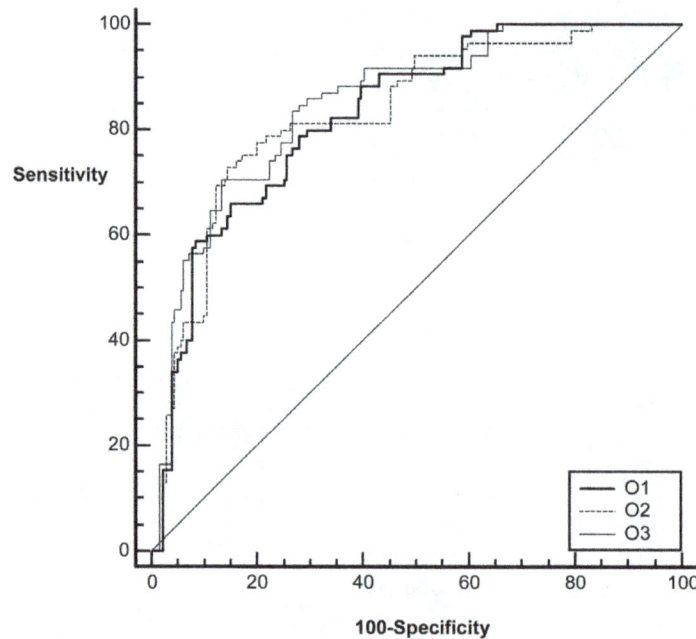

Figure 3. The diagnostic performances of Bayes probabilities estimates from three observations combined with patients' age. O1, O2 and O3 refer to first, second and third observations, respectively.

is comparable to the previously reported values, although the range of κ for individual features in the present study is wider (0.16 - 0.95).

The results of this study also show that the time interval between observations influences observer agreement and there is a steady decrease in κ with time between the observations. The reason for the steady decrease is not completely understood but could be potentially due to the "recall effect" described by Ryan *et al.*, when reviewing the same chest X-ray image repeatedly [18]. When the observations are made close together in time, the user is influenced by the memory of earlier observation, thus creating an unconscious recall bias. As the time between the observations increases, the influence of the earlier observations becomes less pronounced, thus reducing agreement. The results demonstrating a change in agreement with time have not been previously reported and they suggest that the time interval between the observations must be controlled in designing observer agreement studies.

Prior studies evaluating the variability in breast cancer diagnosis with ultrasound have primarily focused on the variability caused by feature selection. While useful, this assessment alone is not complete because the process of diagnostic assessment of a breast lesion is a two-step process where feature selection is followed by weighting of the features to determine the combined probabilities of malignancies. The previous approaches did not take into consideration how the second step of weighting the individual features contributes to observer variability in diagnostic performance. The results of this study show that despite the variability in the individual feature between the three observations, the final diagnostic performances are comparable. These results are further supported by a strong interclass correlation between the probability estimates approaching 0.83. Although there was a notable variation in individual sonographic features between observations, the diagnostic performances did not change. The seeming discrepancy between observations is not surprising because the computer system is trained on the observed features, thus it is able to discount the differences in feature selection by weighting them differently toward assessing probability of malignancies. In essence, the continuous retraining of the computer system on the observed features compensates for the variation in feature selection. Although this study used Bayesian classifiers for computer aided diagnosis, it is reasonable to anticipate that similar patterns should holds for other learning algorithm. It is also conceivable that individual observers may compensate for the variations in features detection by weighting them differently towards the final diagnosis between observations. Thus, the future studies evaluating diagnostic variations between observations should go beyond studying variations in individual BI-RADS features only; they should also include assessment of the diagnostic performances. Although the results presented in this study are encouraging and demonstrate the efficacy of BI-RADS, further studies with multiple readers are needed for a comprehensive understanding of observer variability in breast ultrasound.

In conclusion, ultrasound images of breast masses were analyzed repeatedly using BI-RADS lexicon. When the features were considered together as a group, the observer agreement was moderate to substantial. However, there were notable differences when features were compared individually. Despite differences in the individual sonographic features between readings, the diagnostic performance of computer-aided analysis of malignant and benign breast masses did not change. Through a built-in learning process in the algorithm, the computer-based analysis was able to account for feature variations and thus provided an effective method to differentiate malignant and benign breast masses.

References

[1] Kopans, D.B. (1992) The Positive Predictive Value of Mammography. *American Journal of Roentgenology*, **158**, 521-526. http://dx.doi.org/10.2214/ajr.158.3.1310825

[2] Jiang, Y.L., Nishikawa, R.M., Schmidt, R.A., Metz, C.E., Giger, M.L. and Doi, K. (1999) Improving Breast Cancer Diagnosis with Computer-Aided Diagnosis. *Academic Radiology*, **6**, 22-33. http://dx.doi.org/10.1016/S1076-6332(99)80058-0

[3] Shen, W.C., Chang, R.F., Moon, W.K., Chou, Y.H. and Huang, C.S. (2007) Breast Ultrasound Computer-Aided Diagnosis Using BI-RADS Features. *Academic Radiology*, **14**, 928-939. http://dx.doi.org/10.1016/j.acra.2007.04.016

[4] Shen, W.C., Chang, R.F. and Moon, W.K. (2007) Computer Aided Classification System for Breast Ultrasound Based on Breast Imaging Reporting and Data System (BI-RADS). *Ultrasound in Medicine & Biology*, **33**, 1688-1698. http://dx.doi.org/10.1016/j.ultrasmedbio.2007.05.016

[5] Moon, W.K., Lo, C.M., Chang, J.M., Huang, C.S., Chen, J.H. and Chang, R.F. (2012) Computer-Aided Classification of Breast Masses Using Speckle Features of Automated Breast Ultrasound Images. *Medical Physics*, **39**, 6465-6473. http://dx.doi.org/10.1118/1.4754801

[6] Moon, W.K., Lo, C.-M., Chang, J.M., Huang, C.-S., Chen, J.-H. and Chang, R.-F. (2013) Quantitative Ultrasound Analysis for Classification of BI-RADS Category 3 Breast Masses. *Journal of Digital Imaging*, **26**, 1091-1098. http://dx.doi.org/10.1007/s10278-013-9593-8

[7] Bouzghar, G., Levenback, B.J., Sultan, L.R., Venkatesh, S.S., Cwanger, A., Conant, E.F. and Sehgal, C.M. (2014) Bayesian Probability of Malignancy with Breast Ultrasound BI-RADS Features. *Journal of Ultrasound in Medicine*, **33**, 641-648. http://dx.doi.org/10.7863/ultra.33.4.641

[8] American College of Radiology (2013) Breast Imaging Reporting and Data System: BI-RADS Atlas. 5th Edition, American College of Radiology, Reston.

[9] Stavros, A.T., Thickman, D., Rapp, C.L., Dennis, M.A., Parker, S.H. and Sisney, G.A. (1995) Solid Breast Nodules: Use of Sonography to Distinguish between Benign and Malignant Lesions. *Radiology*, **196**, 123-134. http://dx.doi.org/10.1148/radiology.196.1.7784555

[10] Cohen, J. (1960) A Coefficient of Agreement for Nominal Scales. *Educational and Psychological Measurement*, **20**, 37-46. http://dx.doi.org/10.1177/001316446002000104

[11] Landis, J.R. and Koch, G.G. (1977) The Measurement of Observer Agreement for Categorical Data. *Biometrics*, **33**, 159-174. http://dx.doi.org/10.2307/2529310

[12] Cary, T.W., Cwanger, A., Venkatesh, S.S., Conant, E.F. and Sehgal, C.M. (2012) Comparison of Naive Bayes and Logistic Regression for Computer-Aided Diagnosis of Breast Masses Using Ultrasound Imaging. In: Bosch, J.G. and Doyley, M.M., Eds., *Medical Imaging: Ultrasonic Imaging, Tomography, and Therapy*, SPIE, Bellingham.

[13] DeLong, E.R., DeLong, D.M. and Clarke-Pearson, D.L. (1988) Comparing the Areas under Two or More Correlated ROC Curves: A Nonparametric Approach. *Biometrics*, **44**, 837-845. http://dx.doi.org/10.2307/2531595

[14] Abdullah, N., Mesurolle, B., El-Khoury, M. and Kao, E. (2009) Breast Imaging Reporting and Data System Lexicon for US: Interobserver Agreement for Assessment of Breast Masses. *Radiology*, **252**, 665-672.

[15] Calas, M.J., Almeida, R.M., Gutfilen, B. and Pereira, W.C. (2009) Intra-Observer Interpretation of Breast Ultrasonography Following the BI-RADS Classification. *European Journal of Radiology*, **74**, 525-528. http://dx.doi.org/10.1016/j.ejrad.2009.04.015

[16] Park, C.S., Lee, J.H., Yim, H.W., Kang, B.J., Kim, H.S., Jung, J.I., Jung, N.Y. and Kim, S.H. (2007) Observer Agreement Using the ACR Breast Imaging Reporting and Data System (BI-RADS)-Ultrasound. *Korean Journal of Radiology*, **8**, 397-402.

[17] Lee, H.J., Kim, E.K., Kim, M.J., Youk, J.H., Lee, J.Y., Kang, D.R. and Oh, K.K. (2008) Observer Variability of Breast

Imaging Reporting and Data System (BI-RADS) for Breast Ultrasound. *European Journal of Radiology*, **65**, 293-298. http://dx.doi.org/10.1016/j.ejrad.2007.04.008

[18] Ryan, J.T., Haygood, T.M., Yamal, J.M., Evanoff, M., O'Sullivan, P., McEntee, M. and Brennan, P.C. (2011) The "Memory Effect" for Repeated Radiologic Observations. *American Journal of Roentgenology*, **197**, W985-W991. http://dx.doi.org/10.2214/AJR.10.5859

11

Magnetic Resonance Imaging for Screening of Woman at High-Risk of Breast Cancer

Reham G. Garout, Howayda M. Ahmed, Saddig D. Jastaniah*, Ibrahim A. Awad

Department of Diagnostic Radiology, Faculty of Applied Medical Sciences, King Abdulaziz University, Jeddah, KSA
Email: *sjastaniah@kau.edu.sa

Abstract

MRI is an excellent option for detection of breast cancer for some selected groups, including those patients with a high probability to hit the disease. However, the high costs and low availability of the device have led to a decline in the application of imaging MRI. The aim of this study was to review usefulness of MRI as a new complementary way to detect breast cancer in routine annual checkup for women breasts of certain ages and breast mass. A cross-sectional Descriptive MRI study was performed on 105 asymptomatic women with a mean age of 49 years. The study group with at least one risk factor of breast cancer were presenting for routine annual screening or follow up at King Abdulaziz University Hospital in Jeddah. It has been found that, 48 patients had biopsy, they were recommended by magnetic resonance imaging and only 14 had positive results, while magnetic resonance imaging suggested 16 and mammography had 62 positive results. Magnetic resonance imaging is not recommended for the average-risk or the general population either; it had been advised for screening the high-risk women of breast cancer. Sensitivity of magnetic resonance imaging has been found to be much higher than of mammography but specificity was generally lower. We propose that it is reasonable to consider MRI as a complement to mammography in screening patients who were at high risk for breast cancer because Magnetic Resonance Imaging can detect small foci that are occult in mammography but we don't advise to check with the general population.

Keywords

MRI, Mammogram, Breast Cancer, Women Breasts

---

*Corresponding author.

1. Introduction

Every year, over a million women worldwide are diagnosed for breast cancer. The best chance for cure is offered by early detection. In average-risk women, mammogram is an effective method for early detection. However, its sensitivity tends to decrease in women at high risk for breast cancer. Because of its better sensitivity over mammogram, multiple investigators have studied the potential role of MRI in screening women at high risk. [1]. Hence, in many cases, the patient may be asked to undergo magnetic resonance imaging [2] [3].

Breast MRI is very sensitive and is useful for assessing invasive carcinomas. It is also used to assess high-risk patients who have more than a 20 percent chance of developing breast cancer in their lifetimes based on genetics (BRCA1 and BRCA2) and strong family history of breast cancer. If a MRI detects a suspicious lesion that isn't recognizable on the mammogram, then a second-look ultrasound is recommended. If visible, the lesion may be biopsied under ultrasound guidance; if not, it may need to be biopsied under MRI guidance [4].

MRI was first widely used in the 1990s to find ruptured breast implants. It began to turn up tumors in dense breast tissue after gadolinium. Since then, MRI with intravenous contrast agent has been used as follow up test for suspicious mammograms. Only in the last few years clinical result suggested that MRI may have role as screening tool for early detection of breast cancer [5]. However, MRI is still considered an investigational technique for surveillance and screening of asymptomatic women with normal conventional imaging findings.

The aim of this study was to demonstrate effectiveness, usefulness and limitations of MRI as a new complementary tool for breast cancer screening of high risk populations at certain ages and breast masses.

2. Materials and Methods

2.1. Study Design

This study was done in the department of diagnostic radiology, King Abdul-Aziz University Hospital situated in Jeddah city, Kingdom of Saudi Arabia (KSA). A cross-sectional observational study was performed during the academic year 2012-2013, after obtaining research ethical approval.

2.2. Patients

The study was performed on women who were asymptomatic presenting for routine annual screening or follow up with at least one risk factor for breast cancer. The collected data was 105 patients ranging in age from 26 to 81 years old with the mean age is 48.94 years and Standard deviation 10.83. Age had been categorized as shown in **Table 1**.

2.3. Methods

Breast MRI was performed using MAGNETOM Version 3 T Siemens machine with the 16-Channel Breast array Coil. Post contrast study was done using a Dotarem contrast with concentration 0.5 and the dose 0.2 ml per kg.

2.4. Patient Preparation

Intravenous lines were introduced into the arm for the administration of contrast material during the test. Renal functions "creatinine level" were checked which must be normal (if GFR < 60 "normal"). Potential subjects were screened for intracranial clips, pacemakers, metal fragments or any other objects that would contraindicate MR imaging. All metallic objects were removed before going to scanner room. Patients were asked to change into hospital gown and last menstrual period (LMP) for pregnancy was checked.

Table 1. Age groping of the sample.

Age group	Frequency	Percent
Less than 35	10	9.5%
Between 35 - 55	66	62.9%
More than 55	29	27.6%
Total	105	100.0%

2.5. Patient Position

Patients were placed in prone position with head first and the breasts were placed directly in the center of each round opening of the 16CH breast array coil and head was placed at the head rest of the coil with the patient's arms at side or extended above the head.

2.6. Patient Instruction

Patient were given instructions not to move during the procedure, how to breath shallow and smoothly. Patients were informed that during the exam, the technologist is monitoring from the window and special camera and they will be able to talk to the technologist through microphone and they were asked to hold the emergency bottom in their hands if they needed any help during the exam. Then earplugs were placed to reduce the noise.

2.7. Protocol Used

The protocol used was shown in **Table 2**.

2.8. Image Interpretation

The images produced were independently evaluated using PACS workstations. MRI images of each patient were reviewed with computer aided analysis for the presence of any malignancy and the radiologist makes comments on points include: the background parenchymal enhancement pattern of the breast, type of lesion (foci, mass & non-mass like), lesion morphology characteristic e.g. shape "round, oval, lobulated or irregular", margin "smooth, irregular or speculated", internal enhancement and distribution. Also, the lesion location is defined, size and kinetic curve characteristic. Associated findings are mentioned either, nipple retraction, skin thickening, edema, cyst and any abnormality of lymph nodes. Post-contrast high-resolution imaging is required to visualize important morphological information if focal enhancement is present. Then, in conclusion the assessments and recommendation is written as:

*Assessments; negative, benign, probably benign, suspicious or highly suggestive of malignancy.

*Recommendation; second look by US or MG, follow up, short interval f/u or for biopsy.

2.9. Data Analysis

Demographic patients' data and medical history were collected which includes hormonal medications, family history of breast disease, family history of other cancers, the phase of menstrual cycle and MRI screening findings. The raw data was tabulated then statistically analyzed with the use of SPSS program for Windows, version 19.0.0.

3. Results

Between Jan, 2012 and Dec, 2012, 280 women were included as a study sample. But 175 patients were excluded from the analysis for the following reasons: symptomatic patients, the contrast-enhanced MRI not completed, results were not available, biopsy not performed, biopsy results were not available or MRI result was not certain and they recommend ultrasound for better assessments. Thus, data from the 280 women was reduced to 105 (37.5%) cases only. 41% of the patients did not perform a mammogram because they were recommended for direct MRI screening or follow up, while 59% had a mammogram with positive result and referred to MRI for further evaluation (**Figure 1**).

3.1. MRI Result

The whole sample had performed MRI and the results were: 67.6% had a benign result (−ve), 17.1% uncertain MRI result (?) and 15.2% the result was malignant (+ve). Accord to age grouping the highest malignant results were on women above 55 y/o and highest benign result on women between 35 - 55 y/o (**Figure 2**).

3.2. Biopsy Findings

Out of 105 patients, only 48 patients had performed biopsy under mammographic and ultrasound guidance.

54.3% did not perform biopsy, 32.4% had biopsy with benign result and 13.3% had biopsy but with malignant result. The highest benign and malignant result is at the age between 35 - 55 y/o (**Figure 3**).

Table 2. Protocol used with the parameters.

Plane	Image series	TR	TE	IT	FA	NEX	SL	Matrix	FOV
	localizer	7.6	3.53	-	20	2	6	256	400
Tra	T2-tse-2mm	3000	89	-	80	1	2	320	400
Tra	T1-tse-2mm	590	15	-	80	1	2	320	400
Tra	T2-tirm-2mm	4060	52	230	70	2	2	256	400
	Diffusion-spair	5000	87	-	-	3	4	192	400
pause				Contrast injection					
Tra	T1-fl3d-pre dyn FS	4.55	1.61	-	10	1	2	480	400
Tra	T1-fl3d-post dyn FS	4.55	1.61	-	10	1	2	480	400
	svs-se-breast-ref	2000	100	-	90	1	-	-	-
	Svs-se-breast	1500	100	-	90	128	-	-	-

Abbreviation: **TR**, repetition time; **TE**, echo time; **IT**, inversion time; **FA**, flip angle; **NEX**, number of excitations; **SL**, slice thickness; **FOV**, field of view; **C.M.**, contrast media; **Tra**, transverse; **tse**, turbo spin echo; **tirm**, turbo inversion recovery magnitude; **dyn**, dynamic; **FS**, fat saturation; **svs**, single voxel spectroscopy; **se**, spin echo; **ref**, reference.

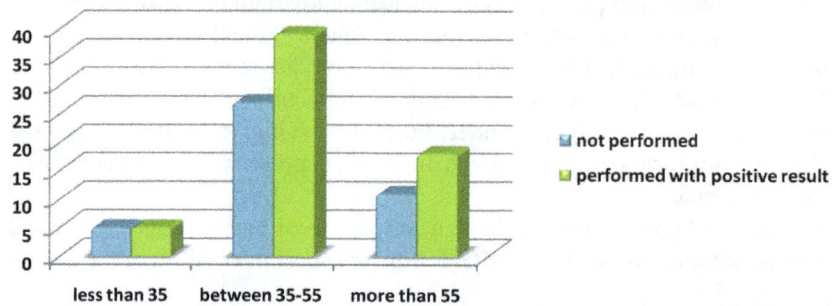

Figure 1. The distribution of mammogram result according to age grouping.

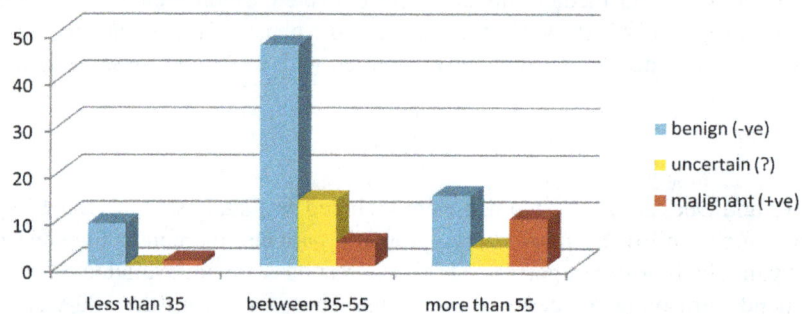

Figure 2. The distribution of MRI result according to type of neoplasm.

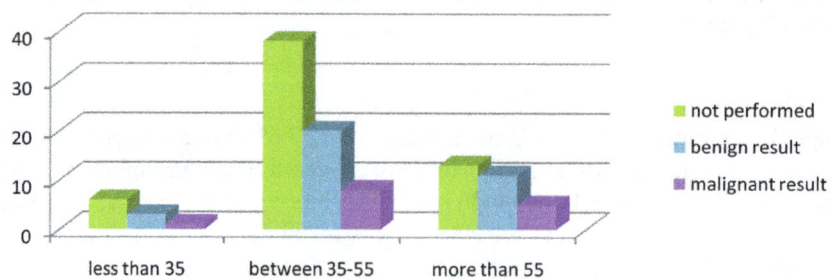

Figure 3. The distribution of biopsy result according to age.

3.3. Correlations between the Family History and the MRI Result

The distribution of the sample according to family history, 71 patients did not have a family history and 34 patients had a family history as shown in **Table 3** while the correlations between the personal history and the MRI result indicated that the personal history risk factor was more common than the family history as shown in **Table 4**. About 44.76% of the sample had different types of personal history (**Figure 4**), while only 32.38% had a family history. The total patients who had a personal history were 47 patients out of 105, and 58 patients did not have a personal history.45% had cancer history on the left breast and 39% on the right breast. This means that 84% had breast cancer before while the other 16% had other different types of personal history risk factor.

3.4. MRI Sensitivity and Specificity

Attribution to biopsy to be as a gold standard to detect the Sensitivity and Specificity of the MRI result. A total 48 patients only of 105 were included in this study, those who performed biopsy, to compare their biopsy result with the MRI result to detect how the Sensitivity and Specificity of MRI is From **Table 5**. The false-negative (FN) results of MRI were 5 patients out of 14 positive result patients (35.7% FN) so, 9 patients were detected as positive result by MRI and biopsy confirmed that. And the false-positive (FP) results were 11 patients out of 34 negative result patients (32.3% FP), this means that the other 23 patients were assigned as negative result (benign) by MRI and the biopsy confirmed benignity of the lesion.

Calculation has been done to know the following the result: Sensitivity of MRI was 64.28% (true positive is highly detected) Specificity of MRI was 67.64% (true negative is higher) Positive predictive value (PPV) 45%. Means if the MRI result was positive, the patient has 45% chance of actually positive result. Negative predictive value (NPV) 82.18%. Means if MRI result was negative, then the patient has 82.18% a chance of not having breast cancer.

3.5. Most Common MRI Findings

The prevalence of different breast diseases detected by MRI for the whole sample was shown in **Figure 5**. Intraductal carcinoma it is also called Ductal carcinoma in situ is the most common malignant (non-invasive) disease as the prevalence in (**Figure 5**) shows. It composes about 10.47% of MRI findings. This type of cancer develops within milk ducts of the breast. One of the most benign findings was fibrocystic changes. Almost 25.71% of the patients had a fibrocystic disease. The following images show breast cancer (**Figure 6**) Ductal carcinoma in situ and invasive ductal carcinoma was diagnosed in 55 years old female and in a 69 years old female patient with family history. They proved to be DCIS and IDC after biopsy had been done. 4.86% of MRI findings were invasive ductal carcinoma which is the most common (invasive) malignant disease. While multiple masses of the right breast was seen in a 65 years old female patient (**Figures 7-9**).

4. Discussion

Mammograms are less likely to find breast tumors in women younger than 50 years than in older women. This is

Table 3. Correlation of MRI results with Family History.

| | | MRI results | | | Total |
		Benign (−ve)	Not Sure (?)	Malignant (+ve)	
Family History	No	44	13	14	71
	Yes	27	5	2	34
Total		71	18	16	105

Table 4. Correlation of MRI results with Personal History.

| | | MRI results | | | Total |
		Benign (−ve)	Not Sure (?)	Malignant (+ve)	
Personal History	No	37	11	10	58
	Yes	34	7	6	47
Total		71	18	16	105

Table 5. Sensitivity and Specificity of MRI according to biopsy result.

		Biopsy		
		+	–	total
MRI	+	9	11	20
	-	5	23	28
	total	14	34	48

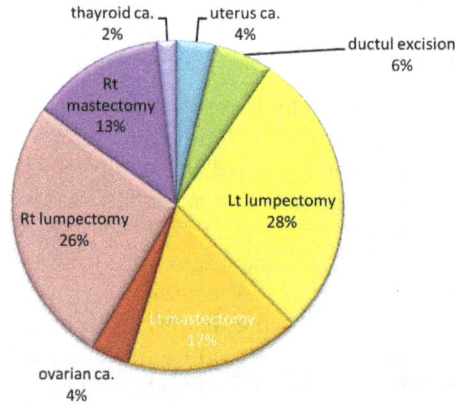

Figure 4. different types of personal history risk factor that the patients had.

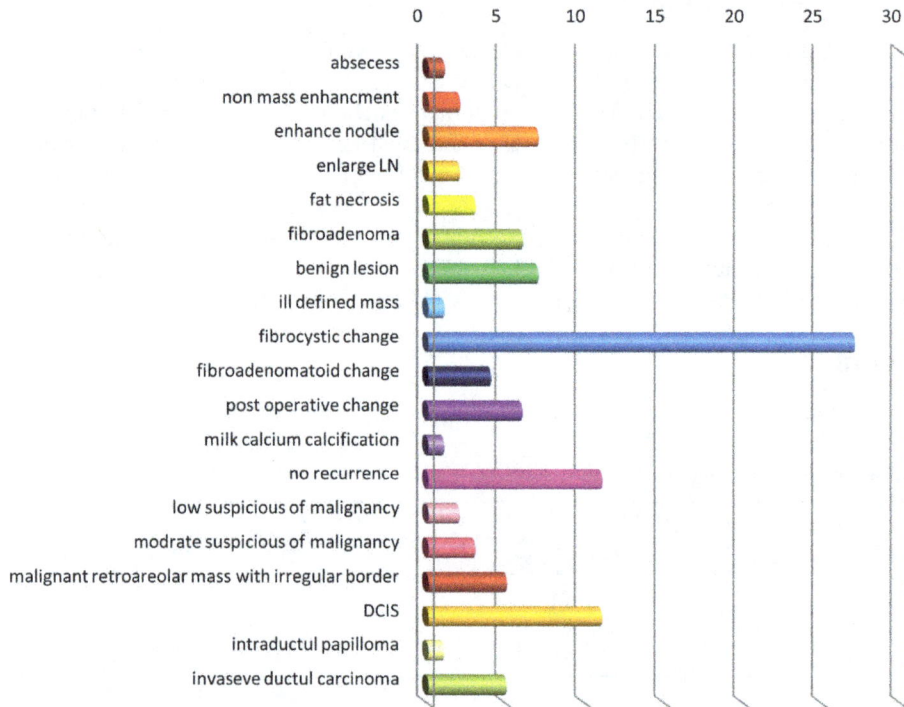

Figure 5. Breast disease finding..

due to the possibility that younger women have denser breast tissue that appears white on a mammogram. Because tumors also appear white on a mammogram, they can be harder to find when there is dense breast tissue [6]. Also MRI found cancer in the other breast that didn't show up yet on mammogram. In addition, after review of more recent studies, the American Cancer Society recently recommended that any woman with a greater than

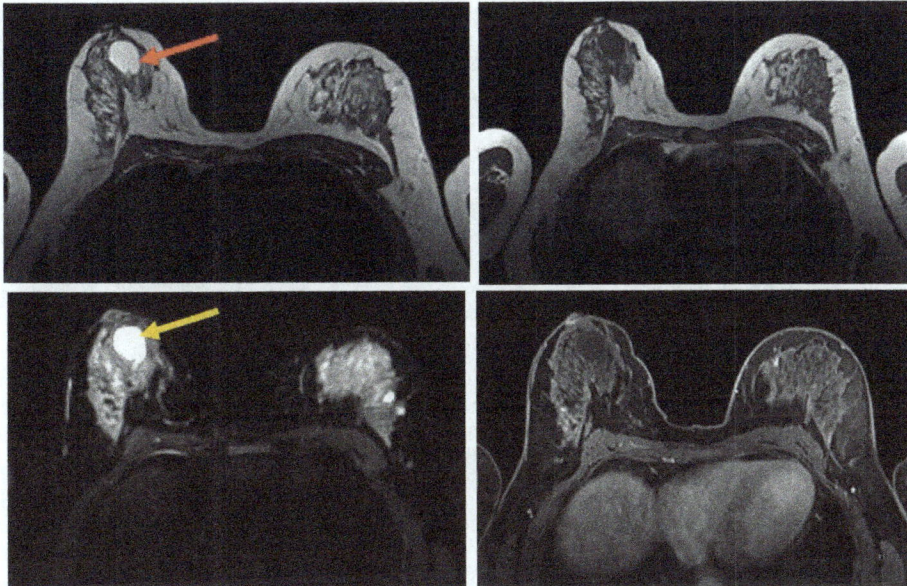

Figure 6. Axial MRI images. Both breast Show prominent glandular tissues with multiple bilateral cysts, the largest one in right breast retroareolarly, Appears as a round mass with smooth margins (well-defined) hyperintense in T2 and hypointense in T1 with very high signal on T2 tirm (fat-suppressed) image. After the injection of gadolinium it appears as hypointense _there is no enhancement_. ˙tirm, turbo inversion recovery.

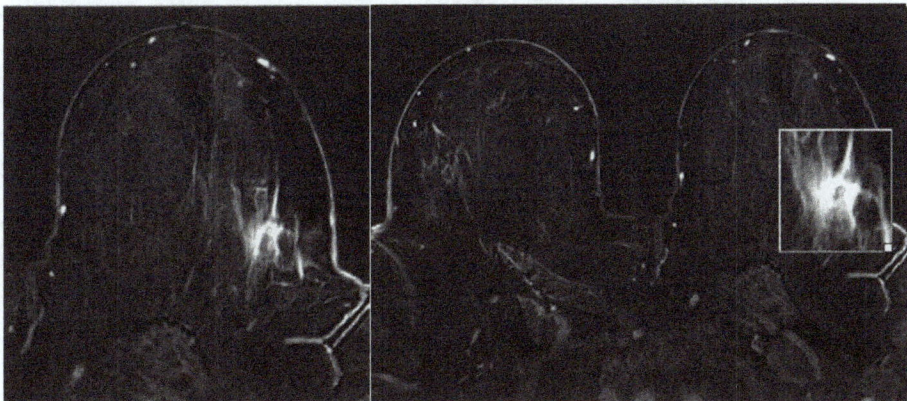

Figure 7. Axial MRI images T1 post contrast shows enlarge ducts in the left breast with high signal after gad injection. They are seen anterior and superior to the main lesion.

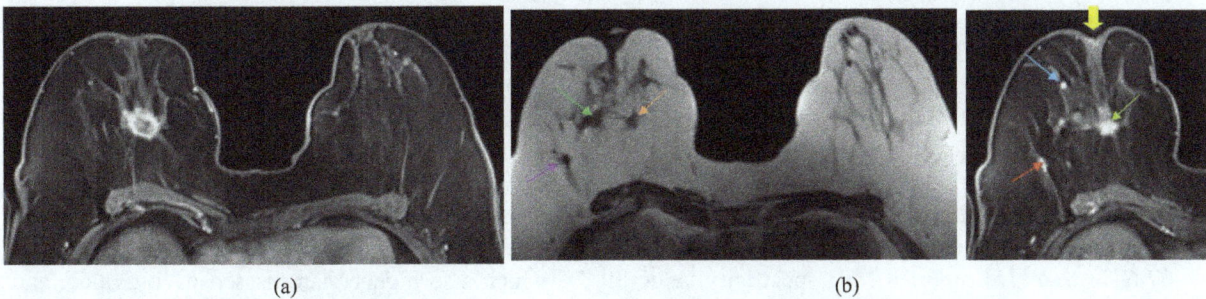

(a)   (b)

Figure 8. (a) Axial MRI T1 post contrast image. It shows a speculated mass enhancing in the right breast centrally. It measures 2 × 1.3 cm in maximum dimension. This proved to be an invasive carcinoma. (b) Axial MRI images. There are multiple speculated peripherally enhancing nodules in the superior lateral aspect of the same breast (right). There is retraction of the nipple (Yellow arrow).

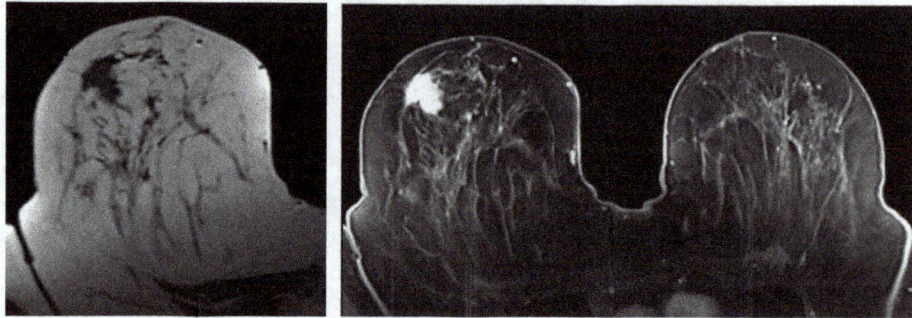

Figure 9. Axial MRI images. Large enhancing irregular mass is noted about 4.5 cm deep and lateral to the nipple, at 10 o'clock of the right breast. In its largest diameter the mass is measuring about 3 × 2.7 cm. it appears hypointense on T1 sequences and after gad injection there is an enhance. For definitive pathology biopsy has been suggested and it is proved to be invasive ductal carcinoma.

20% - 25% lifetime risk for breast cancer should consider undergoing screening with both mammography and breast MRI [7].

The addition of MRI examination of the mammogram in women at increased risk of breast cancer to detect the highest outcome for cancer but also was for false positive results to avoid the harm due to repeated testing or painful biopsies for those who do not have cancer. Therefore, it is advised to use MRI to examine women at high risk of breast cancer [8].

In our study, MRI findings of breast cancer is directly proportional to the age of the patient, where only 15.3% of the whole sample of their findings are malignancy, most of them 10.4% are more than 55 years, 3.8% between 35 - 55 and 0.9% under 35 years. This association is also mentioned by [9]. While another study reported by [10] that is worthwhile to begin screening for women with a high risk from the age of 30 or 35 years old.

The percentage of women recommended by MRI for biopsy in this study is 45.7% and it is a very large percentage comparing to other studies *i.e.* [11] reporting only 2.9% and [12] [13] reporting biopsy procedures with percentages of just over 15%. Also, it was elsewhere mentioned [2] where the range was 6.3% similar to prior studies ranging (from 2.9% to 15.8%) among Screening Women at High Risk for Breast Cancer with Mammography and Magnetic Resonance Imaging.

Breast MRI is not recommended as a routine screening tool for all women. However, it is recommended for screening women who are at high risk for breast cancer, usually due to a strong family history and/or a mutation in genes such as BRCA1 or BRCA2. If you are considered high-risk, you would have breast MRI in addition to your annual mammograms [14].

Family history risk factor in our study composes 32.32%, and from the result 1.91% of the cases have malignancy with positive family history. It is away different from prior studies' results and this is may be due to the large volume of the sample in those studies. In the present study, the personal history risk factor of breast cancer is found in 44.76% of the cases and only 5.7% are diagnosed with breast cancer with MRI and this is very similar to study for Berg W., *et al.*, in Detection of Breast Cancer With Addition of Annual Screening Ultrasound or a Single Screening MRI to Mammography in Women With Elevated Breast Cancer Risk, where only (54%) of participants had a personal history of breast cancer and (4.1%) were diagnosed with cancer [6].

The sensitivity of MRI in our study is 64.28% and this is almost similar to prior studies (71%) mentioned by [15]. In a study of [16] who reported that result of MRI sensitivity level ranging from 57% - 100% due to differences in technical parameters such as the strength of the magnetic field, the type of coil and sequences used, the amount and timing of contrast media, the imaging and the reporting methods.

Specificity of breast MRI in our study is higher than the sensitivity of the MRI, our specificity result is 67.64% also [15] reported MRI specificity value 89.8% which also higher than his sensitivity value, and this differences may be due to the difference in the size of sample.

Although this study is not a comparative study, but we can say that MRI has a better sensitivity than mammogram. From the results of mammography 59% of the whole sample have a positive result, while MRI results say that only 15.2% of the sample have a positive result and after biopsy has performed the actual positive result is

13.3%. In a previous study [17], it was reported that MRI has high sensitivity ranging from 71% to 100% versus 16% to 40% for mammography in a high risk population. Screening mammograms alone, or screening breast ultrasounds alone, each found only a little more than half of the cancers. However, together, screening mammograms and ultrasounds found 82% of the cancers. Breast MRI (after three negative mammogram and ultrasound screenings) found another 8% of breast cancers not detected by the other tests.

In conclusion, from the study we found that the addition of magnetic resonance imaging to mammography in screening women at increased risk of breast cancer resulted in a higher cancer detection due to its high value of sensitivity.

References

[1]   Lehman, C. (2006) Role of MRI in Screening Women at High Risk for Breast Cancer. *Journal of Magnetic Resonance Imaging*, **24**, 964-970. http://dx.doi.org/10.1002/jmri.20752

[2]   Lehman, C., Blume, J., Weatherall, P., Thickman, D., Hylton, N., Warner, E., *et al.* (2005) Screening Women at High Risk for Breast Cancer with Mammography and Magnetic Resonance Imaging. *Cancer*, **103**, 1898-1905. http://dx.doi.org/10.1002/cncr.20971

[3]   Dummin, L.J., Cox, M. and Plant, L. (2007) Prediction of Breast Tumour Size by Mammography and Sonography—A Breast Screen Experience. *The Breast Journal*, **16**, 38-46. http://dx.doi.org/10.1016/j.breast.2006.04.003

[4]   Berg, W., Zhang, Z., Lehrer, D., Jong, R., Pisano, E., Barr, R., *et al.* (2012) Detection of Breast Cancer with Addition of Annual Screening Ultrasound of a Single Screening MRI to Mammography in Women with Elevated Breast Cancer Risk. *JAMA*, **307**, 1394-1404. http://dx.doi.org/10.1001/jama.2012.388

[5]   Gavenonis, S. (2011) Breast MR Imaging: Normal Anatomy. In: Liu, P.S., Ed., *Normal MRI Anatomy from Head to Toe, an Issue of Magnetic Resonance Imaging Clinics*, 1st Edition, Saunders Publisher, 519-507.

[6]   Malur, S., Wurdinger, S., Moritz, A., Michels, W. and Schneide, R. (2001) A Comparison of Written Reports of Mammography, Sonography and Magnetic Resonance Mammography for Preoperative Evaluation of Breast Lesions, with Special Emphasis on Magnetic Resonance Mammography. *Breast Cancer Research*, **3**, 55-60. http://dx.doi.org/10.1186/bcr271

[7]   American Cancer Society (2013) What Are the Risk Factors for Breast Cancer? http://www.cancer.org/cancer/breastcancer/detailedguide/breast-cancer-risk-factors

[8]   Afonso, N. (2009) Women at High Risk for Breast Cancer—What the Primary Care Provider Needs to Know. *JABFM*, **22**, 43-50. http://dx.doi.org/10.3122/jabfm.2009.01.070188

[9]   Sasieni, P., Shelton, J., Ormiston-smith, N., Thomson, C. and Silcocks, P. (2011) Among What Is the Life Time Risk o Developing Cancer? *British Journal of Cancer*, **11**, 460-465.

[10] Urban, L. and Urban, C. (2012) Role of Mammography versus Magnetic Resonance Imaging for Breast Cancer Screening. *Current Breast Cancer Reports*, **4**, 216-223 http://dx.doi.org/10.1007/s12609-012-0085-5

[11] Kriege, M., Brekelmans, C.T., Boetes, C., *et al.* (2004) Efficacy of MRI and Mammography for Breast-Cancer Screening in Women with a Familial or Genetic Predisposition. *The New England Journal of Medicine*, **351**, 427-437. http://dx.doi.org/10.1056/NEJMoa031759

[12] Warner, E., Plewes, D.B., Hill, K.A., *et al.* (2004) Surveillance of BRCA1 and BRCA2 Mutation Carriers with Magnetic Resonance Imaging, Ultrasound, Mammography, and Clinical Breast Examination. *JAMA*, **292**, 1317-1325. http://dx.doi.org/10.1001/jama.292.11.1317

[13] Morris, E., Liberman, L., Ballon, D.J., *et al.* (2003) MRI of Occult Breast Carcinoma in a High-Risk Population. *AJR Am J Roentgenol*, **181**, 619-626. http://dx.doi.org/10.2214/ajr.181.3.1810619

[14] Orel, S.G. and Schnall, M.D. (2001) MR Imaging of the Breast for the Detection, Diagnosis, and Staging of Breast Cancer. *Radiology*, **220**, 13-30. http://dx.doi.org/10.1148/radiology.220.1.r01jl3113

[15] Elmore, J., Armstrong, K., Lehman, C. and Fletcher, S. (2005) Screening for Breast Cancer. *JAMA*, **293**, 1245-1256. http://dx.doi.org/10.1001/jama.293.10.1245

[16] Forrai, G. (2011) Magnetic Resonance Imaging (MRI) in the Screening of High-Risk Patients and in the Detection and Diagnosis of Early Breast Cancer. In: Kahán, Z. and Tot, T., Eds., *Breast Cancer, a Heterogeneous Disease Entity*, Springer, 55-45. http://dx.doi.org/10.1007/978-94-007-0489-3_3

[17] Saslow, D., Boetes, C., Burke, W., Harms, S., Leach, M. and Lehman, C. (2007) American Cancer Society Guidelines for Breast Screening with MRI as an Adjunct to Mammography. *CA: A Cancer Journal for Clinicians*, **57**, 75-89. http://dx.doi.org/10.3322/canjclin.57.2.75

12

Angiogenesis Factors Associated with New Breast Cancer Cell Line AMJ13 Cultured *in Vitro*

Ahmed Majeed Al-Shammari[1]*, Worod Jawad Kadhim Allak[2], Mahfoodha Umran[2], Nahi Y. Yaseen[1], Ayman Hussien[1]

[1]Experimental Therapy Department, Iraqi Center for Cancer and Medical Genetic Research, Al-Mustansiriyah University, Baghdad, Iraq
[2]Biotechnology Department, Collage of Science, Baghdad University, Baghdad, Iraq
Email: *Ahmed.alshammari@iccmgr.org

Abstract

Background: AMJ13 is a new breast cancer cell line that has been established from a 70-year-old Iraqi woman with a histological diagnosis of infiltrating ductal carcinoma. It is the first for an Iraqi population. In breast cancer, angiogenesis provides the tumor tissue, which is rapidly proliferated with oxygen and nutrients, removes wastes and increases the opportunity of cancer cells to invade other organs. Methods: The AMJ13 breast cancer cell line was represented at three different passages and incubated for interval times. Microarray panel of 43 different angiogenesis markers was used to scan the supernatant for the factors. ELISA was used to quantify some of the important angiogenesis factors released in the culture medium and to confirm absence of those who was not detected by the antibody array. RT-PCR was used to confirm the gene expression (mRNA) of studied factors. Results: Microarray analysis showed that TIMP1 and two secreted at highest levels compared to the rest of the factors with low presence of endostatin. Other non-detectable factors by microarray examined by ELISA assay that showed highest expression level of VEGF-A were obtained at earliest passage, while the highest levels of FGF-b were obtained at late passage. The VEGF-D secretion was shown low concentrations at all studied passages. There is no detectable level of EGF protein in different passages and times interval tested. There are no significant differences in secretion of sICAM between different passages and incubation periods. Conclusion is that AMJ13 cell line depends on VEGF-A as main angiogenesis factor to induce micro-vessels supported by low levels of VEGF-D for lymphatic vessels formation. AMJ13 cell line depends on FGF as growth factors as in late passages it was shifted to depend mainly on FGF completely. All of this process may be regulated by TGF-*β*. TIMP-1 has proangiogentic effect and has feedback talk with TIMP-2. Understanding the angiogenesis process for breast cancer can give us better targets for therapy and

more effective treatments.

Keywords

Angiogenesis Factors, Breast Cancer Cell, AMJ13, Tumor Tissue

1. Introduction

Angiogenesis is a process of formation of new blood vessels from a pre-existing vasculature [1]. It is important in number of physiological and pathological events [2]. In cancer, angiogenesis provides the tumor tissue which is rapidly proliferated with oxygen and nutrients and remove wastes [3]. Previous studies demonstrate that the tumor growth reaches a steady state at approximately 2 - 3 mm^2 in diameter due to insufficient nutrients and oxygens and the opportunities of tumor distance metastasis are increased with tumor angiogenesis [3] [4]. It is worth mentioning that the tumor cells may start forming new blood vessels by angiogenesis process to continue growing and invade surrounding tissue. Extensive laboratory data suggest that angiogenesis plays an essential role in breast cancer development, invasion, and metastasis [5]. The new blood vessels increased the opportunity of breast cancer cell to enter the blood stream and invade other organs while the tumor that not vascularized still have high death rate until they switch a new angiogenesis [3]. Angiogenesis mechanisms depend on regulation of biological activity and interactions of two cell main types' endothelial and mural cells forming the vessels [6]. Researchers demonstrated that the tumor cells produce pro-angiogenic factors [7] that induce the endothelial cells proliferation to form a new vessel [8]. Angiogenesis process is regulated by the balance between pro- and anti-angiogenesis factors [7]. Vascular endothelial growth factors [VEGF] and its receptors are the key signaling system that regulates proliferation and migration of endothelial cells forming the basis of any vessel [6]. Hypoxia is the main force that initiates angiogenesis and induces VEGF and its receptors via hypoxia inducing factor-1α (HIF-1α). In addition, hypoxia considers an important component that up regulates the expression of different genes associated with various steps of angiogenesis such as VEGF and FGF [9]. Several oncogenes such as K-ras, v-ras, v-yes, fos, and v-raf may induce the up-regulation of angiogenesis factors, cytokines receptors and proteolytic enzymes [3]. Evidence is accumulating that tumor suppressor genes also play a role in the genetic switch of the angiogenesis [10]. Angiogenesis factors can be classified as: 1) soluble growth factors such as VEGF, FGF-1 and FGF-2 which cause endothelial cell growth and differentiation; 2) factors which inhibit proliferation and induce differentiation like TGF-β and angiogen; 3) extracellular matrix-bound cytokines which regulate angiogenesis such as enodstin and angiostatin. Tumor growth and metastasis can be inhibited by angiogenesis inhibition which was achieved by anti-angiogenesis factors [11]. AMJ13 is a new breast cancer cell line that has been established from an Iraqi breast cancer patient. It is the first for an Iraqi population. The AMJ13 cell line was established from the primary tumor of a 70-year-old Iraqi woman with a histological diagnosis of infiltrating ductal carcinoma. The cells found to be elongated multipolar epithelial-like cells with a population doubling time of 22 hours. The anchorage-independent growth ability test showed that the cells were able to grow in semisolid agarose, confirming their transformed nature. Cytogenetic study of these cells showed chromosomal aberrations with many structural and numerical abnormalities, producing chromosomes of unknown origin called marker chromosomes. Immunocytochemistry showed that the estrogen receptor and the progesterone receptor were not expressed, and a weak positive result was found for HER2/neu gene expression. The cells were positive for BRCA1 and BRCA2, as well as for vimentin [12].

This study aimed to estimate the expression levels of many angiogenesis proteins that are secreted by locally established breast cancer cell line (AMJ13), and to detect the most responsible factors for the angiogenesis process in Iraqi patients to select correct anti-angiogenesis compound in future.

2. Materials and Methods

2.1. Cell Line and Growth Conditions

The AMJ13 breast cancer cell line was supplied by the Iraqi Center for Cancer and Medical Genetic Research (ICCMGR) Experimental Therapy Department, Cell bank Unit. The cells were represented at three different passages 18, 37 and 60 and gown at (150,000 cell/ml) concentration on RPMI-1640 medium (US biological,

USA) supplemented with 10% FBS (Capricorn, Germany) and antibiotics in a humidified atmosphere of 5% CO_2.

2.2. Human Angiogenesis Antibody Array

The Membrane-Based Antibody Arrays (Semi-Quantitative, Sandwich-Based) were used as a tool for screening and comparing expression levels of Angiogenesis cytokines, growth factors and soluble receptors.

The Arrays utilize the sandwich immunoassay principle, wherein a panel of capture antibodies were printed on a nitrocellulose membrane solid support.

The supernatants were collected from AMJ13 cells grown at passage 37 after 24 hrs to scan the expression of several factors related with angiogenesis by Antibody Array. The procedure was according to manufacturer protocol, briefly, the samples were incubated for two hrs on the slides. A cocktail of biotinylated Ab were added after washing the membranes. They further incubated for 2 hrs and washed and incubated for one hour with labled streptavidin. Signal detected using (Epichemi3 Darkroom, UVP, USA) and data analyzed using Labworks software (UVP, USA).

2.3. Quantification of Angiogenesis Factors Release

To quantify angiogenesis factors release, the culture medium were collected at regular intervals (6, 12, 18, 24, 30 and 36 hrs), and it frozen until further analysis. Angiogenesis factors concentrations were determined by using an Enzyme-linked immunosorbent assay (ELISA) kits according to the manufacturer.s protocol VEGF-A, VEGF-D, FGF-b, EGF (Raybiotech, USA) TGF-β and sICAM (IBL, Germany). The GraphPad prism software (GraphPad, San Diego, California, USA) was used to plot the standard curve and calculation the factors concentrations.

2.4. Reverse Transcription-Polymerase Chain Reaction

2.4.1. RNA Extraction
Total RNA was extracted from AMJ13 cells by (Automated total RNA extraction kit, Anatolia, Turkey) according to the manufacturer's protocol and was quantified by nanodrop.

2.4.2. Reverse Transcription-Polymerase Chain Reaction
The expression of mRNAs encoding different polypeptide isoforms of (VEGF-A, VEGF-D, FGF-b, EGF, TGF-β and sICAM) were studied by RT-PCR. Specific primers for the (VEGF-A, VEGF-D, FGF-b, EGF, TGF-β and sICAM) genes (design of primers was based on published sequence on National Center for Biotechnology Information (NCBI). The 20 µl RT-PCR reaction contained 0.27 µg of total RNA, specific primer pair, (IDI DNA, USA), and components of the OneStep RT-PCR kit (KAPA Biosystem, USA). Specific detection of TGF-β gene was achieved with the following primer pairs: forward 5' TGGTGGAAACCCACAACGAA 3' and reverse 5' GAGCAACACGGGTTCAGGTA 3' to detect the TGF-β gene and the following primer pairs: forward 5' CTTCAAGCCATCCTGTGTGC 3' and reverse 5' TCTCTCCTATGTGCTGGCCT 3' to detect the VEGF-A and the following primer pairs: forward 5' CTTCCCCAAGGATTTCAAGATGA 3' and reverse 5' ATGTCTTCA AACCTATAAAACAGCA 3' to detect the FGF-b in AMJ13 cells. The PCR amplification conditions used for TGF-β, VEGF-A and FGF-b amplification were as follows: 42°C for 5 min, 95°C followed by 40 cycles of 43 sec: 3 sec at 95°C, 20 sec at 62°C, and 20 sec at 72°C. Specific detection of VEGF-D gene was achieved with the following primer pairs: forward 5' TCCCATCGGTCCACTAGGTT 3' and reverse 5' CACACAAGGGGGCTT GAAGA 3' to detect the VEGF-D gene in AMJ13 cells. The PCR amplification conditions used for VEGF-D amplification were as follows: 42°C for 5 min, 95°C followed by 40 cycles of 43 sec: 3 sec at 95°C, 20 sec at 55.5°C, and 20 sec at 72°C. Specific detection of EGF gene was achieved with the following primer pairs: forward 5' CCGCATCTGGGGTCAATCAT 3' and reverse 5' GTGCAGGACCCACACAAGTA 3' to detect the EGF gene in AMJ13 cells. The PCR amplification conditions used for TGF-β amplification were as follows: 42°C for 5 min, 95°C followed by 40 cycles of 43 sec: 3 sec at 95°C, 20 sec at 58.5°C, and 20 sec at 72°C. The PCR cDNA product was electrophoresed on a 1.4% agarose gels containing ethidium bromide DNA dye, visualized under UV light, and photographed. Specific amplification was determined by the size of the products on the gel compared to the 100 - 1000 bp DNA ladder (100 bp DNA ladder, KAPA Biosynthesis, USA).

2.5. Statistical Analysis

Statistical analysis of data was performed by using Statistical Package for Social Science (SPSS) version 17 for determination of significant variations by using ANOVA two ways to analysis the data of secretion levels of angiogenesis factors. The differences are considered significant when the probability value is (<0.05).

3. Results

3.1. Scanning for Angiogenesis Factors by Antibody Array

The experiment showed that the highest level of expressions for angiogenesis factors were TIMP1 and TIMP2. Endostatin factor was secreted in low level comparing to the TIMP1 and TIMP2, while other factors secretions were lower than sensitivity level of the kit. The results are shown in (**Figures 1(A)-(C)**).

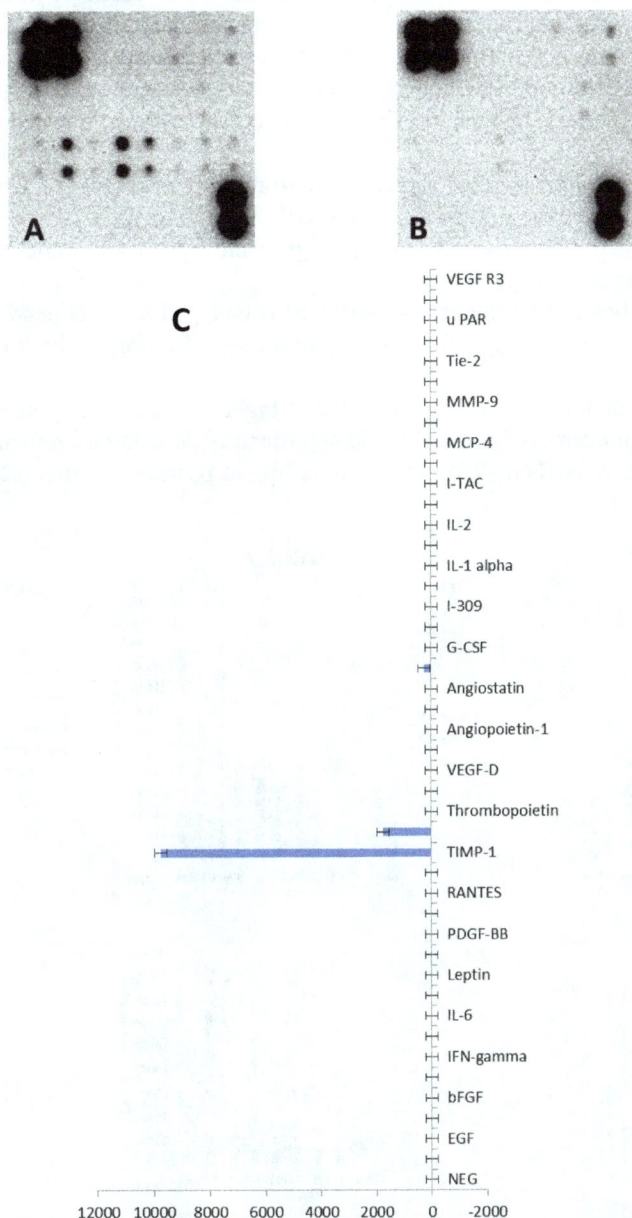

Figure 1. (A) and (B), the membrane with the positive signals. (C), Secretions levels of angiogenesis factors by AMJ13 cultured at passages 37 after 24 hrs incubation at 37°C detected by antibody array.

3.2. Measuring Angiogenesis Factors by ELISA Assay

After screening for 43 potential angiogenesis factors and discovered only 3 factors with very high expression, we went now for more sensitive assay to confirm presence some of the most important factors for angiogenesis and breast cancer growth. The measured angiogenesis factors (VEGF-A, VEGF-D, FGF-b, EGF, TGF-β and sICAM) to confirm if they secreted by human breast cancer cell line (AMJ13) during different time intervals.

The detection of VEGF-A secretion by AMJ13 cell line was significant. It shown to be increased gradually from low to high levels through time to reach highest peak at 36hrs in the three passages tested. From the (**Figure 2**), we can notice that early passages (passage 18) were of higher expression when compared to later passages (passages 36 and 60). The higher concentration was detected at passage 18 after 36 hrs of culture, which was 1982 pg/ml.

The expression of VEGF-D was very low and higher concentrations was 36 pg/ml at passage 60 after 6 hrs and there were no significant differences in secretion levels of the VEGF-D at all interval times and passages measured which indicate that this cancer cell line is not depending on VEGF-D as angiogenesis factors. There is no evidence on EGF protein secretion by the AMJ13 cells at all passages at different intervals. Soluble Intracellular adhesion molecules were detected and its concentrations were increased gradually. There were no significant differences between different passages. The highest secretion levels detected was 1460 pg at passage 60 after 36 hrs.

Fibroblast growth factor were secreted significantly from early passages (18 and 36) at early time (6 hrs) and maintaining good level of expression at all times tested. Surprisingly, the level of expression were changed at passage 60 to show gradual secretion to reach very higher and significant amount especially at 30 and 36 hrs to reach 10,959 and 13,355 pg/ml respectively.

These results may indicates that the breast cancer cells changed to be depend on FGF-b as a growth factor. The expression levels of FGF-b ranged from 395 pg at passage 60 after 12 hrs to 13,355 pg at passage 60 after 36 hrs.

Transforming growth factor beta (TGF-β) secreted at higher levels as early as 6 hrs of incubation at all three studied passages, while it decreased gradually and significantly depending on incubation times (18, 37, and 60). The concentrations of secreted TGF-β ranged from 387 pg at passage 37 after 12 hrs to 2358 pg at passage 37 after 6 hrs (**Figure 2**).

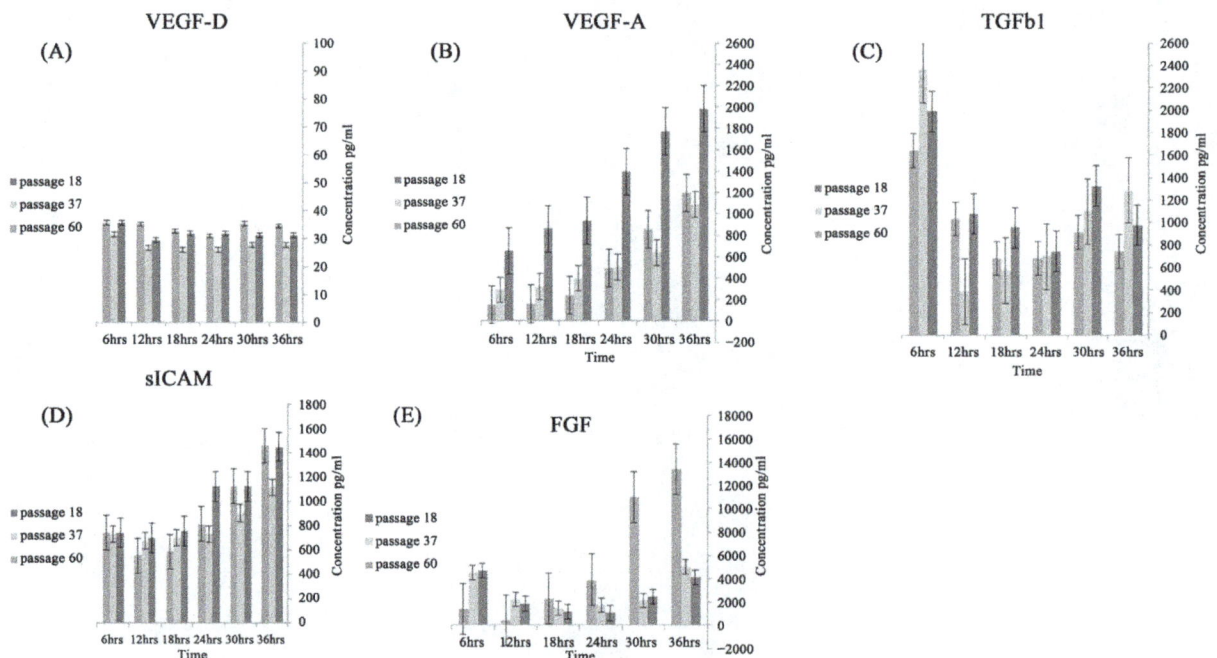

Figure 2. Showing angiogenesis factors concentration secreted by AMJ13 cultured at passages (18, 37 and 60) during (6, 12, 18, 24, 30 and 36) hrs at 37°C measured by ELISA. (A)-showing VEGF-D, (B)-showing VEGF-A, (C)-showing TGF-β, (D)-showing sICAM, (E)-showing FGF-b.

3.3. Reverse Transcriptase Polymerase Chain Reaction RT-PCR

The results illustrated in **Figure 3** showed appearance of sharp bands in 113 bp, 143 bp and 135 bp and the clear bends in 165 bp and 228 bp in **Figures 3(A)-(D)** indicate the expression of VEGF-A, TGF-β, FGF-b, VEGF-D and EGF genes in AMJ13 cells.

4. Discussion

Studying angiogenesis factors that associated to the breast cancer is of important value to developing targeting therapies to block cancer proliferation and invasion and even metastasis. Cancer cells secret many factors that activate angiogenesis process to support themselves for nutrients and waste removal [3]. Our experiment is designed to study newly established breast cancer cell line named AMJ13 [12] in regards to its ability to induce angiogenesis by screening its secretions during cells propagations *in vitro*. This cell line is important as it is first Iraqi breast cancer model and we need to study cancer cells angiogenesis factors and to know which main factor this cancer cells depend on during angiogenesis.

Using microarray technology we screened for the highest levels factors. Tissue inhibitor of metalloproteinases-1 (TIMP-1) was the highest factor that our AMJ13 cell line produce. It is one of new suggested prognostic markers in breast cancer, as a number of studies showed an association between high expression of TIMP-1 protein and a poor prognosis of breast cancer patients, this surprising association is due to a proteolytic activity in cancer cell invasion and metastasis. Tissue inhibitors of metalloproteinases (TIMPs) are a family of endogenous inhibitors associated with the family of enzymes degrades the basement membrane (matrix metalloproteinase MMP) family. Under normal physiologic conditions, the MMPs and TIMPs exist in an exquisite balance and this balance is disrupted during active angiogenesis [5]. However, the recent studies have discovered some other biological functions of TIMP-1 such as growth-stimulating functions, as well as anti-apoptotic and pro-angiogenetic effects [13]. While the *in vitro* studies found TIMP-1 did not affect the proliferation of the endothelial cells (ECs) and tumor cells, suggesting that the TIMP-1 was not cytotoxic protein [14].

The second factor secreted by AMJ13 is the other member of TIMPs family (Tissue inhibitors of metalloproteinase-2 TIMP-2) that is associated with angiogenesis, invasion, and metastasis. TIMP-2 found to inhibit angiogenesis *in vivo* and inhibits endothelial cells proliferation and migration *in vitro* through MMP-dependent mechanisms and MMP-independent mechanisms mediated by endothelial cells proteolysis [15]. This factor may play as feedback to control the other angiogenesis factor and for that, its presence was in low quantities in compare to TIMP-1. The role of TIMP-2 was controversial in breast cancer due to the controversial results in which high TIMP-2 expression was associated either with experienced low cancer recurrence/progression or with a poor prognosis confirming the activating or inhibitory role of TIMP-2 [16].

To establish AMJ13 mechanism for angiogenesis we conducted quantitative study for some of the most important factors that may be associated with angiogenesis and cell growth. We quantitate the secreted VEGF-A factor during first 36 h of the cells propagation. We noticed elevated pattern which can link the VEGF-A secretion levels to several changes in the microenvironment such as hypoxic and/or nutrients deficiency in the culture medium as a variation in physiological conditions [17] that might stimulate the secretion of angiogenic factors to

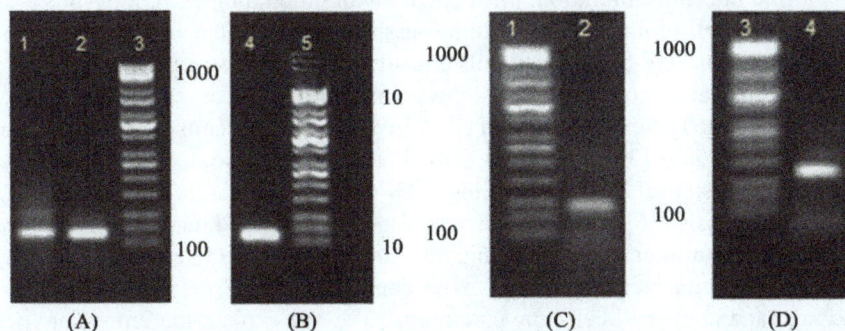

Figure 3. Agarose Gel electrophoresis of RT-PCR products of (A) Lane one and 2 are VEGF-A, FGF-b with size of 143 bp and 135 bp respectively. (B) TGF-β genes with size of 113 bp. Staining with ethidium bromide and visualized under U.V light, Lane 3 and 5 DNA ladder (100 - 1000). (C) VEGF-D gene with size of 165 bp (D) EGF with PCR product size of 228 bp. Lane 1 and 3 DNA ladder (100 - 1000); Lanes 2 VEGF-D Lanes 4 EGF.

increase blood supply in response to nutrient deprivation and hypoxia [18]. Saponaro *et al.* [19] demonstrate that the VEGF-A expression in BRCA1-2 carrier breast cancer tissues was higher than that in BRCAX breast cancer tissues. This confirms what we have in AMJ13 the cell line under investigation which is BRCA1 positive [12]. Furthermore, in both BRCA1-2 carriers and BRCAX the VEGF-A expression was higher than the sporadic group. VEGF-A can be stimulated by other conditions as hypoxia and TGF-β1 [20] and Platelet-derived growth factor (PDGF) [21]. Moreover, we noticed that VEGF-A levels were higher compared to later passages, which was explained by the less need for the factor because culture media is providing sufficient nutrients and less need for angiogenesis *in vitro*.

The secreted levels of VEGF-D by our AMJ13 breast cancer cells were very low in all times tested. This factor showed significant variations in 105 breast cancer patients and it may be completely absent in some breast tumors, as reported by Nakamura *et al.* [22]. Formation of lymphatics within tumors is activated by VEGF-D Stimulation, which also promotes tumor angiogenesis [23]. We suggest that AMJ13 needs less lymphatic vessels which explain the low level of VEGF-D but need higher angiogenesis to deliver nutrients and oxygenation which explain the higher levels for VEGF-A.

Epidermal growth factor is one of the important growth factors and the investigation showed no evidence on EGF protein secretion by the grown cells at all passages at different intervals. Many other human negative estrogen receptor breast cancer cell lines (BT20 and MDA MB 231 cells) showed low or no expression levels of EGF [24]. These data confirm our results, whereas AMJ13 cells are negative estrogen receptor cell line [12]. However, not all estrogen receptor positive cell lines express the EGF as there is no EGF mRNA in MCF 7 cells [24]. Secretions of EGF was observed in (31%) of primary tumors only [25]. Mori *et al.* [26] suggested that MCF-7 human breast cancer cell line synthesize and secrete a polypeptide immunologically related to human EGF into the culture medium. The molecular weight of this poly peptide was similar to that of EGF from human urine. However, in enzyme immunoassay system the dose-response curve of MCF-7 EGF did not show good parallelism with that of standard human EGF. These data may explain why the results of EGF obtained by ELISA differ from that obtained by RT-PCR.

The obtained results from quantitative ELISA assay showed significant increasing in sICAM concentration depending on incubation time and progression of passages. The high expression rate of sICAM-1 in breast cancer patients is associated with tumors at advanced stages and with those with the estrogen receptor negative phenotype [27] and the level of sICAM-1 in the serum of women with breast cancer was significantly higher than that observed in the serum of healthy women. They also found significant differences in sICAM expression between women with metastases to the axillary lymph nodes and women with no metastasis [28]. sICAM-1 concentrations increased in serum of breast cancer patients, and their levels seem to be related to poorer therapy response and prognosis [29]. Angiogenesis and neovascularization could be stimulated by sICAM-1 and promote tumor growth and cell migration [30]. Furthermore, sICAM-I may be involved in the progression of metastasis in certain malignancies [31]. Therefore, sICAM may be considered an important target in breast cancer therapy.

In AMJ13, we can notice shifting in growth factors that regulate cell growth, the increasing of FGF-b secretion levels at the late passage (60) and absence in the EGF secretion can give this impression, whereas FGF-b plays an important role in cell proliferation, differentiation and migration [32]. FGF-b is a critical growth factor in normal and malignant cell proliferation and tumor-associated angiogenesis and there is a significant correlation between the presence of FGF-b in cancer cells and advanced tumor stage [33].

We found that TGF-β peaks immediately as highest concentration recorded at all passages tested were as early as six hours after plating. The expression of TGF-β by breast cancer cells may be influenced by other factors such as estrogen receptor status [34]. Buck and Cornelius [35] demonstrate that the estrogen receptor plays an essential role in the expression of TGF-β signaling. TGF-beta expression is upregulated in breast cancer and it correlates with poor prognosis [36]. TGF-β binds Anaplastic lymphoma kinase5 (ALK5) receptor on endothelial cells resulting in vessel maturation and angiogenic resolution by Smad2/3 activation pathway. Increased expression of TGF-β correlates with increased microvessel density and with poor prognosis in various tumor types, such as breast cancer and non-small cell lung carcinoma [37]. We explain the immediate peak for this factor by its regulatory effect on other growth factors. For example, TGF-β regulates the reactive stroma microenvironment associated with most carcinomas, mediates expression of many stromal derived factors important for tumor progression, including FGF-2 [36], and stimulates VEGF-A [20]. Our conclusion is that AMJ13 cell line depends on VEGF-A as main angiogenesis factor to induce micro-vessels supported by low levels of VEGF-D for lymphatic vessels formation. AMJ13 cell line depends on FGF as growth factors as in late passages it was shifted to depend mainly on FGF completely. All of this process may regulated by TGF-β. TIMP-1 has proangiogenic effect and has feedback talk with TIMP-2. Understanding the angiogenesis process for breast cancer can give us better targets for therapy and more effective treatments.

References

[1]   US Department of Agriculture Animal and Plant Health Services. Info Sheet: Bovine Leukosis Virus (BLV) in U.S. Beef Cattle. February 1999.

[2]   Tonini, T., Rossi, F. and Claudio, P.P. (2003) Molecular Basis of Angiogenesis and Cancer. *Oncogene*, **22**, 6549-6556. http://dx.doi.org/10.1038/sj.onc.1206816

[3]   Liekens, S., De Clercq, E. and Neyts, J. (2001) Angiogenesis: Regulators and Clinical Applications. *Biochemical Pharmacology*, **61**, 253-270. http://dx.doi.org/10.1016/S0006-2952(00)00529-3

[4]   Nishida, N., *et al.* (2006) Angiogenesis in Cancer. *Vascular Health and Risk Management*, **2**, 213-219. http://dx.doi.org/10.2147/vhrm.2006.2.3.213

[5]   Schneider, B.P. and Miller, K.D. (2005) Angiogenesis of Breast Cancer. *Journal of Clinical Oncology*, **23**, 1782-1790. http://dx.doi.org/10.1200/JCO.2005.12.017

[6]   Karamysheva, A.F. (2008) Mechanisms of Angiogenesis. *Biochemistry* (*Moscow*), **73**, 751-762. http://dx.doi.org/10.1134/S0006297908070031

[7]   Carmeliet, P. (2000) Mechanisms of Angiogenesis and Arteriogenesis. *Nature Medicine*, **6**, 389-395. http://dx.doi.org/10.1038/74651

[8]   Jain, R.K. (2003) Molecular Regulation of Vessel Maturation. *Nature Medicine*, **9**, 685-693. http://dx.doi.org/10.1038/nm0603-685

[9]   Pugh, C.W. and Ratcliffe, P.J. (2003) Regulation of Angiogenesis by Hypoxia: Role of the HIF System. *Nature Medicine*, **9**, 677-684. http://dx.doi.org/10.1038/nm0603-677

[10] Van Meir, E.G., *et al.* (1994) Release of an Inhibitor of Angiogenesis upon Induction of Wild Type p53 Expression in Glioblastoma Cells. *Nature Genetics*, **8**, 171-176. http://dx.doi.org/10.1038/ng1094-171

[11] Wu, H.-C., Huang, C.-T. and Chang, D.-K. (2008) Anti-Angiogenic Therapeutic Drugs for Treatment of Human Cancer. *Journal of Cancer Molecules*, **4**, 37-45.

[12] Al-Shammari, A.M., Alshami, M., Umran, M., *et al.* (2015) Establishment and Characterization of a Receptor-Negative, Hormone-Nonresponsive Breast Cancer Cell Line from an Iraqi Patient. *Breast Cancer: Targets and Therapy*, **7**, 223-230. http://dx.doi.org/10.2147/BCTT.S74509

[13] Würtz, S.Ø., *et al.* (2005) Tissue Inhibitor of Metalloproteinases-1 in Breast Cancer. *Endocrine-Related Cancer*, **12**, 215-227. http://dx.doi.org/10.1677/erc.1.00719

[14] Ikenaka, Y., Yoshiji, H., Kuriyama, S., *et al.* (2003) Tissue Inhibitor of Metalloproteinases-1 (TIMP-1) Inhibits Tumor Growth and Angiogenesis in the TIMP-1 Transgenic Mouse Model. *International Journal of Cancer*, **105**, 340-346. http://dx.doi.org/10.1002/ijc.11094

[15] Bourboulia, D., Jensen-Taubman, S., Rittler, M.R., *et al.* (2011) Endogenous Angiogenesis Inhibitor Blocks Tumor Growth via Direct and Indirect Effects on Tumor Microenvironment. *The American Journal of Pathology*, **179**, 2589-2600. http://dx.doi.org/10.1016/j.ajpath.2011.07.035

[16] Têtu, B., Brisson, J., Wang, C., *et al.* (2006) The Influence of MMP-14, TIMP-2 and MMP-2 Expression on Breast Cancer Prognosis. *Breast Cancer Research*, **8**, R28. http://dx.doi.org/10.1186/bcr1503

[17] Elias, A.P. and Dias, S. (2008) Microenvironment Changes (in pH) Affect VEGF Alternative Splicing. *Cancer Microenvironment*, **1**, 131-139. http://dx.doi.org/10.1007/s12307-008-0013-4

[18] Marjon, P.L., Bobrovnikova-Marjon, E.V. and Abcouwer, S.F. (2004) Expression of the Pro-Angiogenic Factors Vascular Endothelial Growth Factor and Interleukin-8/CXCL8 by Human Breast Carcinomas Is Responsive to Nutrient Deprivation and Endoplasmic Reticulum Stress. *Molecular Cancer*, **3**, 5670-5674.

[19] Saponaro, C., Malfettone, A., Ranieri, G., *et al.* (2013) VEGF, HIF-1alpha Expression and MVD as an Angiogenic Network in Familial Breast Cancer. *PLoS ONE*, **8**, e53070. http://dx.doi.org/10.1371/journal.pone.0053070

[20] Darrington, E., Zhong, M., Vo, B.-H., *et al.* (2012) Vascular Endothelial Growth Factor A, Secreted in Response to Transforming Growth Factor-β1 under Hypoxic Conditions, Induces Autocrine Effects on Migration of Prostate Cancer Cells. *Asian Journal of Andrology*, **14**, 745-751. http://dx.doi.org/10.1038/aja.2011.197

[21] Matei, D., Kelich, S., Cao, L.Y., *et al.* (2007) PDGF BB Induces VEGF Secretion in Ovarian Cancer. *Cancer Biology & Therapy*, **6**, 1951- 1959. http://dx.doi.org/10.4161/cbt.6.12.4976

[22] Nakamura, Y., Yasuoka, H., Tsujimoto, M., *et al.* (2003) Prognostic Significance of Vascular Endothelial Growth Factor D in Breast Carcinoma with Long-Term Follow-Up. *Clinical Cancer Research*, **9**, 716-721.

[23] Stacker, S.A., Caesar, C., Baldwin, M.E., Thornton, G.E., *et al.* (2001) VEGF-D Promotes the Metastatic Spread of Tumor Cells via the Lymphatics. *Nature Medicine*, **7**, 186-191. http://dx.doi.org/10.1038/84635

[24] Murphy, L.C. and Dotzlaw, H. (1989) Endogenous Growth Factor Expression in T-47D, Human Breast Cancer Cells, Associated with Reduced Sensitivity to Antiproliferative Effects of Progestins and Antiestrogens. *Cancer Research*, **49**, 599-604.

[25] O'sullivan, C., Lewis, C.E., Harris, A.L., *et al.* (1993) Secretion of Epidermal Growth Factor by Macrophages Associated with Breast Carcinoma. *The Lancet*, **342**, 148-149. http://dx.doi.org/10.1016/0140-6736(93)91348-P

[26] Mori, K., Kurobe, M., Furukawa, S., *et al.* (1986) Human Breast Cancer Cells Synthesize and Secrete an EGF-Like Immunoreactive Factor in Culture. *Biochemical and Biophysical Research Communications*, **136**, 300-305. http://dx.doi.org/10.1016/0006-291X(86)90909-5

[27] El-Sayed, L.H.G., Fadali, G., Saad, A., Hafez, E.S. and Shaaban, S. (2010) Expression of MAGE-A Genes and Soluble ICAM-1 in Egyptian Breast Cancer Patients: Possible Prognostic Impact. *Journal of the Medical Research Institute*, **31**, 7-18.

[28] Thielemann, A., Baszczuk, A., Kopczyński, Z., *et al.* (2014) The Clinical Usefulness of Assessing the Concentration of Cell Adhesion Molecules sVCAM-1 and sICAM-1 in the Serum of Women with Primary Breast Cancer. *Współczesna Onkologia*, **4**, 252-259. http://dx.doi.org/10.5114/wo.2014.43492

[29] Eggeman, H., *et al.* (2011) Influence of a Dose-Dense Adjuvant Chemotherapy on sVCAM-1/sICAM-1 Serum Levels in Breast Cancer Patients with 1-3 Positive Lymph Nodes. *Anticancer Research*, **31**, 2617-2622.

[30] Touvier, M., Fezeu, L., Ahluwalia, N., *et al.* (2013) Association between Prediagnostic Biomarkers of Inflammation and Endothelial Function and Cancer Risk: A Nested Case-Control Study. *American Journal of Epidemiology*, **177**, 3-13. http://dx.doi.org/10.1093/aje/kws359

[31] Lai, L., Kadory, S., Cornell, C., *et al.* (1993) Possible Regulation of Soluble Icam-1 Levels by Interleukin-1 in a Sub-Set of Breast Cysts. *International Journal of Cancer*, **55**, 586-589. http://dx.doi.org/10.1002/ijc.2910550412

[32] Cross, M.J. and Claesson-Welsh, L. (2001) FGF and VEGF Function in Angiogenesis: Signalling Pathways, Biological Responses and Therapeutic Inhibition. *Trends in Pharmacological Sciences*, **22**, 201-207. http://dx.doi.org/10.1016/S0165-6147(00)01676-X

[33] Sahni, A., Simpson-Haidaris, P.J., Sahni, S.K., *et al.* (2008) Fibrinogen Synthesized by Cancer Cells Augments the Proliferative Effect of Fibroblast Growth Factor-2 (FGF-2). *Journal of Thrombosis and Haemostasis*, **6**, 176-183. http://dx.doi.org/10.1111/j.1538-7836.2007.02808.x

[34] MacCallum, J., Bartlett, J.M.S., Thompson, A.M., *et al.* (1994) Expression of Transforming Growth Factor Beta mRNA Isoforms in Human Breast Cancer. *British Journal of Cancer*, **69**, 1006-1009. http://dx.doi.org/10.1038/bjc.1994.197

[35] Buck, M.B. and Knabbe, C. (2006) TGF-Beta Signaling in Breast Cancer. *Annals of the New York Academy of Sciences*, **1089**, 119-126. http://dx.doi.org/10.1196/annals.1386.024

[36] Pardali, E. and ten Dijke, P. (2008) Transforming Growth Factor-Beta Signaling and Tumor Angiogenesis. *Frontiers in Bioscience (Landmark Edition)*, **14**, 4848-4861. http://dx.doi.org/10.2741/3573

[37] Lebrun, J.-J. (2012) The Dual Role of TGF in Human Cancer: From Tumor Suppression to Cancer Metastasis. *ISRN Molecular Biology*, **2012**, Article ID: 381428.

13

Expression of Multidrug Resistance ATP-Binding Cassette (ABC) Transporters in Canine Mammary Tumors

Breno S. Salgado[1,2*], Suely Nonogaki[3], Luisa M. Soares[4], Angela Akamatsu[5], Cristiano R. N. da Silva[5], Thiago P. Anacleto[5], Rodolfo Malagó[5], Rafael M. Rocha[3], Fátima Gärtner[2], Noeme S. Rocha[1,4]

[1]Departamento de Patologia, Faculdade de Medicina de Botucatu, Universidade Estadual Paulista, Campus de Botucatu, Botucatu, Brazil
[2]Instituto de Ciências Biomédicas Abel Salazar, Universidade do Porto (Intitute of Biomedical Sciences Abel Salazar of University of Porto), Oporto, Portugal
[3]Fundação Antônio Prudente, Hospital A.C. Camargo, São Paulo, Brazil
[4]Departamento de Clínica Veterinária, Faculdade de Medicina Veterinária e Zootecnia, Universidade Estadual Paulista, UNESP,. Botucatu, Brazil
[5]Hospital Escola de Medicina Veterinária, Fundação de Ensino e Pesquisa de Itajubá—FEPI, Itajubá, Brazil
Email: *brenosalgado@globo.com

Abstract

Mammary neoplasms are the most common tumors in female dogs. They are usually treated using solely surgical mastectomy—which is recognized as unsatisfactory in many cases. Given this, the benefits of chemotherapy in dogs with mammary cancer need to be further explored. Some drugs that can be used for treating canines with mammary tumors may be substrates of uptake and/or efflux transporters such as the ATP-binding cassette (ABC) transporters. Unfortunately, very little is known regarding the pathobiology of such proteins in canine tumors, including mammary cancer. Accordingly, this study was designed to characterize the expression of ABC transporters P-glycoprotein, MRP1, and MRP2 and their relation with clinicopathologic factors in order to allow a better understanding of their influence in canine mammary cancer. P-glycoprotein was expressed in tumors from 55.8% of patients, while MRP1 and MRP2 were expressed in 37.2% and 39.5% of tumors, respectively. P-glycoprotein expression showed to be related with regional lymph node spread (P = 0.0038), as well as with tumor grade (P = 0.0353) and with a shorter survival (P = 0.0245). MRP1 revealed a strong association with a higher histological grade (P < 0.0001) and overall survival (P = 0.0002). Additionally, MRP1 was determined as prognostic indicator independent of lymph node status using Cox proportional-hazards regression multivariate analysis (P

---

*Corresponding author.

= 0.0216). No relations between MRP2 and clinicopathologic features were observed. We have found that P-glycoprotein and MRP1 are expressed in highly aggressive canine mammary tumors and are related with poor prognosis. Our results suggest that they may play a significant role in the course of canine mammary cancer progression and be promising candidate markers for a validation study on therapy outcome.

Keywords

MDR1, P-Gp, MRP1, MRP2, ABCC2, Mammary Neoplasms, Prognosis, Dog

---

1. Introduction

Mammary tumors represent the most common neoplasm in intact female dogs and approximately half are considered as malignant. Canine mammary carcinomas (CMCs) have heterogeneous features that make it difficult to determine patient prognosis [1] [2]. Studies regarding mammary tumors in dogs aimed at defining a more precise prognosis by evaluating different tumor characteristics such as oncogenes/oncoproteins [3] [4] and tumor growth or suppression related features [5] [6]. However, despite the many achievements regarding the understanding of CMCs pathobiology, much remains unknown.

Treatment for canine mammary tumors usually is restricted to surgical mastectomy—which is recognized as unsatisfactory in many cases [2]. However, there are neither studies with large case series that prove the benefits of chemotherapy for canine cancer nor consensus on which drugs must or may be used. Since different individuals with a similar disease may present different responses to the same drugs due to individual aspects, it is important to understand which cellular components of tumor cells can interfere in drug response. In humans, much has been learned about ATP-binding cassette (ABC) transporters, with different cancers presenting with alterations in such cellular components, leading to failure of cancer chemotherapy [7]-[11]. Initially discovered as chemotherapeutic drug-efflux pumps, ATP-binding cassette (ABC) superfamily of transporters represents the largest family of transmembrane proteins [9]. ABC transporters facilitate translocation of heterogeneous substrates including metabolic products, lipids and sterols, peptides and proteins, saccharides, amino acids, inorganic and organic ions, metals, and drugs across the membrane by using energy from ATP hydrolysis [12].

Since the concept of personalized medicine is being progressively applied to veterinary medicine, we can expect that ABC superfamily members may be increasingly evaluated in small animal oncology in a near future in order to promote a more accurate treatment. However, it is not widely understood whether ABC superfamily members have an influence on canine mammary tumors' pathobiology. Additionally, MRP2 expression was not previously evaluated in canine mammary cancer. Accordingly, in this study we aimed to evaluate the immunoexpression of ABC superfamily members in CMCs in order to address their potential prognostic implications in such tumors.

2. Materials and Methods

2.1. Patients

A prospective series of 43 cases of primary canine mammary tumors in adult females presenting from 2011 to 2013 was used. Surgical specimens were fixed in 10% neutral buffered formalin and embedded in paraffin wax. Sections (3 μm thick) were obtained and stained with hematoxylin and eosin (HE) for histological examination.

2.2. Follow-Up

Patients were followed up for a period of 18 months and overall survival was taken as the time (in months) from the date of the primary surgical treatment to the time of death.

2.3. Histopathological Evaluation

Tumors were classified according to the World Health Organization (WHO) criteria for canine mammary neoplasms [1]. Histological grade [13] and lymph node status were also evaluated.

2.4. Immunohistochemistry

For ABC transporter proteins, 3 μm thick histologic sections were obtained, deparaffinized, and rehydrated. Immunohistochemistry was performed by using a polymeric labeling detection system (Novolink Polymer Detection System, Novocastra Laboratories, Newcastle, UK). Antigen retrieval was carried out by heat treatment in 10 mM citrate buffer pH 6.0 for all primary antibodies. Subsequent endogen peroxidase and protein blockages were performed according manufacturers' instructions. All slides were then overnight incubated at 4°C with the specific primary antibodies. Then, the slides were immersed with the detection systems following the manufacturer's instructions. Subsequently, 3, 3' diaminobenzidine tetrahydrochloride (DAB) was used as chromogen in order to allow the visualization of antigen-antibody reaction. Slides were counterstained using Harris's hematoxylin, dehydrated, and mounted for evaluation and light microscopy. Antibodies data are presented at **Table 1**. All series included know positive cases as positive controls. Negative controls included replacement of the primary antibodies with non-reacting antibodies of the same subclass.

Samples were defined as positive when more than 10% of cells revealed immunoreactivity. Slides were evaluated by two independent observers blinded to patient characteristics and outcome. All cases with discrepant results were discussed during observation with a double-headed microscope, and a consensus was reached.

2.5. Statistical Analysis

Associations between the expression of the different ABC superfamily proteins and with clinicopathologic features were assessed by using Fisher's exact text when compared variables had exactly two groups (2 × 2 contingency tables), such as LN status (positive or negative), and by using the X^2 test for categorical variables such as histological grade and tumor histotype. Survival curves were estimated using Kaplan-Meier product-limit method, and the significance of differences between survival curves was determined using the log rank test. Multivariate analysis was performed by Cox proportional hazards regression modeling. All statistical tests were two sided, and statistical significance was accepted at the $P < 0.05$ level. All analyses were performed using the Prism GraphPad software version 5.0 (San Diego, CA).

3. Results

P-glycoprotein (**Figure 1**) and MRP1 (**Figure 2**) expression was mainly membranous but frequently associated with cytoplasmic positivity, whereas MRP2 expression was weak and mainly cytoplasmic. In all cases they were consistently expressed by luminal mammary cells (**Figure 3**). No associations were observed between ABC transporters and tumor histotype. A positive association between P-glycoprotein and lymph node status ($P = 0.0038$) was found, as well as with tumor grade ($P = 0.0353$). MRP1 revealed a strong association with a higher histological grade ($P < 0.0001$). No relations between MPR2 and clinicopathologic features were observed. Results regarding tumor types, histological grade, and lymph node status according to P-glycoprotein, MRP1, and MRP2 expression are summarized in **Table 2**.

Association between ABC Transporters and Survival

Overall patient survival rates were determined using the log rank test with respect to expression of ABC transporters. P-glycoprotein was found to be significantly associated with a poor outcome ($P = 0.0245$) (**Figure 4(a)**), as well as MRP1 ($P = 0.0002$) (**Figure 4(b)**). However, no significant difference in patient outcome was found with respect to MRP2 (**Figure 4(c)**) ($P = 0.2548$). Additionally, MRP1 was determined as prognostic indicator independent of lymph node status using Cox proportional-hazards regression multivariate analysis ($P = 0.0216$).

Table 1. Primary antibodies used for ABC superfamily immunohistochemistry.

Antibody	Source	Manufacturer	Dilution	Clone
P-glycoprotein	Mouse	Dako	1:100	C494
MRP1	Mouse	Enzo LifeScience	1:200	MRPm6
MRP2	Mouse	Enzo LifeScience	1:200	M$_2$III-6

MRP1, multidrug resistance-associated protein 1; MRP2, multidrug resistance-associated protein 2.

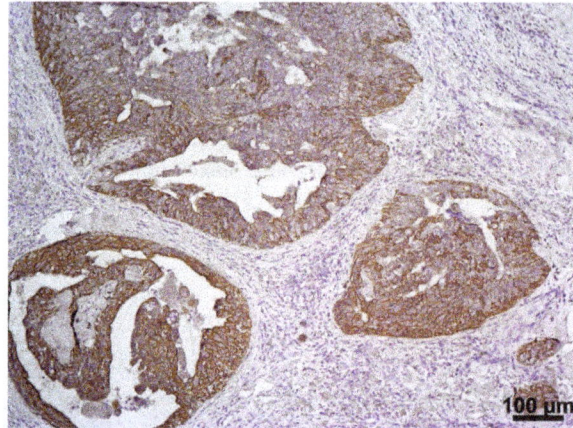

Figure 1. Canine mammary gland carcinoma revealing expression of ABC transporters. (A) Note the P-glycoprotein expression in luminal cells across the membrane and slighter in the cytoplasm (DAB immunohistochemistry, Harris hematoxylin counterstain).

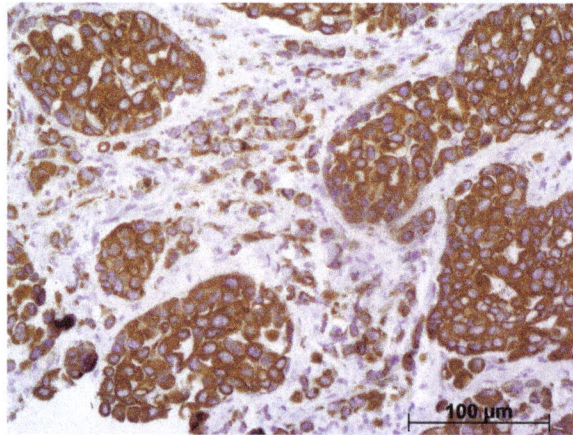

Figure 2. MRP1 strong expression in a mammary tumor with membrane and cytoplasm intense reactivity in canine mammary carcinoma (DAB immunohistochemistry, Harris hematoxylin counterstain).

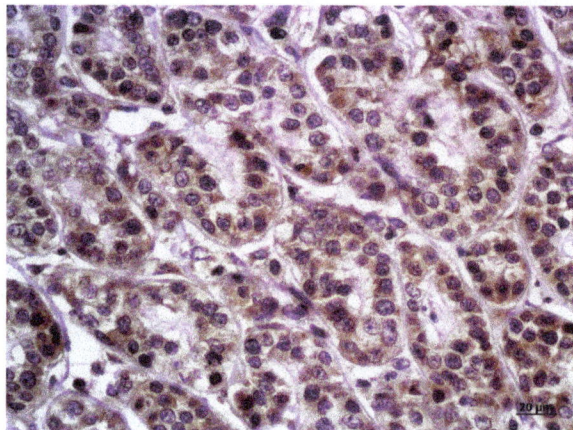

Figure 3. MRP2 expression mainly in the cytoplasm of mammary luminal cells in mammary carcinomas (DAB immunohistochemistry, Harris hematoxylin counterstain).

Table 2. Patients' clinicopathologic characteristics according to ABC transporter protein expression.

Clinical parameters	P-glycoprotein					MRP1					MRP2				
	Negative		Positive		P value	Negative		Positive		P value	Negative		Positive		P value
	N	%	N	%		N	%	N	%		N	%	N	%	
Tumor type															
Tubulo-papillary carcinoma	10	23.3	11	25.6	0.9044	14	32.5	7	16.3	0.112	12	30.3	9	20.9	0.6727
Complex carcinoma	5	11.6	6	13.9		7	16.3	4	9.3		7	16.3	4	9.3	
Carcinoma in mixed tumor	3	7.2	6	13.9		4	9.3	5	11.6		5	11.6	4	9.3	
Others	1	2.3	1	2.3		2	4.7	0	-		2	4.7	0	-	
Histological grade															
I	11	25.6	16	37.2	0.0353	0	-	27	62.8	< 0.0001	12	27.9	15	34.9	0.5721
II	9	20.9	2	4.7		11	25.6	0	-		4	9.3	7	16.3	
III	4	9.3	1	2.3		5	11.6	0	-		1	2.3	4	9.3	
LN status															
+	10	23.3	0	-	0.0038	6	13.9	4	9.3	0.2402	4	9.3	6	13.9	0.1627
-	14	32.5	19	44.2		10	23.3	23	53.5		12	30.3	20	46.5	

N, number; LN, lymph node; MRP1, multidrug resistance-associated protein 1; MRP2, multidrug resistance-associated protein 2.

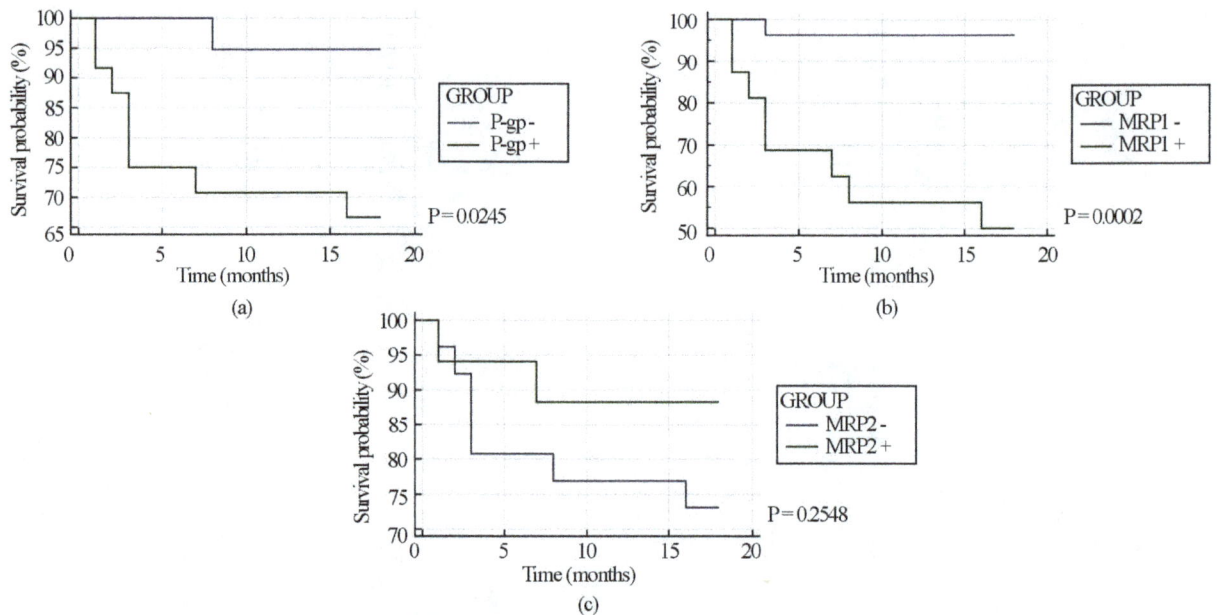

Figure 4. Survival curves and expression of ABC transporters (a) P-glycoprotein, (b) MRP1, and (c) MRP2.

4. Discussion

Several ABC transporters are implicated in multidrug resistance and are recognized causes for failure of cancer chemotherapy [7]-[11]. This is the case of ATP-dependent drug efflux transporter P-glycoprotein (P-gp or ABCB1) whose expression on tumor cells has been identified to be a well-recognized mechanism of cancer multidrug resistance by decreasing intracellular drug accumulation [9].

In the cases herein studied, ABC transporters expression was confined to mammary luminal cells. Other authors [14] revealed immunoexpression of P-glycoprotein in myoepithelial cells, differently from what was observed in this study. This feature probably occurred due to the use of the C219 clone by such authors—an antibody clone which is known to display cross-reactivity with a number of other proteins [15]. In order to avoid such cross-reaction, we used a more specific clone in order to produce more accurate results.

This study addressed the potential prognostic role of ABC transporters P-glycoprotein, MRP1, and MRP2 in a series of 43 canine mammary tumors. Given the function of drug transporters and their capability to extrude toxins, drugs, and physiological substrates from cells [16], a clear definition of their prognostic role is not straightforward to achieve. A possible role of ABC transporters protein expression in canine mammary cancer has previously been studied [6] [14] [17], but the results are not conclusive. In humans, data are also controversial. Some authors reported a loss of MRP1 expression in poorly differentiated histology cases, suggesting that MRP1 loss is associated with loss of differentiation [18] [19]. In contrast, an association of MRP1 and MDR1/P-gp increase with tumor stage had also been suggested [20]-[22], similarly to what was observed in this study and consequently suggesting that MRP1 and P-glycoprotein expression had an implication in disease outcome.

MRP1 and MDR1 have been shown to confer multidrug resistance *in vitro* in human cancer cell lines [23]-[25] and also in canine mammary cell lines [26]. Additionally, they were shown to be associated with poor patient outcomes and/or chemoresistance in different canine tumor types [27] [28] including mammary tumors [6]. In the present study, we had analyzed the protein levels of MDR1/P-gp, MRP1, and MRP2 and found that P-gp and MRP1 levels were higher in tumors with higher histological grade and regional lymph node metastasis, as well as an association with shorter survival, in line with results which characterized P-gp as a prognostic indicator in canine mammary tumors [6].

A number of studies have been carried out on the changes in MRP2 expression in human tumors including colorectal carcinoma [29], lung [30], and breast [31] cancers, which may be associated with their resistance to chemotherapeutic agents. Since MRP2 is involved in the efflux of various anti-neoplastic agents, these findings can indicate that neoplastic cells can acquire drug resistance through the increased MRP2 activity. Since there are no data regarding the expression of MRP2 in canine mammary tumors, it is not possible to directly relate such ABC transporter with drug resistance in the species. When it comes to prognosis, we find no relation of MRP2 with clinicopathologic features. This is in line with studies which evaluate MRP2 expression in human cancers [32] [33].

Overall, our results suggest that P-glycoprotein and MDR1 not only be promising candidate markers for a validation study on therapy outcome but also they may play a significant role in the course of canine mammary cancer progression.

Acknowledgements

B.S.S. thanks the Coordination for the Improvement of Higher Education Personnel (CAPES), Brazil, for financial support and Cleuso Cesário for his help with technical issues.

References

[1] Misdorp, W. (2001) Tumors of the Mammary Gland. In: Meuten, D.J., Ed., *Tumors in Domestic Animals*, Blackweel Publishing Company, Ames, 75-606.

[2] Lana, S.E., Rutteman, G.R. and Withrow, S.J. (2007) Tumors of the Mammary Gland. In: Withrow, S.J. and Vail, D.M., Eds., *Withrow and MacEwen's Small Animal Clinical Oncology*, 4th Edition, Saunders Elsevier, St. Louis, 619-638. http://dx.doi.org/10.1016/b978-072160558-6.50029-0

[3] Gama, A., Gärtner, F., Alves, A. and Schmitt, F. (2009) Immunohistochemical Expression of Epidermal Growth Factor Receptor (EGFR) in Canine Mammary Tissues. *Research in Veterinary Science*, **87**, 432-437. http://dx.doi.org/10.1016/j.rvsc.2009.04.016

[4] Terragni, R., Gardini, A.C., Sabattini, S., Bettini, G., Amadori, D., Talamonti, C., Vignoli, M., Capelli, L., Saunders, J.H., Ricci, M. and Ulivi, P. (2014) EGFR, HER-2 and KRAS in Canine Gastric Epithelial Tumors: A Potential Human Model? *PLoS ONE*, **9**, 1-7. http://dx.doi.org/10.1371/journal.pone.0085388

[5] Lee, C.-H., Kim, W.-H., Lim, J.-H., Kang, M.-S., Kim, D.-Y. and Kweon, O.-K. (2004) Mutation and Overexpression of p53 as a Prognostic Factor in Canine Mammary Tumors. *Journal of Veterinary Science*, **5**, 63-69. http://dx.doi.org/10.1292/jvms.66.63

[6] Koltai, Z. and Valjdovich, P. (2014) Expression of Multidrug Resistance Membrane Transporter (Pgp) and p53 Protein in Canine Mammary Tumours. *Acta Veterinaria Hungarica*, **2**, 194-204. http://dx.doi.org/10.1556/AVet.2014.002

[7] Trock, B.J., Leonessa, F. and Clarke, R. (1997) Multidrug Resistance in Breast Cancer: A Meta-Analysis of MDR1/gp170 Expression and Its Possible Functional Significance. *The Journal of the National Cancer Institute*, **89**, 917-931. http://dx.doi.org/10.1093/jnci/89.13.917

[8] Abolhoda, A., Wilson, A.E., Ross, H., Danenberg, P.V., Burt, M. and Scotto, K.W. (1999) Rapid Activation of MDR1 Gene Expression in Human Metastatic Sarcoma after *in Vivo* Exposure to Doxorubicin. *Clinical Cancer Research*, **5**, 3352-3356.

[9] Wenzel, J.J., Piehler, A. and Kaminski, W.E. (2007) ABC A-Subclass Proteins: Gatekeepers of Cellular Phospho- and Sphin-Golipid Transport. *Frontiers in Bioscience*, **12**, 3177-3193. http://dx.doi.org/10.2741/2305

[10] Amiri-Kordestani, L., Basseville, A., Kurdziel, K., Fojo, A.T. and Bates, S.E. (2012) Targeting MDR in Breast and Lung Cancer: Discriminating Its Potential Importance from the Failure of Drug Resistance Reversal Studies. *Drug Resistance Updates*, **15**, 50-61. http://dx.doi.org/10.1016/j.drup.2012.02.002

[11] Hedditch, E.L., Gao, B., Russel, A.J., Lu, Y., Emmanuel, C., Beesley, J., Johnatty, S.E., Chen, X., Harnett, P., George, J., Williams, R.T., Flemming, C., Lambrechts, D., Despierre, E., Lambrechts, S., Vergote, I., Karlan, B., Lester, J., Orsulic, S., Walsh, C., Fasching, P., Beckmann, M.W., Ekici, A.B., Hein, A., Matsuo, K., Hosono, S., Nakanishi, T., Yatabe, Y., Pejovic, T., Bean, Y., Heitz, F., Harter, P., Du Bois, A., Schwaab, I., Hogdall, E., Kjaer, S.K., Jensen, A., Hogdall, C., Lundvall, L., Engelholm, S.A., Brown, B., Flanagan, J., Metcalf, M.D., Siddiqui, N., Sellers, T., Fridley, B., Cunningham, J., Schidkraut, J., Iversen, E., Weber, R.P., Berchuck, A., Goode, E., Bowtee, D.D., Chenevix-Trench, G., Defazio, A., Norris, M.D., Macgregor, S., Haber, M. and Henderson, M.J. (2014) *ABCA* Transporter Gene Expression and Poor Outcome in Epithelial Ovarian Cancer. *The Journal of the National Cancer Institute*, **7**, 1-11. http://dx.doi.org/10.1093/jnci/dju149

[12] Higgins, C.F. (1992) ABC Transporters: From Microorganisms to Man. *Annual Review of Cell Biology*, **8**, 67-113. http://dx.doi.org/10.1146/annurev.cb.08.110192.000435

[13] Elston, C.W. and Ellis, I.O. (1991) Pathological Prognostic Factors in Breast Cancer. I. The Value of Histological Grade in Breast Cancer: Experience from a Large Study with Long-Term Follow-Up. *Histopathology*, **19**, 403-410. http://dx.doi.org/10.1111/j.1365-2559.1991.tb00229.x

[14] Kim, N.-H., Hwang, Y.-H., Im, K.-S., Kim, J.-H., Chon, S.-K., Kim, H.-Y. and Sur, J.-H. (2012) P-Glycoprotein Expression in Canine Mammary Gland Tumours Related with Myoepithelial Cells. *Research in Veterinary Science*, **93**, 1346-1352. http://dx.doi.org/10.1016/j.rvsc.2012.04.004

[15] van den Elsen, J.M.H., Kuntz, D.A., Hoedemaeker, F.J. and Rose, D.R. (1999) Antibody C219 Recognizes an Alpha-Helical Epitope on P-Glycoprotein. *Proceeding of the National Academy of Sciences of the United States of America*, **96**, 13679-13684. http://dx.doi.org/10.1073/pnas.96.24.13679

[16] Fletcher, J.I., Haber, M., Henderson, M.J. and Norris, M.D. (2010) ABC Transporters in Cancer: More than Just Drug Efflux Pumps. *Nature Reviews Cancer*, **10**, 147-156. http://dx.doi.org/10.1038/nrc2789

[17] Petterino, C., Rossetti, E., Bertoncello, D., Martini, M., Zappulli, V., Bargelloni, L. and Castagnaro, M. (2006) Immunohistochemical Detection of P-Glycoprotein (Clone C494) in Canine Mammary Gland Tumours. *Journal of Veterinary Medicine Series A*, **53**, 174-178. http://dx.doi.org/10.1111/j.1439-0442.2006.00810.x

[18] Beck, J., Bohnet, B., Brugger, D., Bader, P., Dietl, J., Scheper, R.J., Kandolf, R., Liu, C., Niethammer, D. and Gekeler, V. (1998) Multiple Gene Expression Analysis Reveals Distinct Differences between G2 and G3 Stage Breast Cancers and Correlations of PKC Eta with MDR1, MRP and LRP Gene Expression. *British Journal of Cancer*, **77**, 87-91. http://dx.doi.org/10.1038/bjc.1998.13

[19] Ferrero, J.M., Etienne, M.C., Formento, J.L., Francoual, M., Rostagno, P., Peyrottes, I., Ettore, F., Teissier, E., Leblanc-Talent, P., Namer, M. and Milano, G. (2000) Application of an Original RT PCR-ELISA Multiplex Assay for MDR1 and MRP, along with p53 Determination in Node-Positive Breast Cancer Patients. *British Journal of Cancer*, **82**, 171-177.

[20] Filipitis, M., Suchomel, R.W., Dekan, G., Haider, K., Valdimarsson, G., Depisch, D. and Pirker, R. (1996) MRP and MDR1 Gene Expression in Primary Breast Carcinomas. *Clinical Cancer Research*, **2**, 1231-1237. http://dx.doi.org/10.1016/0959-8049(96)84850-7

[21] Nooter, K., Brutel de la Riviere, G., Look, M.P., van Wingerden, K.E., Henzen-Logmans, S.C., Scheper, R.J., Flens, M.J., Klijn, J.G., Stoter, G. and Foekens, J.A. (1997) The Prognostic Significance of Expression of the Multidrug Resistance-Associated Protein (MRP) in Primary Breast Cancer. *British Journal of Cancer*, **76**, 486-493. http://dx.doi.org/10.1038/bjc.1997.414

[22] Sun, S.-S., Hsieh, J.-F., Tsai, S.-C., Ho, Y.-J., Lee, J.-K. and Kao, C.-H. (2000) Expression of Mediated P-Glycoprotein Multidrug Resistance Related to Tc-99m MIBI Scintimammography Results. *Cancer Letters*, **153**, 95-100. http://dx.doi.org/10.1016/S0304-3835(00)00356-6

[23] Goto, H., Keshelava, N., Matthay, K.K., Lukens, J.N., Gerbing, R.B., Stram, D.O., Seeger, R.C. and Reynolds, C.P. (2000) Multidrug Resistance-Associated Protein 1 (MRP1) Expression in Neuroblastoma Cell Lines and Primary Tumors. *Medical and Pediatric Oncology*, **35**, 619-622. http://dx.doi.org/10.1002/1096-911X(20001201)35:6<619::AID-MPO28>3.0.CO;2-H

[24] Ferreira, M.J.U., Gyemant, N., Madureira, A.M., Tanaka, M., Koos, K., Didziapetris, R. and Molnar, J. (2005) The Effects of Jatrophane Derivatives on the Reversion of MDR1- and MRP-Mediated Multidrug Resistance in the MDA-MB-231 (HTB-26) Cell Line. *Anticancer Research*, **25**, 4173-4178.

[25] Nakai, E., Park, K., Yawata, T., Chihara, T., Kumazawa, A., Nakabayashi, H. and Shimizu, K. (2009) Enhanced MDR1 Expression and Chemoresistance of Cancer Stem Cells Derived from Glioblastoma. *Cancer Investigation*, **27**, 901-908. http://dx.doi.org/10.3109/07357900801946679

[26] Pawlowski, K.M., Mucha, J., Majchrzak, K., Motyl, T. and Król, M. (2013) Expression and Role of PGP, BCRP, MRP1 and MRP3 in Multidrug Resistance of Canine Mammary Cancer Cells. *BMC Veterinary Research*, **9**, 119. http://dx.doi.org/10.1186/1746-6148-9-119

[27] Gaspar, L.F.J., Ferreira, I., Colodel, M., Brandão, C.V.S. and Rocha, N.S. (2010) Spontaneous Canine Transmissible venereal Tumor: Cell Morphology and Influence on P-Glycoprotein Expression. *Turkish Journal of Veterinary Animal Science*, **34**, 447-454.

[28] Teng, S.-H., Hsu, W.-L., Chiu, C.-Y., Wong, M.-L. and Chang, S.-C. (2012) Overexpression of P-Glycoprotein, STAT3, Phospho-STAT3 and KIT in Spontaneous Canine Cutaneous Mast Cell Tumours before and after Prednisolone Treatment. *The Veterinary Journal*, **193**, 551-556. http://dx.doi.org/10.1016/j.tvjl.2012.01.033

[29] Hinoshita, E., Uchiumi, T., Taguchi, K., Kinukawa, N., Tsuneyoshi, M., Maehara, Y., Sugimachi, K. and Kuwano, M. (2000) Increased Expression of an ATP-Binding Cassette Superfamily Transporter, Multidrug Resistance Protein 2, in Human Colorectal Carcinomas. *Clinical Cancer Research*, **6**, 2401-2407.

[30] Young, L.C., Campling B.G., Cole, S.P., Deeley, R.G. and Gerlach, J.H. (2001) Multidrug Resistance Proteins MRP3, MRP1, and MRP2 in Lung Cancer: Correlation of Protein Levels with Drug Response and Messenger RNA Levels. *Clinical Cancer Research*, **7**, 1798-1804

[31] Choi, H.-K., Yang, J.-W., Roh, S.-H., Han, C.-Y. and Kang, K.-W. (2007) Induction of Multidrug Resistance Asso-

ciated Protein 2 in Tamoxifen-Resistant Breast Cancer Cells. *Endocrine-Related Cancer*, **14**, 293-303.
http://dx.doi.org/10.1677/ERC-06-0016

[32] Ota, S., Ishii, G., Goto, K., Kubota, K., Kim, Y.-H., Kojika, M., Murata, Y., Yamazi, M., Nishiwaki, Y., Eguchi, K. and Ochiai, A. (2009) Immunohistochemical Expression of BCRP and ERCC1 in Biopsy Specimen Predicts Survival in Advanced Non-Small-Cell Lung Cancer Treated with Cisplatin-Based Chemotherapy. *Lung Cancer*, **64**, 98-104.
http://dx.doi.org/10.1016/j.lungcan.2008.07.014

[33] Tian, C., Ambrosone, C.B., Darcy, K.M., Krivak, T.C., Armstrong, D.K., Bookman, M.A., Davis, W., Zhao, H., Moysich, K., Gallion, H. and DeLoia, J.A. (2012) Common Variants in ABCB1, ABCC2 and ABCG2 Genes and Clinical Outcomes among Women with Advanced Stage Ovarian Cancer Treated with Platinum and Taxane-Based Chemotherapy: A Gynecologic Oncology Group Study. *Gynecologic Oncology*, **124**, 575-581.
http://dx.doi.org/10.1016/j.ygyno.2011.11.022

14

Prognostic Value of CD74 and HLA-DR Expressions in Invasive Ductal Breast Cancer

Muhittin Yaprak[1], Gülgün Erdogan[2], Gulbin Aricic[3], Barış Ozcan[4], Ayhan Mesci[1], Ayhan Dınckan[1], Okan Erdogan[1], Cumhur Arici[1*]

[1]Department of General Surgery, Akdeniz University School of Medicine, Antalya, Turkey
[2]Department of Pathology, Akdeniz University School of Medicine, Antalya, Turkey
[3]Department of Anesthesiology, Akdeniz University School of Medicine, Antalya, Turkey
[4]Department of General Surgery, Medstar Antalya Hospital, Antalya, Turkey
Email: muhittin.yaprak@gmail.com, gerdogan@akdeniz.edu.tr, gulbinarici@yahoo.com, barisozcan2004@yahoo.com, drayhanmesci@yahoo.com, adinckan@akdeniz.edu.tr, oerdogan@akdeniz.edu.tr, *cumarici@yahoo.com

Abstract

Introduction: Despite the presence of many prognostic and predictive factors, overtreatment remains a major problem in patients with breast cancer. The aim of this study is to investigate the effects of CD74 and HLA-DR expressions on the prognosis of patients who have had a mastectomy for the treatment of breast cancer. Materials and Methods: A retrospective search of medical records was carried out for patients who had surgery for breast cancer at the Department of General Surgery, Akdeniz University School of Medicine, between March 1984 and November 1999. Patients with regular follow-up and necessary data for the study (*i.e.* patients' demographics, pathology results, and treatment characteristics) were included in the study. Paraffin blocks of tumor specimens were re-examined with immunohistochemical methods in March 2010 to determine the extent of CD74 and HLA-DR expression and the level of tumor infiltrating lymphocyte (TILs). Results: The mean age and the median duration of follow-up for the 41 participants were 48.29 ± 11.86 years and 125 months (range 115 to 135 months), respectively. Disease-free survival (DFS) in CD74 negative subjects was better than in CD74 positive patients, but the difference was not statistically significant (p = 0.75). Similarly, HLA-DR negative and HLA-DR positive groups showed no statistically significant differences in terms of DFS (p = 0.81). Conclusion: There were positive but insignificant correlations with increased expression of CD74, decreased expression of HLA-DR, and TILs levels. Further studies involving larger sample sizes may provide more insight into these associations.

*Corresponding author.

Keywords

Breast Cancer, Prognosis, CD74 Antigen, HLA-DR Antigens

1. Introduction

Breast cancer is the most common type of cancer and a leading cause of cancer mortality among women, both in developed and developing countries, including Turkey [1]. A multitude of prognostic and predictive factors have been identified in patients with breast cancer in order to assist in prognostic predictions and to guide management strategies [2] [3]. However, despite significant advances in our understanding of tumor biology and genetics, most of the patients continue to be overtreated [4] [5], necessitating novel prognostic and predictive parameters to be defined to further refine our treatment strategies to reduce unnecessary treatments and the associated morbidity.

Tumor-host interactions are known to play an important role in the growth of neoplasms. In this context, the suggested correlation between tumor infiltrating lymphocyte (TIL) grade and prognosis in many tumor types represents a good example for such interactions [6] [7].

A transmembrane glycoprotein with a variety of immunologic functions, CD74 [8], is associated with human leukocyte antigen-DR (HLA-DR) [major histocompatibility complex (MHC) class II] and represents an important chaperone that regulates antigen presentation for the immune response [9]. It also plays a role in assembly, transport, and loading of peptides onto antigen-presenting cells, and is highly expressed by antigen-presenting cells (APCs), including B cells, monocytes, macrophages and dendritic cells in normal tissues [10]. CD74 expression has also been reported in some malignant tumors [6] [8]-[10]. HLA-DR molecules and CD74 interact in the endoplasmic reticulum. Because of this interaction, binding of HLA-DR molecules to endogenous peptides is prevented and the host immune response to tumor cells is suppressed [8]. Therefore, tumor tissues expressing high levels of CD74 may exhibit a worse prognosis as they are able to escape from the host's defenses [6].

Recent research has focused on the assessment of the prognostic and predictive value of CD74 and HLA-DR expression in various types of cancers including colorectal, gastric, pancreatic and breast cancer [6] [8] [9] [11]. For instance, Jiang *et al.* have found an inverse association between the frequency of TILs and CD74 expression, suggesting less immunogenicity and less stimulation of host immune system with increased expression of CD74 [6]. Naga *et al.* established the independent prognostic value of CD74 expression in pancreatic ductal adenocarcinoma [8]. In another study assessing the association between CD74 expression and gastric cancer prognosis along with the clinical and pathological characteristics of CD74-positive gastric cancers, Ishigami *et al.* proposed a useful prognostic role for CD74 expression as an HLA class II-associated prognostic indicator in gastric cancer [9].

In this study, the effects of CD74 and HLA-DR expressions on the prognosis of patients undergoing mastectomy for invasive ductal breast cancer was investigated.

2. Materials and Methods

A retrospective search of medical records was carried out for patients who had surgery for breast cancer at the Department of General Surgery, Akdeniz University School of Medicine (a tertiary care facility in Antalya, Turkey), between March 1984 and November 1999. A total of 41 patients who have completed the 10-year follow-up period with regular attendance to postoperative follow-up visits and adequate data in medical records on the following parameters were included in the study: demographic; pathologic and treatment characteristics including age; duration of follow-up; menopausal status; tumor localization; operation technique; tumor size; lymph node metastasis; nuclear grade; histological grade; hormone receptor status; chemotherapy; radiotherapy; hormonal therapy; presence of local-regional recurrence (LRR); and systemic recurrence (SR). Patients were categorized into two groups as follows: poor prognosis group with LRR and/or SR; and favorable prognosis group with no recurrence.

Patients' paraffin-embedded blocks of tumor tissue were retrieved from the Department of Pathology, Akdeniz University Hospital, and were re-examined using immunohistochemical methods in March 2010. Tissue cross-sections of 4 - 5 mM (micrometer) thickness prepared from paraffin blocks were immunohistochemically treated with Anti-CD74 (clone 1N2, 1/100, Lab vision, Neomarker) and anti-HLA-DR (Clone CR3/43, Dako, 1/50) antibodies using the streptoavidin-biotin complex method. CD74 and HLA-DR expression as well as lymphocyte infiltration were assessed in cancer tissues (**Figure 1(A)** and **Figure 1(B)**).

3. Evaluation of Immunohistochemical Staining

A semi-quantitative assessment was performed using light microscopy. Presence of cytoplasmic staining was considered positive for CD74 and HLA-DR. The level of HLA-DR and CD74 expression and grade of lymphocyte infiltration were evaluated according to Jiang's classification [6]. Accordingly, presence of $\geq 10\%$ positive tumor cell staining was considered positive for CD74 or HLA-DR and presence of $<10\%$ positive tumor cell staining was considered negative for CD74 or HLA-DR. Similarly, patients with numerous large lymphoid aggregates with frequent germinal centers were defined as TILs positive, while those with no or occasional lymphoid aggregates with rare or absent germinal centers comprised the TILs negative group [6] [9]. Then, the association between the results of these assessments and prognostic data obtained from medical records was examined.

SPSS (Statistical Package for Social Sciences) for Windows version 13.0 (SPSS inc. Chicago, IL) program was used for statistical analyses. Chi-square test and Mann-Whitney test were used to analyze the correlation between CD74 and HLA-DR expression and clinical/pathological parameters. The cumulative survival was calculated by Kaplan-Meier method and analyzed by the Log rank test. A P level of less than 0.05 was considered statistically significant.

The study protocol was approved by the Local Ethics Committee, Akdeniz University.

4. Results

The mean age and median follow-up for 41 patients were 48.29 ± 11.86 years and 125 months (range 115 to 135 months), respectively. Only 24% of the patients had Stage I breast cancer. Adjuvant systemic and radiation therapy was administered to 83% and 63% of the subjects, respectively. Hormonal therapy was given to 33 (80%) hormone receptor positive patients. Systemic recurrence (SR) and loco-regional recurrence (LRR) were detected in 18 (43.9%) and 3 (7%) patients during the follow-up period.

Immunohistochemical staining showed a CD74, HLA-DR and TILs positivity rate of 53.7%, 43%, and 41.5%, respectively.

The differences in HLA-DR expression (p = 0.67) and TILs infiltration (p = 0.06) between the CD74 positive and negative groups were not statistically significant. Similarly, there were no significant differences between the HLA-DR positive and negative subjects in terms of lymphocyte infiltration (p = 0.73).

Although the disease-free survival (DFS) was better in CD74 negative subjects than in CD74 positive subjects, the difference was not statistically significant (p = 0.75, **Figure 2(A)**). Similarly, HLA-DR negative and HLA-DR positive patients did not differ significantly in terms of DFS (p = 0.81, **Figure 2(B)**). Also, although DFS

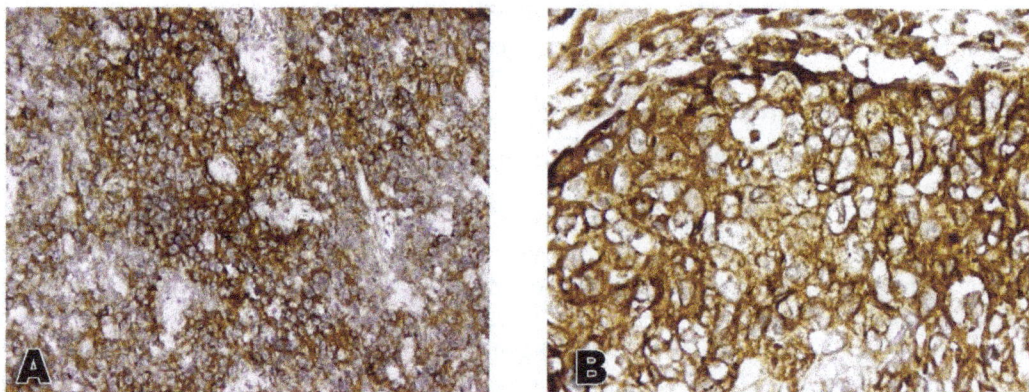

Figure 1. Microscopic sections showing immunohistochemical staining of HLA-DR in invasive ductal carcinoma, DAB ×200 (A); and immunohistochemical staining of CD74 in invasive ductal carcinoma, DAB ×400 (B). Both HLA-DR (A) and CD74 (B) immunoreactivity was identified on the surface and cytoplasm of the tumor cells. Some populations of tumor infiltrating lymphocytes were also immunopositive for those markers.

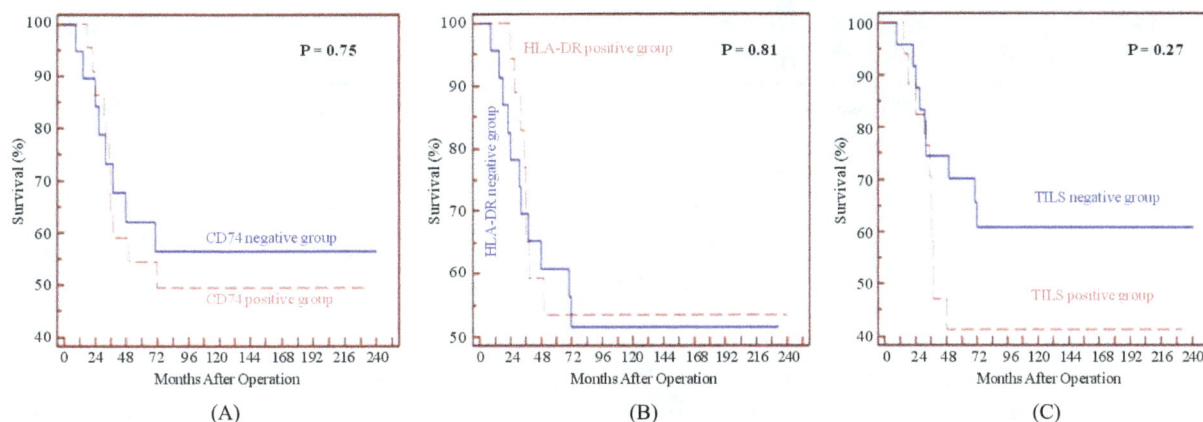

Figure 2. Comparison of CD74 expression rates and disease-free survival (A); HLA-DR expression rates and disease-free survival (B); and TILs infiltration and disease-free survival (C).

was better in TILs negative patients, the difference did not reach statistical significance when compared with TILs positive patients (p = 0.27, **Figure 2(C)**).

Lymph node metastasis was more frequent in HLA-DR negative patients (69.6%) than in positives (55.6%), the difference being insignificant (p = 0.4). However, with respect to the TNM classification, a statistically significant difference was found between the two groups whereby the majority of N3 involvement was in the HLA-DR negative group, while the majority of N2 involvement was in the HLA-DR positive group (p = 0.044).

Differences between the CD74 negative and positive patients with respect to tumor stage (p = 0.9), axillary lymph node metastasis (p = 0.2), nuclear grade (p = 0.3), histological grade (p = 0.4) and presence of distant metastasis (p = 0.8) were insignificant. Also there were no significant differences between HLA-DR negative and positive groups in terms of tumor stage (p = 0.5), nuclear grade (p = 0.2), histological grade (p = 0.5) and presence of distant metastasis (p = 0.6) (**Table 1**).

5. Discussion

As in many other malignant conditions, prognostic and predictive factors play an important role in determining the optimal management strategy for breast cancer. A prognostic factor may be defined as a measurable variable that correlates with the natural history of disease progression, in the absence of systemic therapies. In contrast, a predictive factor is any measurement associated with response to a specific therapy. Some factors, such as hormone receptors and human epidermal growth factor receptor 2 (HER2/neu) overexpression, are both prognostic and predictive [2] [3]. The major prognostic factor for patients with breast cancer is the presence or absence of axillary lymph node involvement [2]. Tumor size, histological grade, and hormone receptor status are other important prognostic factors related to breast cancer [3]. Estrogen and progesterone receptor content in a breast tumor is a well-established predictive factor for response to endocrine treatment [2] [3]. Patient age, lymphatic/vascular invasion, histological subtype, response to neoadjuvant therapy, and HER2/neu overexpression are other recognized prognostic and predictive factors for breast cancer [2] [3]. In addition to those already established indicators, certain other potential prognostic/predictive factors are also being researched including gene expression profile, urokinase plasminogen activator, bone marrow micrometastasis, p53 gene, cathepsin D, microvessel density, and DNA ploidy analysis [3]. Despite the prognostic and predictive value of the currently utilized parameters, their usefulness in determining the best candidates for adjuvant systemic therapy for breast cancer is still limited.

CD74 is a non-polymorphic glycoprotein involved in various immunological functions such as antigen presentation, inflammation, and the behavior of cancer tissues. Among these, the best known is the regulation of the trafficking of HLA-DR proteins in antigen presenting cells. CD74 expression in tumor cells has been suggested to prevent presentation of tumor antigens by HLA-DR molecules [9]. Consequently, poor antigen presentation to intratumoral T-cells may undermine the host immune defense against tumor cells.

CD74 and HLA-DR expressions have been previously found to influence the prognosis of various types of cancers [6] [8] [9] [11]. In the study by Ishigami *et al.*, the association between CD74 expression and prognosis

Table 1. Comparison of the CD74 negative and positive, and HLA-DR negative and positive groups in terms of tumor stage, axillary lymph node metastasis, nuclear grade, histological grade, and presence of distant metastasis.

	CD74 negative Group	CD74 positive Group	p	HLA-DR negative Group	HLA-DR positive Group	p
Tumor stage			0.9			0.5
T1	4 (21%)	6 (27%)		5 (22%)	5 (28%)	
T2	12 (63%)	13 (59%)		13 (56%)	12 (67%)	
T3	2 (11%)	2 (9%)		3 (13%)	1 (5%)	
T4	1 (5%)	1 (5%)		2 (9%)	0	
Axillary lymph						
Node metastasis			0.2			0.4
Positive	10 (53%)	16 (73%)		16 (70%)	10 (56%)	
Negative	9 (47%)	6 (27%)		7 (30%)	8 (44%)	
Nuclear grade			0.3			0.2
Grade 1	5 (26%)	6 (27%)		8 (35%)	3 (17%)	
Grade 2	11 (58%)	16 (73%)		12 (52%)	15 (83%)	
Grade 3	3 (16%)	0		3 (13%)	0	
Histological grade			0.4			0.5
Grade 1	2 (11%)	0		0	1 (6%)	
Grade 2	12 (63%)	17 (77%)		16 (70%)	13 (72%)	
Grade 3	5 (26%)	5 (23%)		7 (30%)	4 (22%)	
Distant metastasis			0.8			0.6
Positive	8 (42%)	10 (45%)		10 (43%)	8 (44%)	
Negative	11 (58%)	12 (55%)		13 (57%)	10 (56%)	

[9] was examined in 126 patients with gastric cancer. Of these patients, 48 were CD74 positive and there was a negative correlation between CD74 expression and the depth of tumor invasion as well as the patient's clinical stage. In addition, CD74 expression negatively correlated with HLA-DR expression. Patients with no CD74 expression had significantly better surgical outcomes than CD74-positive subjects ($p < 0.05$). In the present study, CD74 expression also negatively correlated with HLA-DR expression, but the difference was not significant ($p = 0.67$).

In the study by Nagata *et al.*, CD74 expression emerged as an independent prognostic indicator for pancreatic ductal adenocarcinoma [8]. In their study, 47 (69.1%) and 21 (30.9%) patients showed level I and level II CD74 expression, respectively. Patients with level II CD74 expression showed a higher rate of lymphatic permeation ($p = 0.04$) and perineural invasion ($p = 0.01$) compared with those having level I expression. In addition, patients with level I CD74 expression had a significantly better survival rate than those with level II ($p = 0.003$). Similarly, in our study, survival rate was better in CD74 negative subjects, although the difference was not statistically significant ($p = 0.75$). In Jiang *et al.*'s study, CD74 expression appeared to increase the risk of progression from low- to high-grade colon neoplasms and this effect was most marked in the poorly differentiated carcinomas [6]. These investigators also showed a negative association between CD74 expression and frequency of TILs. A similar observation was made in our study, although this association was not statistically significant ($p = 0.06$).

6. Conclusion

In our study, majority of TNM N3 or N2 lymph node involvement occurred in HLA-DR negative and positive patients, respectively and this difference was significant (p = 0.044). This observation is supportive of the view that low levels of HLA-DR expression may be associated with insufficient host immune response in tumors with low HLA-DR expression. DFS in CD74 negative and HLA-DR positive patients was better when compared with CD74 positive and HLA-DR negative subjects. Lymph node metastasis was more common in CD74 positive and HLA-DR negative groups in comparison with CD74 negative HLA-DR positive subjects. Also, TILs negative patients experienced more frequent metastases than TILs positive patients. This piece of information can generally be regarded as supportive of our view on the effect of these factors on prognosis. However, statistical significance could not be reached, probably due to the inadequate sample size. Further studies with larger sample sizes providing higher statistical power may help elucidate the role of these factors in preventing overtreatment in patients with breast cancer.

Conflict of Interest

There is no conflict of interest.

References

[1]   Ozmen, V. (2008) Breast Cancer in the World and Turkey. *Journal of Breast Health*, **4**, 6-12.

[2]   Aebi, S., Davidson, T., Gruber, G. and Cardoso, F. (2011) Primary Breast Cancer: ESMO Clinical Practice Guidelines for Diagnosis, Treatment and Follow-Up. *Annals of Oncology*, **22**, vi12-vi24. http://dx.doi.org/10.1093/annonc/mdr371

[3]   Subramaniam, D.S. and Isaacs, C. (2005) Utilizing Prognostic and Predictive Factors in Breast Cancer. *Current Treatment Options in Oncology*, **6**, 147-159. http://dx.doi.org/10.1007/s11864-005-0022-1

[4]   Weigel, M.T. and Dowsett, M. (2010) Current and Emerging Biomarkers in Breast Cancer: Prognosis and Prediction. *Endocrine-Related Cancer*, **17**, R245-R262. http://dx.doi.org/10.1677/erc-10-0136

[5]   Knauer, M., Cardoso, F., Wesseling, J., Bedard, P.L., Linn, S.C., Rutgers, E.J.T. and van't Veer, L.J. (2010) Identification of a Low-Risk Subgroup of HER-2-Positive Breast Cancer by the 70-Gene Prognosis Signature. *British Journal of Cancer*, **103**, 1788-1793. http://dx.doi.org/10.1038/sj.bjc.6605916

[6]   Jiang, Z., Xu, M., Savas, L., LeClair, P. and Banner, B.F. (1999) Invariant Chain Expression in Colon Neoplasms. *Virchows Archiv*, **435**, 32-36. http://dx.doi.org/10.1007/s004280050391

[7]   Ohtani, H. (2007) Focus on TILs: Prognostic Significance of Tumor Infiltrating Lymphocytes in Human Colorectal Cancer. *Cancer Immunity*, **7**, 4.

[8]   Nagata, S., Jin, Y.F., Yoshizato, K., Tomoeda, M., Song, M., Iizuka, N., *et al.* (2009) CD74 Is a Novel Prognostic Factor for Patients with Pancreatic Cancer Receiving Multimodal Theraphy. *Annals of Surgical Oncology*, **16**, 2531-2538. http://dx.doi.org/10.1245/s10434-009-0532-3

[9]   Ishigami, S., Natsugoe, S., Tokuda, K., Nakajo, A., Iwashige, H., Aridome, K., *et al.* (2001) Invariant Chain Expression in Gastric Cancer. *Cancer Letters*, **168**, 87-91. http://dx.doi.org/10.1016/S0304-3835(01)00503-1

[10]   Zheng, Y.X., Yang, M., Rong, T.T., Yuan, X.L., Ma, Y.H., Wang, Z.H., Shen, L.S. and Cui, L. (2012) CD74 and Macrophage Migration Inhibitory Factor as Therapeutic Targets in Gastric Cancer. *World Journal of Gastroenterology*, **18**, 2253-2261. http://dx.doi.org/10.3748/wjg.v18.i18.2253

[11]   Lin, X., Wang, X., Capek, H.L., Simone, L.C., Tuli, A., Morris, C.R., *et al.* (2009) Effect of Invariant Chain on Major Histocompatibility Complex Class I Molecule Expression and Stability on Human Breast Tumor Cell Lines. *Cancer Immunology, Immunotherapy*, **58**, 729-736. http://dx.doi.org/10.1007/s00262-008-0595-1

15

Familial versus Sporadic Breast Cancer: Different Treatments for Similar Tumors?

Ellen G. Engelhardt[1], Mieke Kriege[2], Maartje J. Hooning[2], Caroline Seynaeve[2], Rob A. E. M. Tollenaar[3], Christina J. van Asperen[4], Margreet G. E. M. Ausems[5], Lonneke V. van de Poll-Franse[6], Stella Mook[7], Senno Verhoef[8], Matti A. Rookus[1], HEBON Collaborators[9], Marjanka K. Schmidt[1,10]

[1]Division of Psychosocial Research and Epidemiology, Netherlands Cancer Institute, Amsterdam, The Netherlands
[2]Family Cancer Clinic, Department of Medical Oncology, Erasmus MC-Daniel den Hoed Cancer Centre, Rotterdam, The Netherlands
[3]Department of Surgery, Leiden University Medical Centre, Leiden, The Netherlands
[4]Department of Clinical Genetics, Leiden University Medical Centre, Leiden, The Netherlands
[5]Department of Medical Genetics, University Medical Centre Utrecht, Utrecht, The Netherlands
[6]Eindhoven Cancer Registry, Comprehensive Cancer Centre South, Eindhoven, The Netherlands
[7]Department of Radiation Oncology, Netherlands Cancer Institute, Amsterdam, The Netherlands
[8]Family Cancer Clinic, Netherlands Cancer Institute, Amsterdam, The Netherlands
[9]Hereditary Breast and Ovarian Cancer Netherlands (HEBON) Collaborators (see end of article for full list of HEBON collaborators and affiliations)
[10]Division of Molecular Pathology, Netherlands Cancer Institute, Amsterdam, The Netherlands
Email: mk.schmidt@nki.nl

Abstract

Objective: It is unclear if and to what extent family history of breast/ovarian cancer or *BRCA*1/2-mutation carriership influences breast cancer treatment strategy. We investigated whether treatment differed between patients from *BRCA*1/2 families and those unselected for family history. Methods: We included 478 *BRCA*1/2-related patients referred for genetic testing before or after diagnosis. Two references were used: 13,498 population-based and 6896 hospital-based patients. Surgical treatment and adjuvant chemotherapy use was analyzed using logistic regression models, stratified by tumor size, nodal status, age at and period of diagnosis, and estrogen receptor status (ER). Results: *BRCA*1/2 cases aged 35 - 52 years at diagnosis and/or with tumors < 2 cm were more likely to have undergone a modified radical mastectomy (Odd Ratios (OR) ranging from 2.8 to 5.1) compared to the references. This effect was most pronounced in patients treated after 1995 (OR 5.7 to 10.3). Compared to the reference groups, chemotherapy was more often administered to *BRCA*1 and ER-negative *BRCA*1/2-cases irrespective of age and nodal status (OR 1.9

to 24.3). Conclusion: After 1995 treatment of *BRCA*1/2-associated patients consisted notably of more mastectomies and adjuvant chemotherapy than their population-based counterparts with the same tumor characteristics. There is a need to be aware of such differences in daily practice and interpretation of survival studies on *BRCA*1/2 mutation carriers.

Keywords

*BRCA*1/2, Familial, Breast Cancer, Treatment, Adjuvant Chemotherapy, Mastectomy, Breast Conserving Therapy

1. Introduction

*BRCA*1 and *BRCA*2 mutation carriers have an increased risk of developing breast cancer at a young age. These mutations confer a lifetime-risk of 50% - 80% whereas the breast cancer risk of the general Dutch population is 13% [1] [2]. Approximately 2% - 3% of all breast cancer cases can be attributed to a mutation in the *BRCA*1 or *BRCA*2 gene [3].

Nowadays the most important prognosticators of long-term (*i.e.* ≥10-year) survival in sporadic breast cancer patients are still the traditional factors such as tumor size, nodal status, tumor grade, age at diagnosis and ER status [4]. Current evidence suggests that these prognostic factors are also relevant for survival of *BRCA*2-related breast cancer patients, while they are possibly less strong prognosticators for *BRCA*1-related breast cancer [5]-[7]. It is still under debate whether survival in *BRCA*1 carriers is different from that of non-carriers. One out of two reviews based on limited evidence concluded that *BRCA*1 carriers have a worse overall and progression-free survival time compared to non-carriers [8] [9]. Current guidelines on breast cancer treatment do not take genetic status into account [10] [11].

In the Netherlands, breast cancer treatment guidelines for local therapy (surgery/radiotherapy) existed on a regional level as far back as the early 1970's. Breast conserving surgery was introduced in the mid-eighties following the publication of the European Organization for Research and Treatment of Cancer (EORTC) 10801 trial [12], while the first national Dutch guideline regarding adjuvant systemic therapy was implemented by the Dutch Institute for Healthcare Improvement [13] in 1998 following the presentation of the meta-analysis by the Early Breast Cancer Trialists' Collaborative Group (EBCTCG) [14], initiating a wider use of adjuvant systemic therapy most notably for node negative breast cancer [14] [15]. Continuous improvements in breast cancer treatment over the past decades, including local and systemic adjuvant therapy and the introduction of breast cancer screening, have played an important role in improving long-term breast cancer survival [16] [17].

In the Netherlands, Family Cancer Clinics were established in the early 1990's, and after the identification of the breast cancer susceptibility genes *BRCA*1 and *BRCA*2 in 1994 and 1995, respectively, referral for genetic testing and counselling became more frequent. Nowadays, breast cancer genetic counselling has become common practice in the Netherlands. Especially female breast cancer patients diagnosed at a young age (<35 years) or those with a (extensive) family history of breast and/or ovarian cancer are referred for genetic testing [18]. The uptake of preventive surgery by women with a *BRCA*1/2 mutation in the Netherlands—with 35% opting for prophylactic mastectomy and 49% for salpingo-oophorectomy—is relatively high compared to other western countries [19]-[21]. Several studies have shown that preventive salpingo-oophorectomy not only reduces the risk of developing ovarian/fallopian tube cancer, but also reduces the breast cancer risk in *BRCA*1/2-mutation carriers by 50% - 72%; whereas bilateral prophylactic mastectomy reduces the risk of breast cancer by approximately 90% - 95% [21]-[24]. Furthermore, prophylactic salpingo-oophorectomy has been shown to improve the overall and cancer-specific survival, including breast cancer-specific survival, in *BRCA*1/2-mutation carriers [21] [23] [25], while data on a beneficial effect of preventive mastectomy on survival are not yet available.

While the influence of genetic status or family history of breast/ovarian cancer on the decision making regarding prophylactic surgery (*i.e.* prophylactic mastectomy or salpingo-oophorectomy) has been the subject of several studies, it has never been explored whether a family history of breast/ovarian cancer and/or knowledge of *BRCA*1/2-carriership affect choices for breast cancer treatment [26]. Therefore the aim of the current study was to determine whether patients from *BRCA*1 and *BRCA*2 families received more extensive breast cancer treatment compared to sporadic breast cancer cases.

2. Methods

2.1. Patient Selection and Data Collection

For the current case-case study, which was conducted as part of the Hereditary Breast and Ovarian cancer Netherlands (HEBON) Resource study, females in *BRCA*1/2 families diagnosed with breast cancer between 1980 and 2007 were identified through the Gene-Environment Research in Hereditary Breast and Ovarian cancer Netherlands (GEO-HEBON) database [27]. All breast cancer patients who underwent genetic counselling and were (partly) treated at the Antoni van Leeuwenhoek hospital, Amsterdam, Erasmus MC-Daniel den Hoed cancer clinic, Rotterdam, Leiden University Medical Centre or University Medical Centre Utrecht were selected from the GEO-HEBON database (n = 590). Cases with distant metastases at diagnosis or only a ductal carcinoma in situ were excluded (n = 112), leaving 366 *BRCA*1 and 112 *BRCA*2 breast cancer cases for analyses. These 478 breast cancer patients consisted of women who were genotyped as *BRCA*1/2 mutation carrier before breast cancer diagnosis (n = 36), women who were genotyped as *BRCA*1/2 mutation carrier after breast cancer diagnosis (n = 383), and women who had not (yet) undergone genetic testing, but belonged to proven *BRCA*1/2 families and were a first degree family member of a proven mutation carrier (= obligate carrier) (n = 59). These *BRCA*1/2-familial cases are all referred to as *BRCA*1/2 cases in this paper, keeping in mind that the majority of these patients were treated for breast cancer not yet knowing that they were a *BRCA* mutation carrier, as *BRCA*-testing started in 1995 approximately. From July 2009 until January 2010 for all eligible patients detailed information on tumor characteristics, surgical and systemic treatment for the primary breast cancer, and follow-up data regarding local recurrence, distant metastases, other primary tumors and death was extracted from medical records, the GEO-HEBON and other existing (clinical) oncology databases.

We used two reference populations, a general population-based sample of breast cancer cases from the Comprehensive Cancer Centre South database (n = 13,498) [28] and a hospital-based case series from the Antoni van Leeuwenhoek cancer-specialized hospital (NKI-AVL), Amsterdam (n = 6896), applying the same exclusion criteria as for the *BRCA*1/2 cases. The patients from the hospital-based series were diagnosed with breast cancer between 1987-2000 [29]. The cancer hospital-based reference group was included in addition to the population-based reference group (mainly treated in general hospitals), to account for possible differences in treatment strategy between cancer-specialized and general hospitals.

Primary breast cancer treatment included local surgery, consisting of either a modified radical mastectomy or breast conserving therapy aiming at radical excision, followed by adjuvant radiotherapy (on indication after modified radical mastectomy, and always after breast conserving therapy). Also, adequate treatment of the axillary lymph nodes was performed, consisting of either systematic axillary dissection or sentinel lymphadenectomy (SN-procedure, as of the year 2000 approximately). The clinical decision to opt for a modified radical mastectomy or breast conserving surgery was largely based on tumor size (in combination with tumor location and breast volume). Adjuvant systemic therapy (*i.e.* chemotherapy and/or hormonal therapy) was administered after local therapy depending on the patient's age/menopausal status ($\leq$52 years premenopausal, >52 years postmenopausal), tumor stage (tumor size, and nodal status), and later also depending on tumor characteristics (e.g. differentiation grade and hormone receptor status). Since the latter part of the 1990s hormone receptor status, mainly ER status, became an important discriminating factor regarding the type of systemic treatment; a positive ER status was recognized as a predictive factor for efficacy of endocrine therapy, while in case of negative ER status only chemotherapy was considered [13] [30].

2.2. Ethical Standards

The HEBON Resource study was approved by the Review Board of the NKI-AVL, and according to Dutch law, no further institutional Review Board approval was needed. The use of all data in this manuscript, including that of the two control cohorts, complies with Dutch laws and follows the Scientific Codes published by the Dutch federation of Biomedical Scientific Societies [31].

2.3. Statistical Analysis

In order to quantitatively assess breast cancer treatment, we divided treatment into two dichotomous variables, namely 1) type of surgical treatment (modified radical mastectomy versus breast conserving therapy) and 2) use of adjuvant chemotherapy (yes versus no). Only 10% of *BRCA*1/2 cases had received both chemotherapy and hormonal therapy.

Odds ratio's for undergoing a modified radical mastectomy (versus breast conserving therapy) and for receiving chemotherapy were calculated using multivariate logistic regression analyses for *BRCA*1 and *BRCA*2 cases compared to population- and cancer hospital-based reference groups. A priori we expected the *BRCA*1/2 cases to be younger and to have different tumor characteristics. Based on these differences, but also based on covariates, which might influence breast cancer treatment decisions, we decided for which characteristics we would stratify and/or adjust our analyses. Logistic regression models for surgery were stratified for tumor size (≤2 cm and >2 cm) age at breast cancer diagnosis (<35, 35 - 52, >52) and period of breast cancer diagnosis (≤1995, >1995 (introduction of *BRCA*1/2 mutation testing in the Netherlands) and ≤1998, >1998 (paradigm shift in adjuvant treatment). Analyses for chemotherapy were stratified for nodal status (negative, positive), age at breast cancer diagnosis (<35, 35 - 52, >52) and period of breast cancer diagnosis (≤1995, >1995 and ≤1998, >1998). Additionally the logistic models for chemotherapy were also run for ER negative cases only (with *BRCA*1 and *BRCA*2 patients combined due to small numbers). In the logistic regression models for surgery and for chemotherapy, covariates included were differentiation grade (1, 2, 3, and missing), nodal status (node negative, node positive, and missing), tumor size (≤2 cm, >2 cm, and missing), estrogen receptor status (positive, negative, and missing), age at breast cancer diagnosis (<35 years, 35 - 52, and >52), unless the model was stratified for that factor. In the analyses for *BRCA*1 cases versus the reference groups, stratified for multiple factors, only cases with grade 3 tumors were included since grade 1 and grade 2 tumors are rare in *BRCA*1 cases. All statistical analyses were performed using SPSS Inc.18. A two-sided p of <0.05 was considered significant.

3. Results

Of the 478 *BRCA*1/2 breast cancer patients included, 419 were identified as *BRCA*1 (N = 323) or *BRCA*2 (N = 96) mutation carriers themselves, and 59 obligate mutation carrier. Breast cancer was diagnosed before 1995 in 256 (54%) of the *BRCA*1/2 cases and after 1995 in 222 (46%). Of the 222 *BRCA*1/2 cases diagnosed after 1995, 36 (16%) were aware of their own carriership status and 16 (7%) were aware of a *BRCA*1 or *BRCA*2 mutation in their family at breast cancer diagnosis and treatment.

Characteristics of *BRCA*1/2 cases and of the two reference groups are shown in **Table 1**. Mean age at breast cancer diagnosis was 41 and 44 years for *BRCA*1 and *BRCA*2 patients, respectively, compared with 57 years and 55 years for the population-based and hospital-based reference groups, respectively. The majority of the *BRCA*1 and *BRCA*2 patients had grade 3 tumors (88% and 69%, respectively), while this was only 32% and 31% for the population-based and hospital-based reference groups, respectively. The majority of the *BRCA*1 tumors were ER negative (77%) compared with 25% of the *BRCA*2 tumors and 23% of the tumors in both reference groups.

We had data on prophylactic surgery for 408 of the 478 *BRCA*1/2 cases; 24 of them underwent a prophylactic salpingo-oophorectomy and 56 a mastectomy within 1 year of the diagnosis of the primary tumor (no data available for reference groups).

3.1. Type of Surgery

Figure 1 shows unadjusted trends in chemotherapy and surgical treatment per year. Type of surgical treatment by tumor size and nodal status for the two reference groups is shown in **Table 2(a)** and for the *BRCA*1/2 cases in **Table 2(b)**. Within the *BRCA*1/2 cases having a tumor ≤ 2 cm, 64% of those identified as mutation carrier prior to their breast cancer diagnosis underwent a modified radical mastectomy compared to 35% of *BRCA*1/2 cases who had not yet been referred for genetic testing. For the population- and hospital-based reference groups these percentages were 27% and 20%, respectively. *BRCA*1/2 cases with a tumor ≤ 2 cm more often had a mastectomy and received chemotherapy (53%) than the general population- and hospital-based reference groups (<30%) (**Table 2(c)**). So, *BRCA*1/2 cases with tumors ≤ 2 cm underwent a modified radical mastectomy 1.6 to 3.1 times more often than the population- and hospital-based cases, respectively (**Table 3**), while there were no significant differences in type of surgery between *BRCA*1/2 cases and the reference patients with tumors > 2 cm. After stratification for age at diagnosis, *BRCA*1/2 cases aged 35 - 52 years were significantly more likely to undergo a modified radical mastectomy compared to the reference population cases. If we stratified for tumor size and age at diagnosis (only enough cases for the *BRCA*1 subgroup), the higher percentage of modified radical mastectomy in *BRCA*1 cases only remained significant in the subgroup of patients diagnosed between 35 - 52 years and having a tumor ≤ 2 cm. In patients treated before 1995, we did not observe a higher rate of modified radical

Table 1. Population characteristics.

	Clinical genetic centers		Reference groups	
	*BRCA*1	*BRCA*2	Population based	Hospital based
Medical centers, patients (N)				
Antoni van Leeuwenhoek hospital	79	30	NA	6896
Erasmus MC- Daniel den Hoed Cancer Center	212	44	NA	NA
Leiden University Medical Center	51	36	NA	NA
University Medical Center Utrecht	24	2	NA	NA
Comprehensive Cancer Center South	NA	NA	13498	NA
Total (N)	366	112	13498	6896
Diagnosis year (N (%))				
Range	1980-2006	1981-2006	1980-2007	1987-2000
1980-1990	110 (30)	35 (31)	3860 (28)	1541 (22)
1991-2000	202 (55)	49 (44)	5112 (38)	5355 (78)
2001-2010	54 (15)	28 (25)	4526 (34)	0
Age at diagnosis (N (%))				
Mean age (range)	41 (19 - 72)	44 (31 - 81)	57 (20 - 81)	55 (23 - 81)
<35 years	108 (30)	16 (14)	359 (3)	266 (4)
35 - 52 years	211 (58)	76 (68)	4782 (35)	2998 (43)
>52 years	47 (12)	20 (18)	8357 (62)	3632 (53)
Differentiation grade (N (%))				
Grade 1	1 (<1)	4 (6)	1523 (22)	1053 (19)
Grade 2	29 (12)	17 (25)	3091 (46)	2724 (50)
Grade 3	210 (88)	46 (69)	2168 (32)	1727 (31)
Missing	126	45	6716	1392
Tumor diameter (N (%))				
≤2 cm	172 (52)	51 (52)	7064 (54)	3529 (52)
>2 cm	157 (48)	47 (48)	6087 (46)	3320 (48)
Missing	37	14	347	47
Estrogen receptor (N (%))				
Negative	189 (77)	19 (25)	2196 (23)	1050 (23)
Positive	56 (23)	57 (75)	7443 (77)	3536 (77)
Missing	121	36	3859	2310
Nodal status (N (%))				
Negative	225 (66)	49 (47)	6624 (55)	3143 (48)
Positive	115 (34)	56 (53)	5348 (45)	3435 (52)
Missing	26	7	1526	318

NA = not applicable.

mastectomy in *BRCA*1/2 cases with a tumor ≤ 2 cm compared to the reference groups, while *BRCA*1 cases with tumors ≤ 2 cm diagnosed after 1995 had higher odds of undergoing a modified radical mastectomy compared to the population-based (OR = 5.8, 95% CI 3 - 11.2) and the hospital-based cohort (OR = 10.3, 95% CI 4.8 - 22.3) (**Table 3**). The analyses stratified for prior or post 1998 showed similarly increased odds for undergoing modified radical mastectomy in the *BRCA*1/2 cases diagnosed after 1998 (data not shown).

3.2. Adjuvant Chemotherapy

Administration of chemotherapy in relation to negative or positive nodal status is shown in **Table 2(a)** and **Table 2(b)** for the reference and *BRCA*1/2 groups, respectively. Chemotherapy was more often administered in

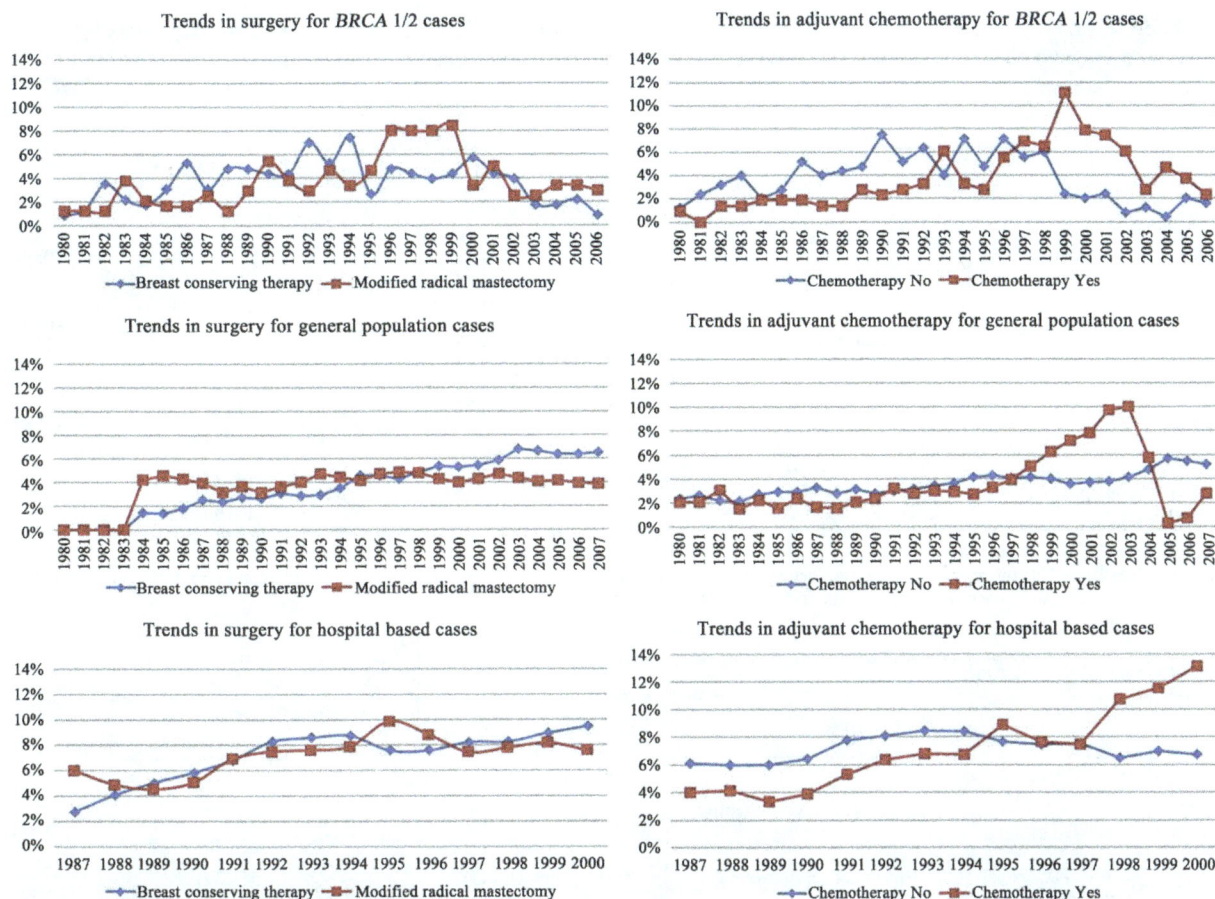

Figure 1. Trends in surgical and adjuvant chemotherapy for population subgroups.

node-negative *BRCA*1/2 patients genotyped prior to their breast cancer diagnosis (73%) compared to *BRCA*1/2 patients who had not yet been tested (17%; **Table 2(b)**); at least partly related to the fact that more chemotherapy was given in later years of diagnosis. *BRCA*1 and ER-negative (*BRCA*1and *BRCA*2 combined) cases across all ages and irrespective of lymph node involvement had higher odds of receiving chemotherapy compared to both reference groups while a higher odds for of receiving chemotherapy in *BRCA*2 cases was especially observed in the node positive subgroup and in the subgroups of 35 - 52 years and >52 years at diagnosis (**Table 4**). The higher odds of receiving chemotherapy in *BRCA*1/2 cases compared with the reference groups was observed in patients treated before as well as after 1995, but numbers were too small for adjusted analyses (**Table 4**). Node positive *BRCA*1 cases treated both prior to and after 1998 had increased odds of receiving chemotherapy compared to the population-based cases (OR = 5,95% CI 2.4 - 10.2; OR = 4.1, 95% CI 1.2 - 14.2). Moreover, node negative *BRCA*1 cases treated after 1998 also showed significantly increased odds of receiving chemotherapy compared to the population reference group (OR = 13.1, 95% CI 5.8 - 29.4) (other data for this comparison not shown). In the current study data regarding hormonal therapy was also collected, however, the numbers of *BRCA*1/2 patients receiving adjuvant hormonal therapy were too small (57 cases) to perform separate analyses.

4. Discussion

Overall we found that *BRCA*1/2 cases more often underwent a modified radical mastectomy, especially *BRCA*1 and *BRCA*2 cases diagnosed after 1995 with tumours ≤ 2 cm, and more often received adjuvant chemotherapy, especially in *BRCA*1 cases and/or ER-negative tumors, compared to unselected breast cancer cases with similar tumor characteristics from hospital- and population-based reference groups. These findings highlight the importance of taking type of treatment into account when comparing survival between mutation carriers and sporadic cases, something which is rarely done by studies published so far, as demonstrated by a recent systematic review

Table 2. (a)Type of surgery and administration of chemotherapy for the reference groups; (b) Type of surgery and administration of chemotherapy by tumor subgroup in relation to timing of DNA testing; (c) Type of surgery and administration of chemotherapy by nodal status for each study population.

(a)

		Population-based[1]	Hospital-based[1]	P[2]
	Type of surgery (N (%))			
≤2 cm	Breast conserving therapy	4758 (73)	2649 (80)	**<0.001**
	Modified radical mastectomy	1836 (27)	643 (20)	
>2 cm	Breast conserving therapy	1803 (35)	1240 (41)	**<0.001**
	Modified radical mastectomy	3324 (65)	1793 (59)	
	Adjuvant chemotherapy (N (%))			
Node negative	Yes	277 (4)	132 (4)	0.967
	No	6347 (96)	3011 (96)	
Node positive	Yes	1773 (33)	1477 (43)	**<0.001**
	No	3575 (67)	1958 (57)	

[1]Numbers of patients varies due to missing values.
[2]P values from Chi-square tests; because these are unadjusted for patient and tumor differences between the references populations, these should not be interpreted as differences in treatment practices between these populations.

(b)

		Clinical Genetic Centers		P[3]
		DNA test pre breast cancer diagnosis[1,2]	DNA test post breast cancer diagnosis[2]	
	Type of surgery (N (%))			
≤2 cm	Breast conserving therapy	10 (36)	106 (65)	**0.011**
	Modified radical mastectomy	18 (64)	57 (35)	
>2 cm	Breast conserving therapy	10 (43)	58 (39)	0.441
	Modified radical mastectomy	13 (57)	89 (61)	
	Adjuvant chemotherapy (N (%))			
Node negative	Yes	24 (73)	34 (17)	**<0.001**
	No	9 (27)	169 (83)	
Node positive	Yes	14 (88)	107 (81)	0.677
	No	2 (12)	25 (19)	

[1]DNA test pre breast cancer diagnosis means that either the case herself or a family member had undergone BRCA genetic testing and received the results of the test prior to the woman included being diagnosed with breast cancer.
[2]Numbers of patients varies due to missing values
[3]P values from Chi-square tests; because these are unadjusted for patient and tumor differences between the pre-and post-breast cancer diagnoses tested carriers, these should not be interpreted as differences in treatment practices between those groups.

(c)

	Treatment		Population			P[1]
	Adjuvant chemotherapy	*Type of surgery (N (%))*	BRCA 1/2 cases	*General population-based*	*Cancer hospital-based*	
Node negative	No	Breast conserving therapy	130 (63)	3488 (62)	2223 (81)	**<0.001**
		Modified radical mastectomy	75 (37)	2114 (38)	531 (19)	
	Yes	Breast conserving therapy	30 (45)	144 (55)	90 (71)	**0.001**
		Modified radical mastectomy	36 (55)	118 (45)	36 (29)	
Node positive	No	Breast conserving therapy	6 (21)	1330 (43)	702 (39)	**0.008**
		Modified radical mastectomy	22 (79)	1799 (57)	1087 (61)	
	Yes	Breast conserving therapy	50 (36)	697 (44)	609 (44)	0.155
		Modified radical mastectomy	90 (64)	884 (56)	780 (56)	

[1]P values from Chi-square test; because these are unadjusted for patient and tumour differences, these should not be interpreted as differences in treatment practices between groups.

Table 3. Odds of undergoing a modified radical mastectomy versus breast conserving therapy for *BRCA1/2* cases compared to population- and cancer hospital-based cases.

Subgroup			N	*BRCA*1/2 cases versus population-based cases		*BRCA*1/2 cases versus hospital-based cases	
				Unadjusted	Adjusted[1]	Unadjusted	Adjusted[1]
				OR (95%-CI)	OR (95%-CI)	OR (95%-CI)	OR (95%-CI)
Cases stratified by tumour diameter							
BRCA 1	≤2 cm		171	1.7 (1.2 - 2.3)	1.6 (1.2 - 2.3)[*]	2.7 (1.9 - 3.7)	2.9 (2.0 - 4.2)[*]
	>2 cm		156	0.7 (0.5 - 0.9)	0.8 (0.6 - 1.1)	0.9 (0.6 - 1.2)	1.5 (1.0 - 2.2)[*]
BRCA 2	≤2 cm		51	2.0 (1.1 - 3.4)	1.9 (1.1 - 3.3)[*]	3.1 (1.8 - 5.5)	3.1 (1.7 - 5.6)[*]
	>2 cm		47	1.2 (0.6 - 2.1)	1.3 (0.7 - 2.4)	1.5 (0.8 - 2.7)	1.9 (1.0 - 3.7)
Cases stratified by age at breast cancer diagnosis							
BRCA 1	<35		107	0.8 (0.5 - 1.3)	0.8 (0.5 - 1.4)	1.0 (0.7 - 1.6)	1.4 (0.8 - 2.4)
	35 - 52		205	1.4 (1.1 - 1.9)	1.5 (1.1 - 2.0)[*]	1.8 (1.4 - 2.4)	2.5 (1.8 - 3.5)[*]
	>52		42	1.3 (0.7 - 2.4)	1.2 (0.6 - 2.3)	1.6 (0.9 - 2.9)	1.8 (0.9 - 3.7)
BRCA 2	<35		16	1.0 (0.4 - 2.8)	1.0 (0.3 - 3.0)	1.3 (0.5 - 3.7)	1.3 (0.4 - 4.1)
	35 - 52		76	2.0 (1.3 - 3.2)	1.9 (1.1 - 3.1)[*]	2.6 (1.6 - 4.1)	2.6 (1.5 - 4.4)[*]
	>52		20	2.3 (0.9 - 5.6)	2.4 (0.9 - 6.8)	2.7 (1.1 - 6.7)	4.4 (1.5 -12.9)[*]
Cases stratified by age at breast cancer diagnosis and tumour diameter							
BRCA 1 *(only grade 3 tumours included)*	<35	≤2 cm	27	2.1 (0.8 - 5.9)	x^2	1.8 (0.7 - 4.9)	x^2
		>2 cm	34	0.4 (0.2 - 0.9)	0.5 (0.2 - 1.4)	0.7 (0.3 - 1.7)	1.4 (0.5 - 4.0)
	35 - 52	≤2 cm	63	2.5 (1.5 - 4.4)	2.8 (1.6 - 4.8)[*]	3.5 (2.0 - 6.2)	5.1 (2.7 - 9.8)[*]
		>2 cm	54	1.2 (0.7 - 2.1)	1.5 (0.8 - 2.6)	1.1 (0.6 - 2.0)	1.9 (1.0 - 3.7)
	>52	≤2 cm	11	0.6 (0.1 - 2.7)	0.6 (0.1 - 2.9)	0.6 (0.1 - 2.7)	0.9 (0.1 - 5.0)
		>2 cm	12	0.8 (0.2 - 2.4)	0.9 (0.3 - 2.9)	0.9 (0.3 - 2.8)	2.4 (0.6 - 9.3)
BRCA 2[2]							
Cases stratified by year of diagnosis and tumour diameter							
BRCA 1 *(only grade 3 tumours included)*	≤1995	≤2 cm	53	0.8 (0.4 - 1.6)	x^2	0.9 (0.4 - 1.7)	x^2
		>2 cm	37	0.5 (0.3 - 1.1)	0.8 (0.4 - 1.8)	1.0 (0.5 - 1.9)	2.4 (1.1 - 5.3)[*]
	>1995	≤2 cm	48	5.7 (3.0 - 10.7)	5.8 (3.0 - 11.2)[*]	6.5 (3.4 - 12.6)	10.3 (4.8 - 22.3)[*]
		>2 cm	63	1.0 (0.6 - 1.8)	1.0 (0.6 - 1.8)	0.9 (0.5 - 1.6)	1.5 (0.8 - 2.8)
BRCA 2[2]							

[1]Model with surgery (modified radical mastectomy versus breast conserving therapy) adjusted for: differentiation grade (grade 1 & 2 (ref), grade 3 and missing), nodal status (node positive (ref), node negative and missing), age at breast cancer incidence (<35 years, 35 - 52 years (ref) and > 52 years, tumour diameter (≤2 cm (ref), >2 cm, missing). All models were adjusted for the above-mentioned factors, unless the model was stratified for that factor.
[2]Insufficient cases to run the model.
[*]Statistically significant (P < 0.05) (indicated only for adjusted ORs).

that found that of 66 studies assessing the survival of *BRCA*1/2 mutation carriers, only 8 corrected for confounding by adjuvant treatment [32]. Current evidence suggests that contrary to currently held beliefs, if confounding by treatment is taken into account, differences in survival between *BRCA*1/2 mutation carriers and sporadic breast cancer patients if any are likely to be small.

The Dutch guidelines for breast cancer treatment do not differ specifically for *BRCA*1/2 cases and sporadic breast cancer cases. Breast conserving surgery was introduced in 1986 following the EORTC 10,801 trial [12]. Age by itself and tumor size have been shown to be important factors in the choice of type of breast cancer surgery, but even within the Netherlands there is variance between hospitals [33]. In our analysis, we found an increased probability of more extensive surgery in *BRCA*1/2 cases with a tumor ≤ 2 cm, both compared to the NKI-AVL cancer hospital-based (where 22% of the *BRCA*1/2 cases had also been treated) as well as to the

Table 4. Odds of receiving chemotherapy for *BRCA*1/2 cases compared to population-based and cancer hospital-based cases.

Subgroup			N	BRCA1/2 cases versus population-based cases		BRCA1/2 cases versus hospital-based cases	
				Unadjusted	Adjusted[1]	Unadjusted	Adjusted[1]
				OR (95%-CI)	OR (95%-CI)	OR (95%-CI)	OR (95%-CI)
Cases stratified by nodal status							
BRCA 1		Negative	223	8.8 (6.4 - 12.1)	1.9 (1.3 - 2.7)*	8.8 (6.2 - 12.4)	2.5 (1.7 - 3.8)*
		Positive	115	9.6 (5.9 - 15.6)	4.3 (2.4 - 7.6)*	6.3 (3.9 - 10.2)	2.7 (1.4 - 5.3)*
BRCA 2		Negative	49	2.6 (1.0 - 6.6)	0.9 (0.3 - 2.4)	2.6 (1.0 - 6.6)	1.2 (0.5 - 3.4)
		Positive	56	9.3 (4.7 - 18.4)	4.4 (2.0 - 9.7)*	6.1 (3.1 - 12.1)	2.7 (1.1 - 6.5)*
ER-negative only BRCA 1/2 *combined*		Negative	142	4.6 (3.1 - 6.8)	2.0 (1.3 - 3.1)*	24.3 (15.2 - 38.9)	x[b]
		Positive	65	8.4 (4.1 - 17.1)	3.8 (1.8 - 8.3)*	8.4 (4.1 - 17.0)	2.6 (1.0 - 6.7)
Cases stratified by age at breast cancer diagnosis							
BRCA 1		<35	108	1.6 (1.1 - 2.5)	3.2 (1.8 - 5.8)*	1.1 (0.7 - 1.7)	2.4 (1.2 - 4.7)*
		35 - 52	205	1.6 (1.2 - 2.2)	2.5 (1.8 - 3.6)*	1.0 (0.8 - 1.3)	2.5 (1.6 - 3.7)*
		>52	44	5.4 (2.7 - 10.7)	3.7 (1.7 - 8.0)*	6.0 (3 - 12.1)	7.8 (3.5 - 17.7)*
BRCA 2		<35	16	1.2 (0.4 - 3.2)	1.0 (0.3 - 3.3)	0.8 (0.3 - 2.2)	0.3 (0.1 - 1.1)
		35 - 52	76	2.3 (1.5 - 3.6)	2.5 (1.4 - 4.5)*	1.4 (0.9 - 2.2)	1.9 (1.0 - 3.7)
		>52	19	5.4 (2.7 -10.7)	3.5 (1.0 - 12.2)	4.8 (1.6 - 14.6)	7.4 (2.1 - 26.0)*
ER-negative only BRCA 1/2 *combined*		<35	69	2.0 (1.1 - 3.6)	3.8 (1.8 - 8.2)*	1.3 (0.7 - 2.5)	3.8 (1.2 - 12.1)*
		35 - 52	122	1.5 (1.0 - 2.2)	2.1 (1.3 - 3.3)*	1.3 (0.9 - 1.8)	4.1 (2.3 - 7.3)*
		>52	20	2.4 (0.9 - 6.2)	2.7 (1.0 - 7.7)	8.6 (3.2 - 22.8)	39.1 (8.9 - 173)*
Cases stratified by year of diagnosis and nodal status							
BRCA 1(*only grade* 3 *tumours included*)	≤1995	Negative	64	2.6 (0.8 - 9.0)	x[2]	1.9 (0.6 - 5.9)	x[2]
		Positive	28	11.2 (4.1-30.3)	10.3 (2.3 - 46.7)*	7.1 (2.7 - 18.9)	8.6 (1.8 - 40.6)*
	>1995	Negative	68	7.8 (4.5 - 13.5)	x[2]	4.3 (2.4 - 7.8)	2.8 (1.5 - 5.2)*
		Positive	37	12.9 (3.9 - 42.3)	6.6 (1.9 - 22.3)*	6.7 (2 - 22.2)	x[2]
BRCA 2[b]							
ER-negative only BRCA 1/2 *combined*	≤1995	Negative	62	4.5 (1.1 - 18.3)	1.2 (0.2 - 5.9)	4.8 (1.3 - 18.2)	x[2]
		Positive	27	8.5 (3.2 - 22.9)	3.8 (1.1 - 13.0)*	7.0 (2.6 - 18.5)	1.9 (0.5 - 7.1)
	>1995	Negative	80	5.8 (3.5 - 9.6)	3.0 (1.7 - 5.2)*	38.8 (21.5 - 70.2)	x[2]
		Positive	38	8.3 (2.9 - 23.7)	5.0 (1.7 - 14.9)*	9.9 (3.5 - 28.1)	x[2]

[1]Model with surgery (modified radical mastectomy versus breast conserving therapy) adjusted for: differentiation grade (grade 1 & 2 (ref), grade 3 and missing), nodal status (node positive (ref), node negative and missing), age at breast cancer incidence (<35 years, 35 - 52 years (ref) and >52 years, tumour diameter (≤2 cm (ref), >2 cm, missing). All models were adjusted for the above-mentioned factors, unless the model was stratified for that factor.
[2]Insufficient cases to run the model.
*Statistically significant (P < 0.05) (indicated only for adjusted ORs).

population-based reference group. It seemed that particularly after 1995, the *BRCA*1/2 cases were more likely to receive a modified radical mastectomy for smaller tumors, but we lacked power to investigate the effects of knowledge of *BRCA*-carriership. It is known that a part of the affected *BRCA*1/2 cases also choose for a contralateral preventive mastectomy (in combination with a modified radical mastectomy of the affected breast) to prevent contralateral breast cancer [20], which might play a role in the higher rate of modified radical mastectomies observed in *BRCA*1/2 cases in this study. Unfortunately, in the current study it is unknown how many *BRCA*1/2 cases underwent a contralateral mastectomy. Our observations also may reflect the (early) perception of many physicians that more extensive surgery for mutation carriers would be better in the long term. Possibly, effects of a general time trend of increased use of modified radical mastectomy in patients < 50 years also played a role [33].

Both node positive and node negative *BRCA*1/2 cases were more likely to receive chemotherapy for ER-negative tumors. Until the publication of the EBCTCG review results in 1997 [14] and the implementation of the first Dutch guidelines on adjuvant systemic breast cancer treatment in 1998, adjuvant systemic treatment was rarely used in node-negative breast cancer in the Netherlands. Since then adjuvant systemic therapy in node negative patients has become more commonplace and included in the guideline for those patients from whom a 10-year survival gain of at least 3% - 5% is expected [13] [14]. This might partly explain our observation that node negative *BRCA*1/2 cases were more likely to receive chemotherapy especially after 1998. Another explanation for this observation might be the growing awareness that *BRCA*-associated breast cancer frequently metastasized and was possibly more sensitive to chemotherapy [34] [35].

The current study confirmed the high prevalence of high-grade tumors in *BRCA*1 and *BRCA*2 cases (88% and 69%) described in the literature [9]. Nowadays differentiation grade is a factor of consideration regarding the use of adjuvant systemic therapy in node-negative breast cancer given the fact that the cumulative 10-year survival of high grade tumors has been estimated to be 30% - 78% compared to 90% - 94% for breast cancers with the lowest differentiation grade tumors [4]. However, in the current Dutch treatment guidelines a high-grade tumor alone is not considered sufficient justification for prescribing adjuvant systemic therapy [13], and effects we found were consistent also when only comparing grade 3 tumors. Moreover, in the period that the majority of the included cases were diagnosed, grade was not yet a relevant factor used in clinical decision-making. Unfortunately, we do not have information on other tumor markers such as EGFR, E-cadherin and ki67. Also, the majority of patients were treated before the nationwide introduction of Trastuzumab.

Despite the unique results of the current study, we are aware of some limitations. Ideally we would have compared *BRCA*1/2 cases to sporadic cases from the same hospitals. Young women (<40 years) treated at a general hospital were more likely to undergo breast conserving therapy compared to those treated at a teaching or academic hospital [36]. Also, a pronounced difference in the use of adjuvant systemic therapy at a hospital level was found though this did not appear to be associated with type of hospital [36]. The variations in treatment observed could be due to a delayed introduction of new techniques or implementation of new scientific insights. Importantly, overall we observed similarly increased odds, or at least overlapping confidence intervals, for the *BRCA*1/2 cases for receiving more extensive treatment compared to both the population-based and the cancer hospital-based reference groups. Secondly, the current multicenter study included a sizeable study population and had a long follow up; the treatment data is largely complete, yet a large proportion of tumor characteristics, such as tumor differentiation grade and ER-status are missing, partly due to the work-up and the factors considered during the period of treatment. Also, possibly just a few of the 59 obligate *BRCA*1/2 carriers (obligate based on mendelian inheritance) might have turned out to be *BRCA*1/2 mutation negative would they have been tested individually. Further, since no testing was performed in the reference population, there might have been some mutation carriers in these populations. However, it is unlikely that this affected the results given the large number of patients in the reference groups and the small proportion of mutation carriers expected. In addition, selection bias may have occurred as patients who were included in the GEO-HEBON cohort if they had responded to a mailed questionnaire. This could have led to the selection of those in better physical condition or the more motivated patients. If a more extensive treatment has led to a better survival, this is overrepresented in the selected cohort. Further, another draw-back of our study was the small numbers in specific subgroup analyses, producing wide confidence intervals. Also, a proportion of the *BRCA*1/2 mutation carriers were not aware of their *BRCA* status at the time of diagnosis and treatment. However, it is worth noting that although they were not aware of their *BRCA* status, family history was known and was considered an important prognostic factor. Finally, reasons driving treatment decisions were not clearly identifiable in this study, given the retrospective study design.

Currently, as far as we know, there is little information available regarding the influence of having breast cancer in the family or being a *BRCA*1/2 mutation carrier on the clinical breast cancer treatment decision process. Most studies evaluated factors influencing the decision whether or not to undergo additional preventive surgery in high risk populations, showing that *BRCA* test results are one of the most important factors in combination with the carrier's age and personal circumstances (e.g. marital status, having children) for this decision [19]. It is unknown whether these factors also play a role in decisions on breast cancer treatment for *BRCA*1/2 mutation carriers, additionally, we do not know whether the differences in treatment for *BRCA*1/2 cases observed in this study were driven by the choice of the patient or the physician. Over the last decades shared decision-making has been promoted in clinical practice and a large proportion of patients favors this trend [37]. Yet, exploration of whether breast cancer surgeons and oncologists who shared decision-making with their patients, felt comfortable with this approach, and whether they perceived any barriers to implementation, showed a substantial gap between the high self-reported comfort levels with shared decision-making (87% - 89%) and the self-reported use (56% - 69%) [38] [39]. The physicians reported that time constraints and patient's knowledge and psychological state were the most important factors inhibiting shared decision-making [38] [39].

Conclusion

In conclusion, we found evidence of different breast cancer treatment strategies in *BRCA*1/2-associated compared to sporadic cases with similar tumor characteristics, including more mastectomies and administration of adjuvant chemotherapy among *BRCA*1/2 cases. Although it is unknown which factors exactly played a role in the treatment decision among *BRCA*1/2 mutation carriers and sporadic patients, respectively, and whether treatment choice was driven by the patient or the physician, the results of the current analyses highlight the importance of the need to be aware of such differences in daily practice and interpretation of survival studies on *BRCA*1/2 mutation carriers.

Acknowledgements

We would like to thank all patients and Esther Janssen, Kiki Jeanson, GittyJaanen, Petra Bos, Jannet Blom and Twiggy van Cronenburg for their assistance with data collection.

Authors' Contributions

MKS, MJH and CS designed the study; EGE, MKS, MJH, MK, CJvA, MGEMA, LVvdPF, SM and MAR collected the data; EGE and MKS performed the data analyses; EGE, MKS, MJH, MK and CS interpreted the data and wrote the paper; EGE, MKS, MK, MJH, CS, RAEMT, CJvA, MGEMA, LVvdPF, SM, SV, MAR read and approved the final version of the manuscript.

Funding

Dutch Cancer Society grants NKI2009-4363 and DDHK 2009-4318; NWO 184.021.007 (BBMRI-NL); Netherlands Organization of Scientific Research grant NWO/Zon-MW 91109024 (HEBON Resource).

Conflict of Interest

The authors declare that they have no conflict of interest.

Full List of HEBON Collaborators and Affiliations

The Hereditary Breast and Ovarian Cancer Research Group Netherlands (HEBON) consists of the following Collaborating Centers: Coordinating center: Netherlands Cancer Institute, Amsterdam, NL: M.A. Rookus, F.B.L. Hogervorst, F.E. van Leeuwen, S. Verhoef, M.K. Schmidt, J.L. de Lange; Erasmus Medical Center, Rotterdam, NL: J.M. Collée, A.M.W. van den Ouweland, M.J. Hooning, C. Seynaeve, C.H.M. van Deurzen, I.M. Obdeijn; Leiden University Medical Center, NL: C.J. van Asperen, J.T. Wijnen, R.A.E.M. Tollenaar, P. Devilee, T.C.T.E.F. van Cronenburg; Radboud University Nijmegen Medical Center, NL: C.M. Kets, A.R. Mensenkamp; University Medical Center Utrecht, NL: M.G.E.M. Ausems, R.B. van der Luijt; Amsterdam Medical Center, NL: C.M. Aalfs, T.A.M. van Os; VU University Medical Center, Amsterdam, NL: J.J.P. Gille, Q. Waisfisz, H.E.J. Meijers-Heijboer; University Hospital Maastricht, NL: E.B. Gómez-Garcia, M.J. Blok; University Medical Center Groningen, NL: J.C. Oosterwijk, A.H. van der Hout, M.J. Mourits, G.H. de Bock. The Netherlands Foundation for the detection of hereditary tumours, Leiden, NL: H.F. Vasen.

References

[1]   Antoniou, A., Pharoah, P., Narod, S., Risch, H., Eyfjord, J., Hopper, J., *et al.* (2003) Average Risks of Breast and Ovarian Cancer Associated with *BRCA*1 or *BRCA*2 Mutations Detected in Case Series Unselected for Family History: A Combined Analysis of 22 Studies. *The American Journal of Human Genetics*, **72**, 1117-1130.
       http://dx.doi.org/10.1086/375033

[2]   Kiemeney, L., Lemmers, F., Verhoeven, R., Aben, K., Honing, C., de Nooijer, J., *et al.* (2008) De kans op kanker voor Nederlanders. *Nederlands Tijdschrift voor Geneeskunde*, **152**, 2233-2241.

[3]   Boyle, P. and Levin, B., Eds. (2008) World Cancer Report 2008. International Agency for Research on Cancer (IARC), Geneva, 1-6-2010.

[4]   Soerjomataram, I., Louwman, M., Ribot, J., Roukema, J. and Coebergh, J. (2008) An Overview of Prognostic Factors for Long-Term Survivors of Breast Cancer. *Breast Cancer Research and Treatment*, **107**, 309-330. http://dx.doi.org/10.1007/s10549-007-9556-1

[5]   Brekelmans, C., Seynaeve, C., Menke-Pluymers, M., Brüggenwirth, H., Tilanus-Linthorst, M., Bartels, C., *et al.* (2006) Survival and Prognostic Factors in BRCA1-Associated Breast Cancer. *Annals of Oncology*, **17**, 391-400. http://dx.doi.org/10.1093/annonc/mdj095

[6]   Foulkes, W., Reis-Filho, J. and Narod, S. (2010) Tumor Size and Survival in Breast Cancer—A Reappraisal. *Nature Reviews Clinical Oncology*, **7**, 348-353. http://dx.doi.org/10.1038/nrclinonc.2010.39

[7]   Tutt, A., Robson, M., Garber, J., Domchek, S., Audeh, M., Weitzel, J., *et al.* (2010) Oral Poly(ADP-Ribose) Polymerase Inhibitor Olaparib in Patients with *BRCA*1 or *BRCA*2 Mutations and Advanced Breast Cancer: A Proof-of-Concept Trial. *The Lancet*, **376**, 235-244. http://dx.doi.org/10.1016/S0140-6736(10)60892-6

[8]   Bordeleau, L., Panchal, S. and Goodwin, P. (2010) Prognosis of BRCA-Associated Breast Cancer: A Summary of Evidence. *Breast Cancer Res Treat*, **119**, 13-24. http://dx.doi.org/10.1007/s10549-009-0566-z

[9]   Lee, E., Park, S., Park, B., Kim, S., Lee, M., Ahn, S., *et al.* (2010) Effect of *BRCA*1/2 Mutation on Short-Term and Long-Term Breast Cancer Survival: A Systematic Review and Meta-Analysis. *Breast Cancer Research and Treatment*, **122**, 11-25. http://dx.doi.org/10.1007/s10549-010-0859-2

[10]   Goldhirsch, A., Ingle, J., Gelber, R., Coates, A., Thürlimann, B., Senn, H., *et al.* (2009) Thresholds for Therapies: Highlights of the St Gallen International Expert Consensus on the Primary Therapy of Early Breast Cancer 2009. *Annals of Oncology*, **20**, 1319-1329. http://dx.doi.org/10.1093/annonc/mdp322

[11]   Maughan, K., Lutterbie, M. and Ham, P. (2010) Treatment of Breast Cancer. *American Family Physician*, **81**, 1339-1346.

[12]   Litiere, S., Werutsky, G., Fentiman, I.S., Rutgers, E., Christiaens, M.R., Van Limbergen, E., *et al.* (2012) Breast Conserving Therapy versus Mastectomy for Stage I-II Breast Cancer: 20 Year Follow-Up of the EORTC 10801 Phase 3 Randomised Trial. *The Lancet Oncology*, **13**, 412-419. http://dx.doi.org/10.1016/S1470-2045(12)70042-6

[13]   NABON (2012) Breast Cancer, Dutch Guideline, Version 2.0. http://www.oncoline.nl/mammacarcinoom

[14]   Early Breast Cancer Trialists' Collaborative Group (1998) Polychemotherapy for Early Breast Cancer: An Overview of the Randomised Trials. *The Lancet*, **352**, 930-942. http://dx.doi.org/10.1016/S0140-6736(98)03301-7

[15]   Vervoort, M., Draisma, G., Fracheboud, J., Poll-Franse, L. and de Koning, H. (2004) Trends in the Usage of Adjuvant Systemic Therapy for Breast Cancer in the Netherlands and Its Effect on Mortality. *British Journal of Cancer*, **91**, 242-247. http://dx.doi.org/10.1038/sj.bjc.6601969

[16]   Vos, E., Linn, S. and Rodenhuis, S. (2006) Effects and Costs of Adjuvant Chemotherapy for Operable Lymph Node Positive Breast Cancer with HER2/Neu Overexpression. *Nederlands Tijdschrift voor Geneeskunde*, **150**, 776-780.

[17]   Early Breast Cancer Trialists' Collaborative Group (2005) Effects of Chemotherapy and Hormonal Therapy for Early Breast Cancer on Recurrence and 15-Year Survival: An Overview of the Randomised Trials. *The Lancet*, **365**, 1687-1717. http://dx.doi.org/10.1016/S0140-6736(05)66544-0

[18]   Devilee, P., Tollenaar, R. and Cornelisse, C. (2012) From Gene to Disease; from BRCA1 or BRCA2 to Breast Cancer. *Nederlands Tijdschrift voor Geneeskunde*, **144**, 2549-2551.

[19]   Klitzman, R. and Chung, W. (2010) The Process of Deciding about Prophylactic Surgery for Breast and Ovarian Cancer: Patient Questions, Uncertainties, and Communication. *American Journal of Medical Genetics*, **152A**, 52-66. http://dx.doi.org/10.1002/ajmg.a.33068

[20]   Meijers-Heijboer, H., Brekelmans, C., Menke-Pluymers, M., Seynaeve, C., Baalbergen, A., Burger, C., *et al.* (2003) Use of Genetic Testing and Prophylactic Mastectomy and Oophorectomy in Women with Breast or Ovarian Cancer from Families with a *BRCA*1 or *BRCA*2 Mutation. *Journal of Clinical Oncology*, **21**, 1675-1681.

[21]   Rebbeck, T., Kauff, N. and Domchek, S. (2009) Meta-Analysis of Risk Reduction Estimates Associated with Risk-Reducing Salpingo-Oophorectomy in BRCA1 or BRCA2 Mutation Carriers. *Journal of the National Cancer Institute*, **101**, 80-87. http://dx.doi.org/10.1093/jnci/djn442

[22]   Domchek, S., Friebel, T., Neuhausen, S., Wagner, T., Evans, G., Isaacs, C., *et al.* (2006) Mortality after Bilateral Salpingo-Oophorectomy in BRCA1 and BRCA2 Mutation Carriers: A Prospective Cohort Study. *The Lancet Oncology*, **7**, 223-229. http://dx.doi.org/10.1016/S1470-2045(06)70585-X

[23]   Rebbeck, T., Friebel, T., Lynch, H., Neuhausen, S., van't Veer, L., Garber, J., *et al.* (2004) Bilateral Prophylactic Mas-

tectomy Reduces Breast Cancer Risk in BRCA1 and BRCA2 Mutation Carriers: The PROSE Study Group. *Journal of Clinical Oncology*, **22**, 1055-1062.

[24] Graves, K., Peshkin, B., Halbert, C., DeMarco, T., Isaacs, C. and Schwartz, M. (2007) Predictors and Outcomes of Contralateral Prophylactic Mastectomy among Breast Cancer Survivors. *Breast Cancer Research and Treatment*, **104**, 321-329. http://dx.doi.org/10.1007/s10549-006-9423-5

[25] Domchek, S., Friebel, T. and Singer, C. (2010) Association of Risk-Reducing Surgery in *BRCA*1 or *BRCA*2 Mutation Carriers with Cancer Risk and Mortality. *Japan Automobile Manufacturers Association*, **304**, 967-975. http://dx.doi.org/10.1001/jama.2010.1237

[26] Klaren, H., van't Veer, L., van Leeuwen, F. and Rookus, M. (2003) Potential for Bias in Studies on Efficacy of Prophylactic Surgery for *BRCA*1 and *BRCA*2 Mutation. *Journal of the National Cancer Institute*, **95**, 941-947. http://dx.doi.org/10.1093/jnci/95.13.941

[27] Pijpe, A., Manders, P., Brohet, R., Collée, J., Verhoef, S., Vasen, H., *et al*. (2010) Physical Activity and the Risk of Breast Cancer in BRCA1/2 Mutation Carriers. *Retreats—Breast Cancer Recovery*, **120**, 235-244. http://dx.doi.org/10.1007/s10549-009-0476-0

[28] Sukel, M., van de Poll-Franse, L., Nieuwenhuijzen, G., Vreugdenhil, G., Herings, R., Coebergh, J., *et al*. (2008) Substantial Increase in the Use of Adjuvant Systemic Treatment for Early Stage Breast Cancer Reflects Changes in Guidelines in the Period 1990-2006 in the Southeastern Netherlands. *European Journal of Cancer*, **44**, 1846-1854. http://dx.doi.org/10.1016/j.ejca.2008.06.001

[29] Mook, S., Schmidt, M., Rutgers, E., van de Velde, A., Visser, O., Rutgers, S., *et al*. (2009) Calibration and Discriminatory Accuracy of Prognosis Calculation for Breast Cancer with the Online Adjuvant! Program: A Hospital-Based Retrospective Cohort Study. *The Lancet Oncology*, **10**, 1070-1076. http://dx.doi.org/10.1016/S1470-2045(09)70254-2

[30] Bontenbal, M., van Putten, W., Burghouts, J., Baggen, M., Ras, G., Stiegelis, W., *et al*. (2000) Value of Estrogenic Recruitment before Chemotherapy: First Randomized Trial in Primary Breast Cancer. *Journal of Clinical Oncology*, **18**, 734.

[31] Council of the Dutch Federation of Medical Scientific Societies Code of Conduct for Medical Research. http://www.federa.org/sites/default/files/bijlagen/coreon/code_of_conduct_for_medical_research_1.pdf

[32] van den Broek, A., Schmidt, M., van't Veer, L., Tollenaar, R. and van Leeuwen, F (2015) Worse Breast Cancer Prognosis BRCA1/BRCA2 Mutation Carriers: What's the Evidence? A Systematic Review with Meta-Analysis. *PLoS ONE*, **10**, e0120189. http://dx.doi.org/10.1371/journal.pone.0120189

[33] Siesling, S., van de Poll-Franse, L.V., Jobsen, J.J., Repelaer van Driel, O.J. and Voogd, A.C. (2005) Trends and Variation in Breast Conserving Surgery in the Southeast and East of the Netherlands over the Period 1990-2002. *Nederlands Tijdschrift voor Geneeskunde*, **149**, 1941-1946.

[34] Bayraktar, S. and Glück, S. (2012) Systemic Therapy Options in BRCA Mutation-Associated Breast Cancer. Breast *Cancer Research and Treatment*, **135**, 355-366. http://dx.doi.org/10.1007/s10549-012-2158-6

[35] Kriege, M., Seynaeve, C., Meijers-Heijboer, H., Collee, J., Menke-Pluymers, M., Bartels, C., *et al*. (2009) Sensitivity to First-Line Chemotherapy for Metastatic Breast Cancer in *BRCA*1 and *BRCA*2 Mutation Carriers. *Journal of Clinical Oncology*, **27**, 3764-3771.

[36] van Steenbergen, L., Poll-Franse, L., Wouters, M., Jansen-Landheer, M., Coebergh, J., Struikmans, H., *et al*. (2010) Variation in Management of Early Breast Cancer in the Netherlands, 2003-2006. *European Journal of Surgical Oncology*, **36**, S36-S43. http://dx.doi.org/10.1016/j.ejso.2010.06.021

[37] Degner, L., Kristjanson, L., Bowman, D., Sloan, J., Carriere, K., O'Neil, J., *et al*. (1997) Information Needs and Decisional Preferences in Women with Breast Cancer. *Journal of the American Medical Association*, **277**, 1485-1492. http://dx.doi.org/10.1001/jama.1997.03540420081039

[38] Step, M., Siminoff, L. and Rose, J. (2009) Differences in Oncologist Communication across Age Groups and Contributions to Adjuvant Decision Outcomes. *Journal of the American Geriatrics Society*, **57**, S279-S282. http://dx.doi.org/10.1111/j.1532-5415.2009.02512.x

[39] Charles, C., Gafni, A. and Whelan, T. (2004) Self-Reported Use of Shared Decision-Making among Breast Cancer Specialists and Perceived Barriers and Facilitators to Implementing This Approach. *Health Expectations*, **7**, 338-348. http://dx.doi.org/10.1111/j.1369-7625.2004.00299.x

16

Expression of the Epidermal Growth Factor Receptors and Ligands in Paired Samples of Normal Breast Tissue, Primary Breast Carcinomas and Lymph Node Metastases

Anja Brügmann[1,2]*, V. Jensen[3], J. P. Garne[4], E. Nexo[2], B. S. Sorensen[2]

[1]Institute of Pathology, Aalborg Hospital, Aalborg, Denmark
[2]Department of Clinical Biochemistry, Aarhus University Hospital, Aarhus, Denmark
[3]Institute of Pathology, Aarhus University Hospital, Aarhus, Denmark
[4]Department of Breast Surgery, Aalborg Hospital, Aalborg, Denmark
Email: *ahb@rn.dk

Abstract

Purpose: In breast cancer, the EGF receptors host an increasing number of therapeutic targets and the interactive mechanisms of actions of the receptors and their ligands justify investigation of the EGF family as an entity. Experimental design: Paired tissue samples of normal breast tissue and primary breast carcinomas were examined in a prospective study of 163 patients. A third sample was obtained from the paired ipsilateral metastatic lymph node from 58 of these patients. The mRNA expression of four EGF receptors (HER1 - HER4) and 11 activating ligands was quantified with real-time RT-PCR. Results: Expression of HER2, HER3, and HER4 mRNA was upregulated in primary carcinomas compared to normal breast tissue while HER1 was downregulated. The mRNA expression of HER3 and HER4 differed between primary breast carcinomas and lymph node metastases whereas there was no difference in the expression of HER1 and HER2. The combination of low HER3 and low HER4 expression in the primary carcinoma was significantly more frequent in lymph node-negative patients as compared to lymph node positive patients. Distinct correlation patterns of the receptors and their corresponding activating ligands appeared in both normal breast tissue and in carcinomas, notably for the HER3 and HER4 receptors and their 3 specific ligands: HB-EGF, NRG2, and NRG4. Conclusion: HER2, HER3, and HER4 showed increased mRNA expression in carcinomas and were positively correlated to each other and to specific activating ligands. Furthermore, low HER3 and HER4 expression in the carcinomas correlated to the absence of lymph node metastases.

---

*Corresponding author.

Keywords

Breast Cancer, Lymph Node Metastases, EGF Receptors, EGF Ligands, RT-PCR

1. Introduction

In breast cancer, the family of epidermal growth factor (EGF) receptors is the target of an increasing number of therapeutic drugs [1] [2]. Traditionally, the biomarkers decisive for targeted treatment are evaluated in the primary breast carcinoma although the target is the metastatic cells and the minimal residual disease. Axillary lymph node metastases are the detectable clinical manifestation of metastatic cells.

The primary route for the metastatic spread of breast carcinoma is via the lymphatic system, and the axillary lymph node status remains the best prognostic factor [3] [4]. Assuming that the lymph node metastases represent a migrated fraction of the primary tumor cells, the metastatic cells would, conceivably, share an identical molecular profile [5]. Recent research has shown that the heterogeneity and clonal diversity seen in breast cancer contradict this notion [6]-[11].

In view of these findings, we analyzed the expression of all the human epidermal growth factor (EGF) receptors and their activating ligands in primary breast carcinoma and correlated it with their expression in the axillary lymph node metastasis and with normal breast tissue.

The EGF family comprises four structurally similar tyrosine kinases known as human epidermal growth factor receptor 1 to 4 (HER1-4). The receptors are abundant in numerous epithelia where their normal cell functions involve proliferation, differentiation, apoptosis, migration, and angiogenesis [1] [12]. In several epithelial cancers, including breast cancer, dysregulation of EGF receptors and their functions promotes carcinogenesis [13]-[15]. EGF receptors are transmembrane glycoproteins with an extracellular ligand-binding domain. The activating ligands are receptor specific [16]. The Epidermal growth factor (EGF), amphiregulin (AMPH), and transforming growth factor-α (TGF-α) activate HER1. Heparin-binding EGF-like growth factor (HB-EGF), epiregulin (EPR), and betacellulin (BTC) activate both HER1 and HER4. The neuregulins (NRG) activate HER3 and HER4 [17] [18]. HER2 has no activating ligand, but possesses a constitutively active conformation activated upon dimerization. Ligand binding facilitates hetero- or homodimerization between two EGF receptors. This dimerization leads to cross phosphorylation of intracellular tyrosine kinase domains, and docking sites for signaling proteins are created.

Conceptually, the complex and interactive mechanisms of actions of the EGFR family, justifies investigation of all four receptors of the EGF family as an entity [18]-[20] as a supplement to the studies describing the receptors individually. Comparative studies exist on the HER2 expression in the primary tumors, lymph node metastases, and distant metastases [21]-[24]. In these studies semi-quantitative methods were used and the samples collected at different time points during the disease, primarily from distant metastases. Overall HER2 tends to correlate well between primary tumors and metastatic sites but significant variations in discordance rates have been reported (2% - 27%) [25]. Cardoso *et al.* studied the correlation of HER2 in primary breast carcinoma and lymph node metastases in a large archival material (n = 370) [11]. In this study the overall percentage of discordant marker status was 2%; however, for the tumors that were lymph-node positive, 15% were negative in the primary tumor. The HER2 study by Santiago *et al.* of 52 breast carcinomas and matched axillary metastasis showed an 88.5% concordance using IHC and 98% using FISH [26]. They concluded that HER2 status is stable during axillary metastatic progression.

In this study, we made a point in determining correlation using a quantitative method (real-time RT-PCR) at the time of primary surgery. At this point in the time course of the disease, the clinical decisions regarding adjuvant therapies are taken for each individual patient. We correlated the expression of the EGF receptors and their ligands in paired samples of primary breast carcinomas and corresponding lymph node metastases. Furthermore, we investigated whether their expression in the primary carcinomas could predict the metastatic status of the axillary lymph node.

2. Materials and Methods

The Regional Ethics Committee Northern Jutland, Denmark, approved this prospective cohort study, and signed informed consent was obtained from each patient (N-20070047).

2.1. Patients

One hundred and seventy-nine women with primary operable breast cancer treated at the Department of Breast Surgery, Aalborg Hospital, participated in the study. Inclusion took place during the prevalent screening phase. Patients with a medical history of cancer and patients treated with neoadjuvant therapy were not included. Patients with multicentric cancers were excluded (n = 12). Furthermore, 4 patients were excluded because they had a noninvasive lesion (ductal carcinoma in situ) or the invasive focus was less than 3 mm. Tissue specimens were successfully examined in 163 patients (**Figure 1**). The clinicopathological characteristics of the cohort are listed in **Table 1**.

2.2. Tissue Specimens

Breast tissue specimens were obtained from primary breast cancer surgical procedures. The samples were prospectively collected from November 2008 to May 2010 from unfixed mastectomy or lumpectomy specimens. All tissue specimens were transported on ice from the operating room to the Institute of Pathology, Aalborg Hospital. The normal breast tissue, tumor specimens, and lymph node samples were all frozen in liquid nitrogen within a mean period of 40 (95% c.i.: 39 to 42 min, range 20 to 79) minutes after surgical removal. A pilot study performed on samples from 10 patients showed stable mRNA quantities of HER1-4 at 15, 30, and 60 minutes after surgical removal (unpublished data), and similar results have been published by Ohashi *et al.* [27].

Normal breast tissue was sampled during macroscopic pathoanatomical examination by experienced breast pathologists. The distance between the location for tumor sampling and normal breast tissue sampling was measured in the surgical resections (n = 158). The mean distance was 48 mm (95% c.i.: 43 to 53 mm, range: 4 to 150 mm).

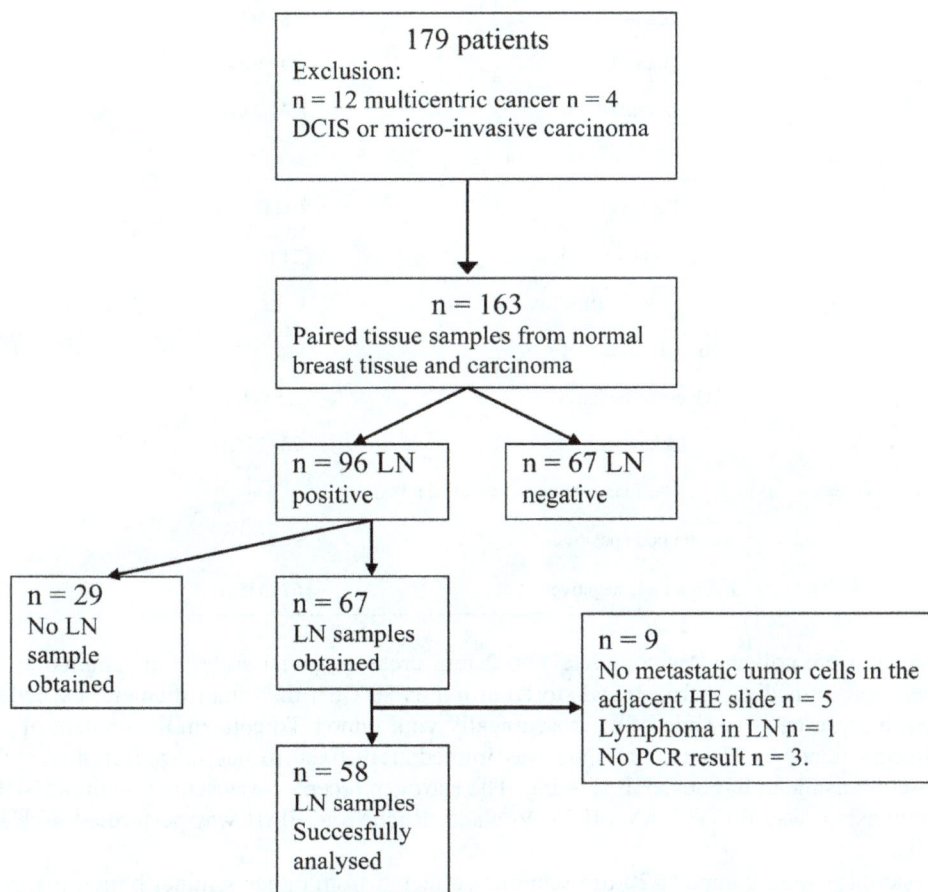

Figure 1. Flow diagram showing included and excluded patients with breast carcinoma, and lymph node status, and the tissue samples obtained. LN: Lymph node.

Table 1. Clinicopathological characteristics for 163 patients with breast carcinomas. Estrogen and HER2 status was determined by routine diagnostic immunohistochemistry/FISH (see methods section).

Total number of patients	163
Gender	Female
Age at diagnosis mean, (range) years	63 (32 - 85)
Histology, n (%)	
Invasive ductal carcinoma	129 (79%)
Invasive lobular carcinoma	23 (14%)
Other	11 (7%)
Tumor size, n (%)	
<20 mm	89 (55%)
20mm ≤ size < 50mm	70 (43%)
≥50mm	4 (2%)
Malignancy grade, n (%)	
Grade 1	53 (32%)
Grade 2	58 (36%)
Grade 3	49 (30%)
Not graded	3 (2%)
Estrogen receptor status, n (%)	
Positive	142 (87%)
Negative	21 (13%)
HER2 status, n (%)	
Normal expression	126 (77%)
Overexpression	15 (9%)
Unknown	22 (14%)
Axillary lymph node status, n (%)	
Lymph node positive	96 (59%)
Lymph node negative	67 (41%)

Tumor specimens were collected as complete 1 to 2 mm cross sectional slides and sampled at random into RNase free tubes, and immediately frozen and stored at minus 80°C. If the tumor diameter exceeded 5 cm, the pathologist chose a representative slide of macroscopically vital tumor. To confirm the content of invasive carcinoma, the adjacent tumor cross sectional slide was immediately fixed in neutral-buffered formalin and prepared for microscopy using an in-house HE staining. The estrogen receptor was stained with the SP1 clone. The IHC HER2 immunostain was PATHWAY (4B5), Ventana, Roche and FISH was performed with HER2 FISH pharmDx, DAKO.

Lymph node samples were complete 20-μm sections collected from either sentinel lymph nodes (n = 23) or axillary dissections (n = 35). The adjacent slide was used as a control to confirm the content of metastatic carcinoma.

2.3. RNA Extraction from Tissue Samples

Total RNA was extracted from frozen tissue samples by the principles described by Chomczynski and Sacchi [28]. Due to the adipose nature of breast tissue, optimal RNA extraction was performed using a lipid tissue kit (RNeasy Lipid Tissue Kit, Qiagen). Depending on the individual tissue sample weight, we used the RNeasy midi or mini kits following the manufacturer's instructions. In brief, the tissue samples were homogenized in QIAzol Lysis Reagent on ice. After incubation for 5 minutes at room temperature, 1 ml chloroform was admixed by shaking followed by 5 min centrifugation (5000 × g) at 4°C. The aqueous phase, now containing the RNA, was transferred to a fresh tube. An equal volume of 70% ethanol was added and the suspended RNA was transferred to an RNeasy spin column and centrifuged for 5 min at 5000 ×g. Flow-through was discarded and the membrane washed followed by centrifugation (5000 × g). While RNA remained bound to the RNeasy membrane, the DNA was removed by DNA digestion. The DNases were removed by buffer washings, each followed by centrifugation ensuring that no residual ethanol was carried over. In a fresh tube, the RNA was finally eluated in RNase free water with 2 centrifugations (5000 × g).

The yield of total RNA was determined by UV spectrophotometry (absorbance at 260 nm).

2.4. Reverse Transcription

cDNA was transcribed from the RNA extracted from the tissue samples using oligo (dT) priming. The HER2 analysis was a template specific fluorescent probe assay (taqman®).

A total RNA amount of 0.1 μg was reversely transcribed in a 20 μL reaction mixture containing 2 μL 10× PCR buffer (Applied Biosystems, Foster City, CA., USA), 5 μL MgCl$_2$ (6.3 mmol/L), 8 μL of deoxyribonucleoside triphosphates (dATP, dTTP, dGTP, and dCTP, 25 mmol/L), 2.5 mmol/L 16mer oligo dT nucleotide, 20 units RNase inhibitor (Applied Biosystems), 50 units reverse transcriptase (Applied Biosystems), and 1 μL nuclease free-water.

Reverse transcription was performed in a thermocycler (Gene Amp PCR system 9700, Applied Biosystems) at 42°C for 30 minutes followed by 98°C for 1 minute, and finally at 4°C for 5 minutes. The resulting cDNA was immediately used for RT-PCR, or stored at minus 20°C.

Analyses of all target genes were performed on the same cDNA preparation, thereby minimizing variation.

2.5. Real-Time PCR

The EGF system including HER1-4, CYT1-2, and their activating ligands and the household genes were quantified by real-time PCR with the primers and reaction conditions (**Table S1**). One μL of the cDNA was used as template and 5 μL Light Cycler 480 SYBR green I master mix (Roche Mannheim, GE) supplemented with 0.5 μL sense and antisense primers and probes (Primers and conditions as shown in **Table S1**). The volume was adjusted to 10 μL with nuclease-free water.

The samples were amplified in the Light Cycler 480 system (Roche, Light Cycler software, version 1.5.0), and PCR performed with an initial denaturation step at 95°C, immediately followed by annealing (annealing temperatures given in **Table S1**) for 15 seconds. Quantification was done with the second derivate max method by the Light Cycler software.

2.6. The Calibration Curve

The LightCycler software constructs calibration curves based on serial dilutions of the individual calibrators in water (calibrators listed in **Table S1**). The fitted regression line of the calibrator dilution provides the read of the sample concentration. The results are expressed relative to the mRNA content in the calibrator used for generating the calibration curve.

The interassay coefficient of variation (CV) for HER1-HER4 and HMBS was 7% - 12%, calculated for 10 real-time PCR runs. For CYT1 and CYT2 and the ligands, it was 4% - 28% in 10 runs.

2.7. Normalization

In order to standardize initial RNA quantities in different samples, an endogenous reference gene was used for normalization. We used the Microsoft Excel add-in application Norm Finder [29] to rank the gene expression stability of 5 household genes. Analyzing the 3 investigated tissue types, normal breast tissue, breast carcinoma, and lymph nodes, for 5 household genes enabled us to identify the most stable reference gene.

2.8. Identification of the Reference gene

To determine a stable expressed household gene we examined 85 samples from 35 patients comprising 35 normal specimens, 35 carcinomas, and 15 lymph node samples. The mRNA expressions of hydroxymethylbilane synthase (HMBS), β-Actin (ACTB), glyceraldehyde-3-phosphate dehydrogenase (GAPDH), tyrosine 3-monooxygenase/tryptophan 5-monooxygenase activation protein zeta polypeptide (YWHAZ) and beta-2-microglobulin (B2M) were quantified with real-time PCR. The household gene with the most stable expression was identified as HMBS with the NormFinder application [29]. The candidate genes are ranked by the NormFinder application according to their stability values. Based on the results, we employed HMBS as the reference gene for analyses of the EFG receptors and ligands.

2.9. Statistics

Data were analyzed using STATA version 10 (StataCorp LP, Texas, USA) and graphic statistic illustrations using GraphPad Prism 5 statistical software package (GraphPad Software Inc., San Diego, CA., USA). A non-parametric test was used to analyze the data. Two-sided P-values less than 0.05 were considered to be significant. Paired analyses of the paired samples were done by Wilcoxon matched-pairs signed-rank test. The correlations of the receptors and their ligands were performed by Spearman non-parametric correlation. Comparison of the lymph node-negative patients and the lymph node-positive patients was performed by Mann-Whitney U-test and Fisher's exact test.

3. Results

We examined the mRNA expressions of the four EGF receptors (HER1-HER4) including the 2 HER4 isomeric splicevariants (CYT1 and CYT2), and 11 of their activating ligands in paired samples of normal breast tissue and carcinoma specimens from 163 patients. In 58 of these patients a corresponding metastatic lymph node was obtained for analyses. The clinicopathological characteristics of the patients are described in **Table 1**.

3.1. The Receptors

There was a significant difference in mRNA expression of all four HER receptors comparing normal breast tissue with carcinoma. HER2, HER3, and HER4 (including the two isomeric splicevariants of HER4, CYT1 and CYT2 (data not shown)) were upregulated in carcinomas (**Figure 2**). In contrast, HER1 showed a significantly higher mRNA expression in the normal breast tissue specimens compared with the carcinomas.

The paired analyses of breast carcinoma versus lymph node metastases showed a significant difference regarding HER3 and HER4, whereas there was no difference in the expression of HER1 and HER2 between the 2 locations (**Figure 2**).

3.2. Receptor Correlations between the 3 Locations

The receptors were individually correlated between the 3 different locations from which the tissue samples had been obtained. Significant correlations between primary carcinoma and the lymph node metastases were found for all receptors except HER3 (**Table 2**). Between normal breast tissue and carcinoma, only HER1 showed a significant correlation.

3.3. Combinations of Receptors Were Correlated within the 3 Locations

The mRNA expressions of any combination of HER2, HER3, and HER4 were all highly significantly correlated (P < 0.05) in normal breast tissue as well as in carcinoma (**Table 3**), while any combinations of receptors involving HER1 did not show significant correlations.

Interestingly, in the lymph node metastases the expression of HER3-HER4 was the only receptor combination that showed a significant correlation.

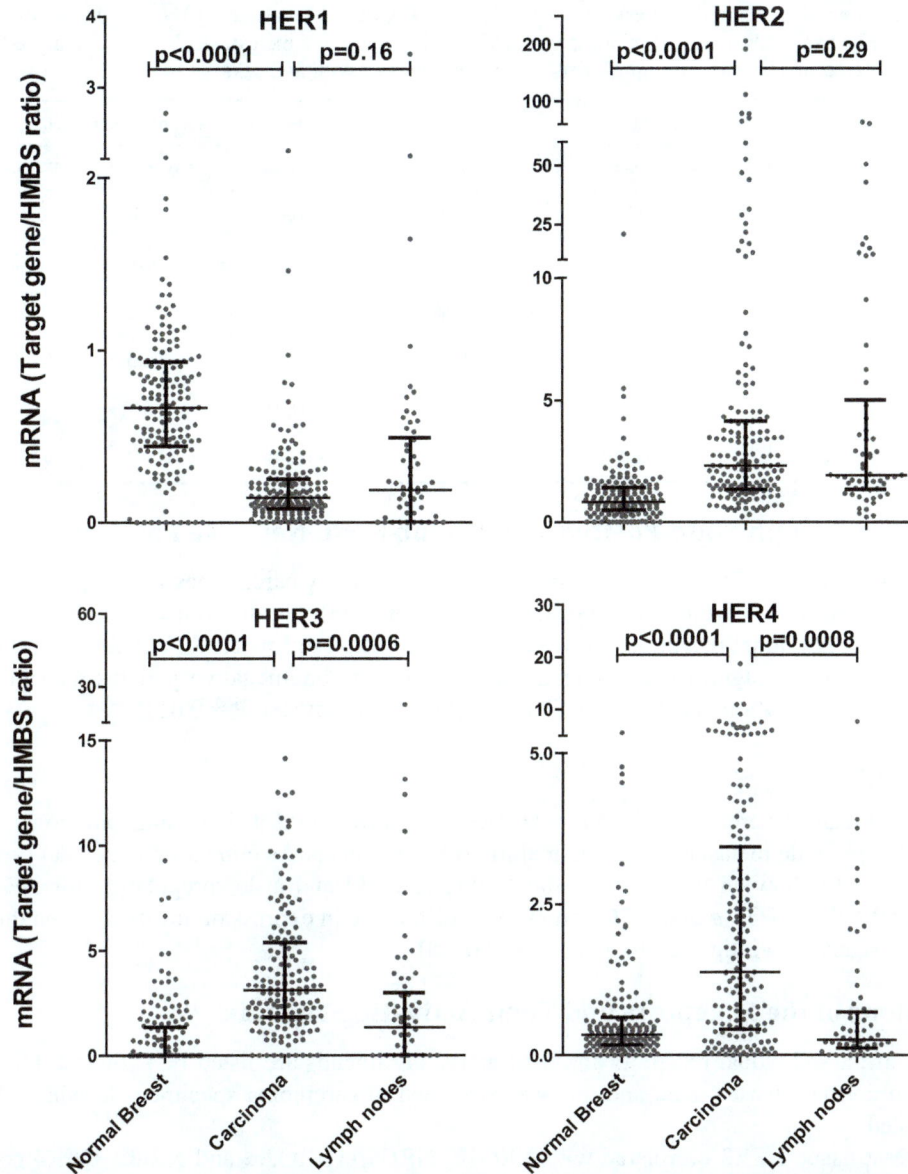

Figure 2. Paired expression of HER1–4 at 3 locations in breast cancer patients: Normal breast tissue (n = 163), breast carcinoma (n = 163), and lymph node metastases (n = 58). All data are the ratio of the target gene and the household gene, HMBS, given in arbitrary units. Medians with interquartile ranges are presented. P values were determined by Wilcoxon matched-pairs signed-rank test. Note: units are non-comparable between receptors.

Table 2. Correlations of the expression of the EGF receptors between the 3 locations by Spearman non-parametric correlation. Significant P values are marked with asterisks.

	Normal breast-carcinoma (n = 163)		Carcinoma-lymph node metastasis (n = 58)	
	Correlation	P value	Correlation	P value
HER1	0.19	0.013[*]	0.48	<0.0001[*]
HER2	0.083	0.29	0.58	<0.0001[*]
HER3	0.14	0.073	0.15	0.28
HER4	0.12	0.14	0.29	0.026[*]

Table 3. Correlations of the paired expressions of HER1-HER4 within 3 locations in breast cancer patients: Normal breast tissue (n = 163), breast carcinoma (n = 163), and lymph node metastases (n = 58). Analysed by Spearman non-parametric correlation. Significant P values are marked with asterisks.

	Normal breast tissue		Breast carcinoma		Lymph node metastases	
	Correlation	P value	Correlation	P value	Correlation	P value
HER1-HER2	0.085	0.28	−0.063	0.42	−0.12	0.36
HER1-HER3	−0.007	0.93	0.079	0.31	0.16	0.22
HER1-HER4	0.012	0.88	0.020	0.80	0.12	0.35
HER2-HER3	0.39	<0.0001*	0.28	0.0003*	0.23	0.081
HER2-HER4	0.49	<0.0001*	0.16	0.041*	0.062	0.64
HER3-HER4	0.47	<0.0001*	0.50	<0.0001*	0.54	<0.0001*

3.4. Receptors in Lymph Node-Positive and Lymph Node-Negative Patients

We explored the difference in EGF receptor expressions in the primary carcinomas for lymph node-negative patients (n = 67) as compared to lymph node-positive patients (n = 96). No difference was observed between the groups for any of the individual receptors. However, the combination of low HER3 and low HER4 expression in the primary carcinoma was significantly more frequent in lymph node-negative patients than in lymph node-positive patients, the distribution is indicated in **Table 4** (Fisher's exact test, P = 0.011).

3.5. The Ligands

We observed significant different expression levels between normal breast tissue and carcinoma, and between carcinoma and lymph node metastases, for the majority of the ligands. As compared to normal breast tissue we found breast tumors to show an upregulation for AMPH and EPI and a downregulation for HB-EGF and all neuregulins except NRG3. TGF-α and NRG3 showed no difference in expression levels between the 3 locations.

Data for all the ligands investigated are given in **Figure S1**.

3.6. Correlations of the Receptors and Their Activating Ligands

The correlation of the individual receptors and their activating ligands are listed in **Table S2**. HER1 correlated with HB-EGF in normal breast tissue, and this was also seen in carcinoma specimens in which AMPH/HER1 was also correlated.

In normal breast tissue HER3 correlated with NRG1α, NRG1β, NRG2α, and NRG3. HER4 correlated with NRG1α, NRG1β, NRG2α, NRG2β, and NRG3.

In carcinoma both HER3 and HER4 correlated with NRG2α and NRG4. Additionally, HER4 correlated with HB-EGF and NRG2β.

Notably, we could demonstrate correlation patterns for the ligands in both normal breast tissue and in the carcinoma. As a HER1 and HER4 activator, HB-EGF proved to be correlated to HER1 in both locations, even though HER1 showed a low mRNA expression in carcinomas. Furthermore, HB-EGF and HER4 correlations appeared in the carcinomas. Likewise, NRG2α and NRG4 remained correlated to both of the 2 receptors that these ligands can activate (HER3 and HER4), and for HER4 the NRG2β correlation was also retained.

The correlations of NRG1α, 1β, and NGR3 with both HER3 and HER4 were not repeated in the carcinoma specimens or in the metastatic lymph nodes.

4. Discussion

In this prospective cohort study of tissue samples from breast cancer patients, we have investigated the expression patterns of receptors and ligands of the EGF system. Comparison of normal breast tissue and carcinoma showed a significant upregulation in the mRNA expression of HER2, HER3, and HER4, whereas HER1 was downregulated in carcinomas. HER2 and HER3 mRNA overexpression in carcinomas is supported by previous

Table 4. Distribution of patients with the combination of low mRNA expression of HER3/HER4 and their lymph node status in patients with breast cancer (n=163). *Fisher's exact test (P = 0.011).

	Low HER3 and low HER4		
	Low	High	Total
+LN metastases	25	71	96*
−LN metastases	31	36	67*
Total	56	107	163

reports describing co-expression, high prevalence, and potent mitogenic signaling of this particular heterodimer in breast cancer [31]-[33]. HER3 stands out as the only EGF receptor lacking intracellular tyrosine kinase activity, but recent evidence from experimental models suggest that its non-catalytic functions are critical for cancers driven by the EGF receptor partners [34] [35]. Therefore, the importance of HER3 is being revisited [36] [37]. In a study of 278 tissue samples from breast cancer patients correlating IHC and FISH to survival, Sassen *et al.* found HER3 to have a negative impact on disease-free survival [19]. We confirm that HER2 and HER3 are overexpressed and significantly co-expressed in breast carcinomas; a prerequisite to be the most prevalent heterodimer [38]. Also, HER3 was significantly correlated to the mRNA expression of the HER3 activating ligands, NRG2α and NRG4, in breast carcinoma. Considering this to indicate a high protein expression of both receptors and ligands these findings imply that an active signaling network using these 2 ligands and HER2 and HER3 is present.

We report HER4 overexpression in primary carcinomas, in accord with previous results [33]. The functional significance of this is controversial [39]. The HER4 receptor appears to possess divergent functions demonstrated *in vitro* to depend on the isoform of the receptor [40] [41]. The HER4 response can also depend on the activating ligand [42], or the localization in the cell compartments (membrane bound, cytoplasmatic or in the nucleus) [43]. Changes in HER4 expression during the metastatic process [10] [44] lead to the conclusion that the HER4 receptor is adaptable and that the cell response can be different depending on the stimuli.

The HER1 receptor was the only of the EGF receptors in our study that showed a lower expression in the carcinomas compared with the normal breast tissue. Low HER1 mRNA expression in breast carcinoma has also been reported by Witton *et al.* [33]. Witton reports that patients with mRNA overexpression of HER1 and a HER1 positive IHC staining (16% of all cases) had reduced overall survival. The role of HER1 as a carcinogenic driver in breast cancer is well established [45] but the apparent carcinoma downregulation and presumed alternation in function has yet to be explored.

Our paired analyses between primary carcinoma and lymph node metastases showed that HER1 and HER2 were not significantly altered in expression but highly correlated. These findings provide important support for the current clinical practice for evaluating HER2 in the primary breast carcinomas on the assumptions that the protein expressions are identical to those in the minimal residual disease. In other words, the targets of the postoperative adjuvant therapy with Herceptin and Lapatinib are assumed to be present in the minimal residual disease when overexpressed in the primary carcinoma. Obviously this conclusion based on our quantitative mRNA measurements will have to be further validated in clinical trials.

Although, the mRNA expression of HER3 and HER4 are significantly lower in normal breast tissue than in the primary carcinoma, the expression of the receptors are significantly correlated at both sites. Interestingly, this correlation pattern of HER3 and HER4 was the only one to reoccur in the lymph node metastases. Combined with the mRNA expressions of the HER3 and HER4 activating ligands we describe plausible transformations of the EGF system during neoplastic progression.

The carcinomas maintain and increase several of the EGF expression patterns of normal breast tissue (**Figure 2** and **Table 2**). Only bipotent ligands (HB-EGF, NRG2α, 2β, and NRG4) capable of activating more than one receptor type and AMPH (the only ligand showing a highly significant increase in mRNA expression (**Figure S1**)) correlated to the receptors they activate in breast cancer. These findings regarding HB-EGF, AMPH, and NRG2 expression in breast cancer concur with the ligand study by Révillion *et al.* [46], but the correlation to the receptors they can activate has not been described previously.

The numerous described characteristics of normal breast tissue that are also seen in carcinoma specimens are not present in the lymph node metastases, with the exception of the HER3-HER4 correlation. The expression levels of the neuregulins cover a considerably wider range in the lymph node metastases than in the carcinomas, exemplified by NRG2α and NRG3 in **Figure S1**. We assume that in the lymph node metastases the activating ligands would either come from the tumor cells or from the blood supply because stromal cells are not always present. The alterations of the expression of the EGF system in the lymph node metastases point to the carcinoma surroundings as the most obvious physical difference between the carcinoma of the breast and the lymph node metastases. Stromal-epithelial interactions are characteristic of breast carcinomas, but juxtacrine signaling mechanisms are also a possible alternative way of receptor activation [47].

The expression of the individual EGF receptors in the primary tumor could not discriminate lymph node-positive patients from lymph node-negative patients. However, the combination of low expression of HER3 and HER4 in the primary carcinomas could distinguish the 2 groups. The combination of low HER3 and HER4 expression in the primary carcinoma was significantly more frequent in lymph node-negative patients than in lymph node-positive patients, and we interpret this as a positive prognostic indicator. On the other hand, in the primary carcinoma HER3 and HER4 could promote tumor growth by ligand specific activation of NRG2α and NRG4.

In conclusion, HER2, HER3, and HER4 showed increased mRNA expression in carcinoms and were positively correlated to each other and to specific activating ligands. The combination of low HER3 and low HER4 expression in the primary carcinoma was significantly more frequent in lymph node-negative patients as compared to lymph node positive patients.

Conflicts of Interest

The authors declare that they have no conflict of interest.

Acknowledgments

The authors thank Ann Skjødt Pedersen and Birgit Nielsen, Institute of Pathology, Aalborg Hospital, and Lene Dabelstein Petersen and Birgit Westh Mortensen, Department of Clinical Biochemistry, Aarhus University Hospital, for their excellent technical assistance.

The dedication of the breast team surgeons has been exceptional; our appreciation goes to Liselotte Jeppesen, Karen Haugaard and Hanne Bygbjerg and the staffs at the breast surgery ward and in the operating room.

Grant Support

Breast Friends, Roche; Region Midtjyllands Health Research Foundation; Henny Sophie Clausen og Møbelarkitekt Axel Clausens Foundation; Nordjyllands Lægekredsforenings Research Foundation; Aalborg Hospital Foundation for Young Doctors; Danish Agency for Science, Technology and Innovation; Grant from North Denmark Region; Ebba og Aksel Shølins Foundation; Dr. Heinrich Kopp's Grant.

References

[1] Zahnow, C.A. (2006) ErbB Receptors and Their Ligands in the Breast. *Expert Reviews in Molecular Medicine*, **23**, 1-21.

[2] Kalous, O., Conklin, D., Desai, A.J., O'Brien, N.A., Ginther, C., Anderson, L., *et al.* (2012) Dacomitinib (PF-00299804), an Irreversible Pan-HER Inhibitor, Inhibits Proliferation of HER2-Amplified Breast Cancer Cell Lines Resistant to Trastuzumab and Lapatinib. *Molecular Cancer Therapeutics*, **9**, 1978-1987.
http://dx.doi.org/10.1158/1535-7163.MCT-11-0730

[3] McGuire, W.L. (1987) Prognostic Factors for Recurrence and Survival in Human Breast Cancer. *Breast Cancer Research and Treatment*, **1**, 5-9. http://dx.doi.org/10.1007/BF01806129

[4] Carter, C.L., Allen, C. and Henson, D.E. (1989) Relation of Tumor Size, Lymph Node Status, and Survival in 24, 740 Breast Cancer Cases. *Cancer*, **1**, 181-187.
http://dx.doi.org/10.1002/1097-0142(19890101)63:1<181::AID-CNCR2820630129>3.0.CO;2-H

[5] Li, J., Gromov, P., Gromova, I., Moreira, J.M., Timmermans-Wielenga, V., Rank, F., *et al.* (2008) Omics-Based Profiling of Carcinoma of the Breast and Matched Regional Lymph Node Metastasis. *Proteomics*, **23-24**, 5038-5052.
http://dx.doi.org/10.1002/pmic.200800303

[6] Santinelli, A., Pisa, E., Stramazzotti, D. and Fabris, G. (2008) HER-2 Status Discrepancy between Primary Breast Cancer And Metastatic Sites. Impact on target therapy. *International Journal of Cancer*, **5**, 999-1004.

[7] Vecchi, M., Confalonieri, S., Nuciforo, P., Vigano, M.A., Capra, M., Bianchi, M., *et al.* (2008) Breast Cancer Metastases Are Molecularly Distinct from their Primary Tumors. *Oncogene*, **15**, 2148-2158. http://dx.doi.org/10.1038/sj.onc.1210858

[8] Feng, Y., Sun, B., Li, X., Zhang, L., Niu, Y., Xiao, C., *et al.* (2007) Differentially Expressed Genes between Primary Cancer and Paired Lymph Node Metastases Predict Clinical Outcome of Node-Positive Breast Cancer Patients. *Breast Cancer Research and Treatment*, **3**, 319-329. http://dx.doi.org/10.1007/s10549-006-9385-7

[9] Pandit, T.S., Kennette, W., Mackenzie, L., Zhang, G., Al-Katib, W., Andrews, J., *et al.* (2009) Lymphatic Metastasis of Breast Cancer Cells Is Associated with Differential Gene Expression Profiles That Predict Cancer Stem Cell-Like Properties and the Ability to Survive, Establish and Grow in a Foreign Environment. *International Journal of Oncology*, **2**, 297-308.

[10] Fuchs, I.B., Siemer, I., Buhler, H., Schmider, A., Henrich, W., Lichtenegger, W., *et al.* (2006) Epidermal Growth Factor Receptor Changes during Breast Cancer Metastasis. *Anticancer Research*, **6B**, 4397-4401.

[11] Cardoso, F., Di, L.A., Larsimont, D., Gancberg, D., Rouas, G., Dolci, S., *et al.* (2001) Evaluation of HER2, p53, bcl-2, Topoisomerase II-Alpha, Heat Shock Proteins 27 and 70 in Primary Breast Cancer and Metastatic Ipsilateral Axillary Lymph Nodes. *Annals of Oncology*, **5**, 615-620. http://dx.doi.org/10.1023/A:1011182524684

[12] Stern, D.F. (2003) ErbBs in Mammary Development. *Experimental Cell Research*, **1**, 89-98. http://dx.doi.org/10.1016/S0014-4827(02)00103-9

[13] Paez, J.G., Janne, P.A., Lee, J.C., Tracy, S., Greulich, H., Gabriel, S., *et al.* (2004) EGFR Mutations in Lung Cancer, Correlation with Clinical Response to Gefitinib Therapy. *Science*, **5676**, 1497-1500. http://dx.doi.org/10.1126/science.1099314

[14] Bang, Y.J, Van, C.E., Feyereislova, A., Chung, H.C., Shen, L., Sawaki, A., *et al.* (2010) Trastuzumab in Combination with Chemotherapy versus Chemotherapy Alone for Treatment of HER2-Positive Advanced Gastric or Gastro-Oesophageal Junction Cancer (ToGA): a Phase 3, Open-Label, Randomised Controlled Trial. *Lancet*, **9742**, 687-697. http://dx.doi.org/10.1016/S0140-6736(10)61121-X

[15] Siena, S., Sartore-Bianchi, A., Di, N.F., Balfour, J. and Bardelli, A. (2009) Biomarkers Predicting Clinical Outcome of Epidermal Growth Factor Receptor-Targeted Therapy in Metastatic Colorectal Cancer. *Journal of the National Cancer Institute*, **19**, 1308-1324. http://dx.doi.org/10.1093/jnci/djp280

[16] Riese, D.J. and Stern, D.F. (1998) Specificity within the EGF Family/ErbB Receptor Family Signaling Network. *Bioessays*, **1**, 41-48. http://dx.doi.org/10.1002/(SICI)1521-1878(199801)20:1<41::AID-BIES7>3.0.CO;2-V

[17] Citri, A. and Yarden, Y. (2006) EGF-ERBB Signalling: Towards the Systems Level. *Nature Reviews Molecular Cell Biology*, **7**, 505-516. http://dx.doi.org/10.1038/nrm1962

[18] Wilson, K.J., Gilmore, J.L., Foley, J., Lemmon, M.A. and Riese, D.J. (2009) Functional Selectivity of EGF Family Peptide Growth Factors: Implications for Cancer. *Pharmacology & Therapeutics*, **1**, 1-8. http://dx.doi.org/10.1016/j.pharmthera.2008.11.008

[19] Sassen, A., Rochon, J., Wild, P., Hartmann, A., Hofstaedter, F., Schwarz, S., *et al.* (2008) Cytogenetic Analysis of HER1/EGFR, HER2, HER3 and HER4 in 278 Breast Cancer Patients. *Breast Cancer Research*, **1**, R2. http://dx.doi.org/10.1186/bcr1843

[20] McIntyre, E., Blackburn, E., Brown, P.J., Johnson, C.G. and Gullick, W.J. (2010) The Complete Family of Epidermal Growth Factor Receptors and Their Ligands Are Co-Ordinately Expressed in Breast Cancer. *Breast Cancer Research and Treatment*, **1**, 105-110. http://dx.doi.org/10.1007/s10549-009-0536-5

[21] Carlsson, J., Nordgren, H, Sjostrom, J., Wester, K., Villman, K. and Bengtsson, N.O., *et al.* (2004) HER2 Expression in Breast Cancer Primary Tumours and Corresponding Metastases. Original Data and Literature Review. *British Journal of Cancer*, **12**, 2344-2348.

[22] Gancberg, D., Di, L.A., Cardoso, F., Rouas, G., Pedrocchi, M. and Paesmans, M., *et al.* (2002) Comparison of HER-2 Status between Primary Breast Cancer and Corresponding Distant Metastatic Sites. *Annals of Oncology*, **7**, 1036-1043. http://dx.doi.org/10.1093/annonc/mdf252

[23] Gong, Y., Booser, D.J. and Sneige, N. (2005) Comparison of HER-2 Status Determined by Fluorescence *in Situ* Hybridization in Primary and Metastatic Breast Carcinoma. *Cancer*, **9**, 1763-1769. http://dx.doi.org/10.1002/cncr.20987

[24] Tapia, C., Savic, S., Wagner, U., Schonegg, R., Novotny, H. and Grilli, B., *et al.* (2007) HER2 Gene Status in Primary Breast Cancers and Matched Distant Metastases. *Breast Cancer Research*, **3**, 31. http://dx.doi.org/10.1186/bcr1676

[25] Zidan, J., Dashkovsky, I., Stayerman, C., Basher, W., Cozacov, C. and Hadary, A. (2005) Comparison of HER-2 Overexpression in Primary Breast Cancer and Metastatic Sites and Its Effect on Biological Targeting Therapy of Me-

tastatic Disease. *British Journal of Cancer*, **5**, 552-556. http://dx.doi.org/10.1038/sj.bjc.6602738

[26] Santiago, M.P., Vazquez-Boquete, A., Fernandez, B., Masa, C., Antunez, J.R. and Fraga, M., *et al.* (2009) Whether to Determine HER2 Status for Breast Cancer in the Primary Tumour or in the Metastasis. *Histology and Histopathology*, **6**, 675-682.

[27] Ohashi, Y., Creek, K.E., Pirisi, L., Kalus, R. and Young, S.R. (2004) RNA Degradation in Human Breast Tissue after Surgical Removal: A Time-Course Study. *Experimental and Molecular Pathology*, **2**, 98-103. http://dx.doi.org/10.1016/j.yexmp.2004.05.005

[28] Chomczynski, P. and Sacchi, N. (1987) Single-Step Method of RNA Isolation by Acid Guanidinium Thiocyanate-Phenol-Chloroform Extraction. *Analytical Biochemistry*, **1**, 156-159. http://dx.doi.org/10.1016/0003-2697(87)90021-2

[29] Andersen, C.L., Jensen, J.L. and Orntoft, T.F. (2004) Normalization of Real-Time Quantitative Reverse Transcription-PCR Data: A Model-Based Variance Estimation Approach to Identify Genes Suited for Normalization, Applied to Bladder and Colon Cancer Data Sets. *Cancer Research*, **15**, 5245-5250. http://dx.doi.org/10.1158/0008-5472.CAN-04-0496

[30] Holbro, T., Beerli, R.R., Maurer, F., Koziczak, M., Barbas III, C.F. and Hynes, N.E. (2003) The ErbB2/ErbB3 Heterodimer Functions as an Oncogenic Unit: ErbB2 Requires ErbB3 to Drive Breast Tumor Cell Proliferation. *Proceedings of National Academy of Science of the United States of America*, **15**, 8933-8938. http://dx.doi.org/10.1073/pnas.1537685100

[31] Gasparini, G., Gullick, W.J., Maluta, S., Dalla, P.P., Caffo, O. and Leonardi, E., *et al.* (1994) c-*erb*B-3 and c-*erb*B-2 Protein Expression in Node-Negative Breast Carcinoma—An Immunocytochemical Study. *European Journal of Cancer*, **1**, 16-22. http://dx.doi.org/10.1016/S0959-8049(05)80010-3

[32] Travis, A., Pinder, S.E., Robertson, J.F., Bell, J.A., Wencyk, P. and Gullick, W.J., *et al.* (1996) C-erbB-3 in Human Breast Carcinoma: Expression and Relation to Prognosis and Established Prognostic Indicators. *British Journal of Cancer*, **2**, 229-233. http://dx.doi.org/10.1038/bjc.1996.342

[33] Witton, C.J., Reeves, J.R., Going, J.J., Cooke, T.G. and Bartlett, J.M. (2003) Expression of the HER1-4 Family of Receptor Tyrosine Kinases in Breast Cancer. *The Journal of Pathology*, **3**, 290-297. http://dx.doi.org/10.1002/path.1370

[34] Amin, D.N., Campbell, M.R. and Moasser, M.M. (2010) The Role of HER3, the Unpretentious Member of the HER Family, in Cancer Biology and Cancer Therapeutics. *Seminars in Cell & Developmental Biology*, **9**, 944-950. http://dx.doi.org/10.1016/j.semcdb.2010.08.007

[35] Garrett, J.T., Olivares, M.G., Rinehart, C., Granja-Ingram, N.D., Sanchez, V. and Chakrabarty, A., *et al.* (2011) Transcriptional and Posttranslational Up-Regulation of HER3 (ErbB3) Compensates for Inhibition of the HER2 Tyrosine Kinase. *Proceedings of National Academy of Science of the United States of America*, **12**, 5021-5026. http://dx.doi.org/10.1073/pnas.1016140108

[36] Garrett, J.T., Sutton, C.R., Kuba, M.G., Cook, R.S. and Arteaga, C.L. (2013) Dual Blockade of HER2 in HER2-Overexpressing Tumor Cells Does Not Completely Eliminate HER3 Function. *Clinical Cancer Research*, **3**, 610-619. http://dx.doi.org/10.1158/1078-0432.CCR-12-2024

[37] Vaught, D.B., Stanford, J.C., Young, C., Hicks, D.J., Wheeler, F. and Rinehart, C., *et al.* (2012) HER3 is Required for HER2-Induced Preneoplastic Changes to the Breast Epithelium and Tumor Formation. *Cancer Research*, **10**, 2672-2682. http://dx.doi.org/10.1158/0008-5472.CAN-11-3594

[38] Citri, A., Skaria, K.B. and Yarden, Y. (2003) The Deaf and the Dumb: The Biology of ErbB-2 and ErbB-3. *Experimental Cell Research*, **1**, 54-65. http://dx.doi.org/10.1016/S0014-4827(02)00101-5

[39] Earp III, H.S., Calvo, B.F. and Sartor, C.I. (2003) The EGF Receptor Family—Multiple Roles in Proliferation, Differentiation, and Neoplasia with an Emphasis on HER4. *Transactions of the American Clinical and Climatological Association*, 315-333.

[40] Jones, F.E. (2008) HER4 Intracellular Domain (4ICD) Activity in the Developing Mammary Gland and Breast Cancer. *Journal of Mammary Gland Biology and Neoplasia*, **2**, 247-258. http://dx.doi.org/10.1007/s10911-008-9076-6

[41] Muraoka-Cook, R.S., Sandahl, M.A., Strunk, K.E., Miraglia, L.C., Husted, C. and Hunter, D.M., *et al.* (2009) ErbB4 Splice Variants Cyt1 and Cyt2 Differ by 16 Amino Acids and Exert Opposing Effects on the Mammary Epithelium *in Vivo*. *Molecular and Cellular Biology*, **18**, 4935-4948.

[42] Sartor, C.I., Zhou, H., Kozlowska, E., Guttridge, K., Kawata, E. and Caskey, L., *et al.* (2001) Her4 Mediates ligand-Dependent Antiproliferative and Differentiation Responses in Human Breast Cancer Cells. *Molecular and Cellular Biology*, **13**, 4265-4675.

[43] Thor, A.D., Edgerton, S.M. and Jones, F.E. (2009) Subcellular Localization of the HER4 Intracellular Domain, 4ICD, Identifies Distinct Prognostic Outcomes for Breast Cancer Patients. *American Journal of Pathology*, **5**, 1802-1809.

[44] Das, P.M., Thor, A.D., Edgerton, S.M., Barry, S.K., Chen, D.F. and Jones, F.E. (2010) Reactivation of Epigenetically

Silenced HER4/ERBB4 Results in Apoptosis of Breast Tumor Cells. *Oncogene*, **37**, 5214-5219.

[45] Foley, J., Nickerson, N.K., Nam, S., Allen, K.T., Gilmore, J.L. and Nephew, K.P., *et al.* (2010) EGFR Signaling in Breast Cancer: Bad to the Bone. *Seminars in Cell & Developmental Biology*, **9**, 951-960.

[46] Revillion, F., Lhotellier, V., Hornez, L., Bonneterre, J. and Peyrat, J.P. (2008) ErbB/HER Ligands in Human Breast Cancer, and Relationships with Their Receptors, the Bio-Pathological Features and Prognosis. *Annals of Oncology*, **1**, 73-80.

[47] Dong, J., Opresko, L.K., Chrisler, W., Orr, G., Quesenberry, R.D. and Lauffenburger, D.A., *et al.* (2005) The Membrane-Anchoring Domain of Epidermal Growth Factor Receptor Ligands Dictates Their Ability to Operate in Juxtacrine Mode. *Molecular Biology of the Cell*, **6**, 2984-2998.

Supplementary Tables and Figures

Table S1. Primers and conditions used for RT-PCR of EGF receptors and ligands.

Assay	Forward	Reverse	Primer conc./Annealing temp	Amp. size	Cali-brator
HER1	5'-GAG AAC GCC TCC CTC A-3'	5'-GGT ACT CGT CGG CAT C-3'	5 pmol/54°C	261 bp	HCV
HER2*	5'-CCA GGA CCT GCT GAA CTG GT-3'	5'-TGT ACG AGC CGC ACA TCC-3'	5 pmol/59°C	209 bp	HCV
HER3	5'-GGT GCT GGG CTT GCT TTT-3'	5'-CGT GGC TGG AGT TGG TGT TA-3'	5 pmol/65°C	365 bp	HEC1A
HER4	5'-ACA GCA GTA CCG AGC CTT TGC G-3'	5'-GCC ACT AAC ACG TAG CCT GTG AC-3'	5 pmol/64°C	141 bp	KLE
CYT1	5'-GAT GAT CGT ATG AAG CTT CCC A-3'	5'-AGG AGG AGG GCT GTG TC-3'	5 pmol/60°C	221 bp	CYT1
CYT2	5'-GAT GAT CGT ATG AAG CTT CCC A-3'	5'-CGG TAT ACA AAC TGG TTC CTA TTC-3'	5 pmol/60°C	194 bp	CYT2
EGF	5'-GAC TTG GGA GCC TGA GCA GAA-3'	5'-CAT GCA CAA GTG TGA CTG GAG GT-3'	5 pmol/66°C	90 bp	KLE
HB-EGF	5'-GGT GGT GCT GAA GCT CTT TC-3'	5'-CCC CTT GCC TTT CTT CTT TC-3'	5 pmol/61°C	282 bp	HCV
TGF-α	5'-GCC CGC CCG TAA AAT GGT CCC CTC-3'	5'-GTC CAC CTG GCC AAA CTC CTC CTG G-3'	5 pmol/70°C	528 bp	HCV
Epiregulin	5'-AAA GTG TAG CTC TGA CAT G-3'	5'-CTG TAC CAT CTG CAG AAA TA-3'	10 pmol/60°C	238 bp	KLE
Amphiregulin	5'-GGC TCA GGC CAT TAT GC-3'	5'-ACC TGT TCA ACT CTG ACT GA-3'	10 pmol/58°C	266 bp	HCV
NRG1-α	5'-ATC CAC CAC TGG GAC A-3'	5'-TTT GGA TCA TGG GCA-3'	5 pmol/60°C	179 bp	KLE
NRG1-β	5'-TAG GAA ATG ACA GTG CCT C-3'	5'-CGT AGT TTT GGC AGC GA-3'	5 pmol/65°C	321 bp	KLE
NRG2-α	5'-AAA TAT GGC AAC GGC AG-3'	5'-CGC AAA GGC AGT TTC T-3'	5 pmol/60°C	308 bp	RT4
NRG2-β	5'-GTC TTA CGT CAA CAG CG-3'	5'-CCG GTG TAT CCC ACA G-3'	5 pmol/63°C	236 bp	PANC
NRG3	5'-ACA GTG CAA GCG AAA AC-3'	5'-CAC TAT GAT ATG AGG GCG-3'	5 pmol/61°C	256 bp	KLE
NRG4	5'-CTG TTG TCT GCG GTA TTC-3'	5'-TCA TTC TTG GTC AAG AGA GT-3'	5 pmol/61°C	107 bp	RT4
HMBS	5'-CGG TAC CCA CGC GAA TCA C-3'	5'-GGG TAC CCA CGC GAA TCA C-3'	5 pmol/59°C	64 bp	HCV
GAPDH	5'-TGA TGA CAT CAA GAA GGT GGT GAA G-3'	5'-TCC TTG GAG GCC ATG TGG GCC AT-3'	5 pmol/68°C	240 bp	HCV
B2M	5'-TGA CTT TGT CAC AGC CCA AGA TA-3'	5'-AAT CCA AAT GCG GCA TCT TC-3'	15 pmol/64°C	84 bp	HCV
ACTB	5'-AGG GGC CGG ACT CGT CAT ACT-3'	5'-GGC GGC ACC ACC ATG TAC CCT-3'	10 pmol/68°C	202 bp	HCV
YWHAZ	5'-ACT TTT GGT ACA TTG TGG CTT CAA-3'	5'-CCG CCA GGA CAA ACC AGT AT-3'	5 pmol/59°C	71 bp	HCV

*The HER2 analysis was a template specific fluorescent probe 5'-CAG ATT GCC AAG GGG ATG AGC TAC CTG-3' (taqman®) 10 pmol. HCV (HCV29): Non-malignant bladder cancer cell line; HEC1A: Endometrial cancer cell line; KLE: Endometrial cancer cell line; CYT1: Human urothelial cancer cell line T24 transfected with the CYT1 variant of HER4; CYT2: Human urothelial cancer cell line T24 transfected with the CYT2 variant of HER4; RT4: Urothelial cell line; PANC (PANC1): Human pancreatic cancer cell line.

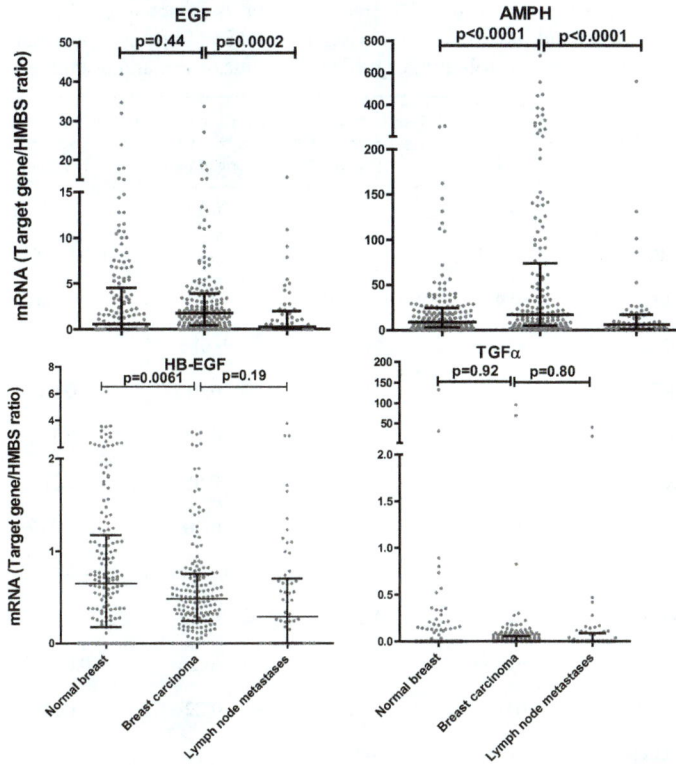

(a)

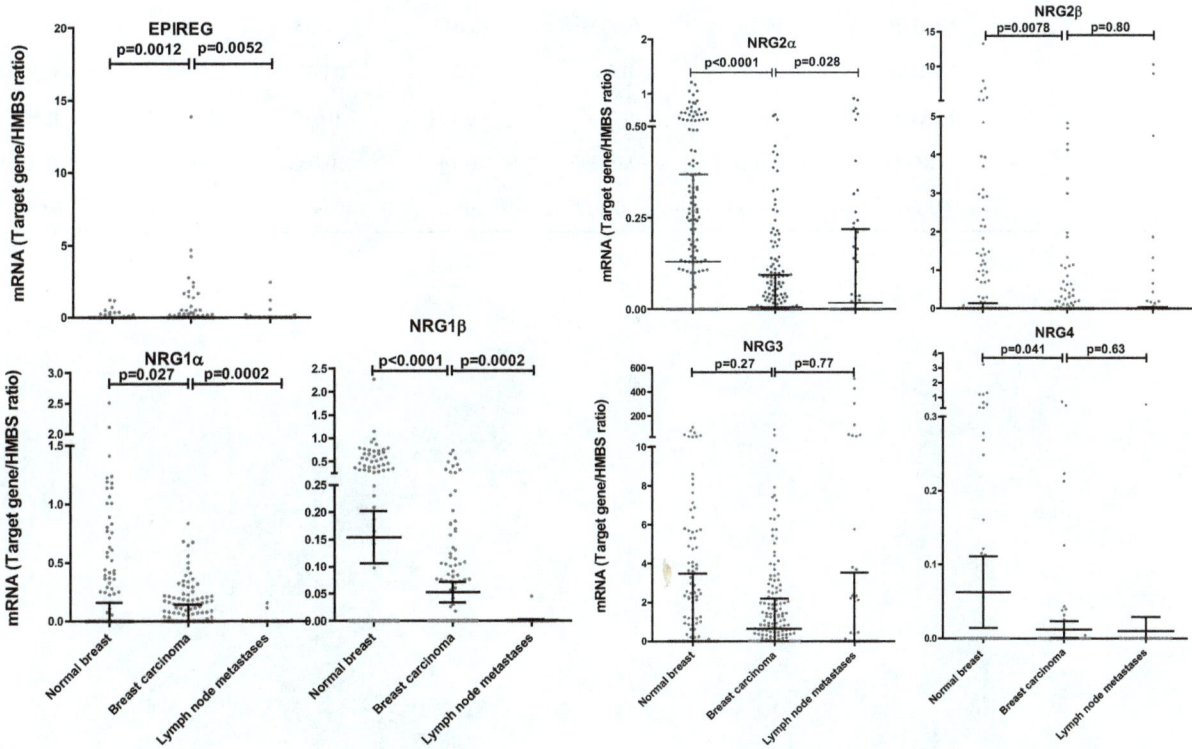

(b)   (c)

Figure S1. Expression of 11 EGFR family ligands in 3 locations in breast cancer patients: Normal breast tissue (n = 163), breast carcinoma (n = 163), and lymph node metastases (n = 58). All data are the ratio of the target gene and HMBS given in arbitrary units. Medians with interquartile ranges are presented. P values determined by Wilcoxon matched-pairs signed-rank test.

Table S2. Correlations of the expression of the EGF receptors and their activating ligands in normal breast tissue (n = 163, breast carcinomas (n = 163) and lymph node metastases (n = 58) of breast cancer patients. The correlations are determined by Spearman non-parametric correlation. Significant P values are marked with asterisks.

Receptor	Activating ligand	Normal breast tissue		Breast carcinoma		Lymph node metastases	
		Correlation	P value	Correlation	P value	Correlation	P value
HER1	EGF	−0.052	0.51	0.11	0.17	0.019	0.89
	AMPH	0.092	0.25	0.27	0.0005*	0.073	0.59
	HB-EGF	0.42	<0.0001*	0.43	<0.0001*	0.23	0.09
	TGF-α	−0.12	0.13	0.086	0.27	0.099	0.46
	EPIREG	0.025	0.75	−0.017	0.83	0.062	0.64
HER3	NRG1α	0.42	<0.0001*	0.12	0.11	0.11	0.42
	NRG1β	0.18	0.021*	−0.086	0.28	0.16	0.23
	NRG2α	0.23	0.0027*	0.20	0.011*	0.12	0.38
	NRG2β	0.011	0.89	0.061	0.44	−0.041	0.76
	NRG3	0.23	0.0036*	0.022	0.78	−0.071	0.59
	NRG4	−0.064	0.42	−0.26	0.0010*	0.14	0.29
HER4	HB-EGF	0.099	0.21	0.22	0.0048*	0.25	0.055
	EPIREG	0.15	0.054	0.11	0.17	−0.014	0.92
	NRG1α	0.23	0.0037*	0.11	0.16	−0.090	0.50
	NRG1β	0.20	0.0093*	0.047	0.55	0.13	0.33
	NRG2α	0.32	<0.0001*	0.24	0.0017*	0.14	0.30
	NRG2β	−0.19	0.017*	0.19	0.019*	−0.07	0.60
	NRG3	0.023	0.0029*	0.14	0.083	0.013	0.92
	NRG4	−0.073	0.36	−0.22	0.0046*	−0.22	0.096

17

Determinants of Malignant Transformation in Fibrocystic Disease of Breast

Ketan Vagholkar

Department of Surgery, Dr. D. Y. Patil Medical College, Navi Mumbai, India
Email: kvagholkar@yahoo.com

Abstract

Background: Fibrocystic disease of the breast in one of the commonest diseases in women above 30 years of age. The assumption of it being innocuous and benign is questionable with increased incidence of malignancies developing in these women. Introduction: Understanding the pathophysiology of fibrocystic disease is essential for identifying determinants of malignant change. Case Report: A case of carcinoma of breast developing in a longstanding and recurrent fibrocystic disease is reported. Discussion: The pathological changes including the influence of hormones on the natural history of the disease are discussed to identify the determinants of malignant transformation. Conclusion: Breast cyst fluid, patterns of cellular lining of the cysts, multiplicity, recurrence and patterns of cellular morphology are important determinants of malignant change.

Keywords

Fibrocystic Disease Breast Carcinoma

1. Introduction

Fibrocystic disease of breast is one of the commonest diseases affecting women in age group of 30 - 50 yrs. Traditionally the disease has always been described as benign in nature with very low or almost no potential to develop into a malignant lesion. However, studies now reveal that not all cases of fibrocystic disease are absolutely benign but a select few can progress to malignant transformation [1]. The disease has been reported to be present and undergo malignant change even in males [2].

A case of a 52-year-old lady who underwent surgery for fibrocystic disease on two separate occasions on the same breast and later developed carcinoma in same breast is presented with a brief review of literature.

2. Case Report

52-year-old lady presented with history of an irregular mass in the right breast since 3 months. She gave history of a lump in same breast 9 years back. Investigations then revealed the lump to be cystic in nature. Fluid was aspirated and did not reveal any malignant cells. Subsequently she was asymptomatic for quite some time.

In 2008, she developed 2 small lumps in the same breast which were excised. Histopathological examination of these lesions revealed fibrocystic disease. The cyst was fibrous with flattened epithelium, lining with foci of dilated ducts. One of these ducts showed intraductal epitheliosis. Nuclei were morphologically normal with some amount of perilobularinfiltration by lymphocytes. These details were mentioned on the report. Slides were unfortunately not available for detailed appraisal.

Patient was asymptomatic for a short period of time but again noticed lumps in the same breast. The lumps were excised surgically in 2012. Histological examination revealed fibrocystic disease of the breast with no further details.

3 months subsequent to this excision she again noticed similar lumps in right breast. These increased in size over a period of 1 year which she neglected until she was finally referred to my surgical facility.

On examination vital parameters were within normal limits. Physical examination did not reveal cervical lymphadenopathy, jaundice or bony tenderness. Abdominal examination did not reveal hepatomegaly or ascites.

Local examination of right breast revealed extensive scarring of whole breast, with an ulcerative lesion at superior aspect of right areola approximately 2.5 cm diameter with a deformed nipple (**Figure 1**).

Palpation revealed a large mass measuring 10 cm diameter involving entire right breast. The mass was adherent to the underlying pectoral muscles. Axillary lymph nodes were impalpable.

Multiple FNAC's revealed an intraductal carcinoma. Ultrasound examination of the abdomen did not reveal any metastases in the liver or any ascites.

In view of a locally advanced lesion two cycles of chemotherapy were administered preoperatively (CMF regimen) which led to regression of the lesion by approximately 25%.

Subsequently she underwent right modified radical mastectomy with axillary clearance. At surgery the mass was found to be involving almost the entire pectoral is major muscle which was resected. (**Figure 2**) Axillary lymph nodes were not palpable. Axillary clearance was done (**Figure 3**) and the wound was closed with good approximation of flaps. Post-operative recovery was uneventful (**Figure 4**).

Histopathological evaluation of the specimen revealed the mass to be an infiltrating ductal carcinoma. Theresection margins were free of tumour. However lymphovascular invasion with involment of 5 axillary lymph nodes was detected. The hormonal receptor status was positive for oestrogen receptors. She is presently under go completion of chemotherapy followed by tamoxifen therapy.

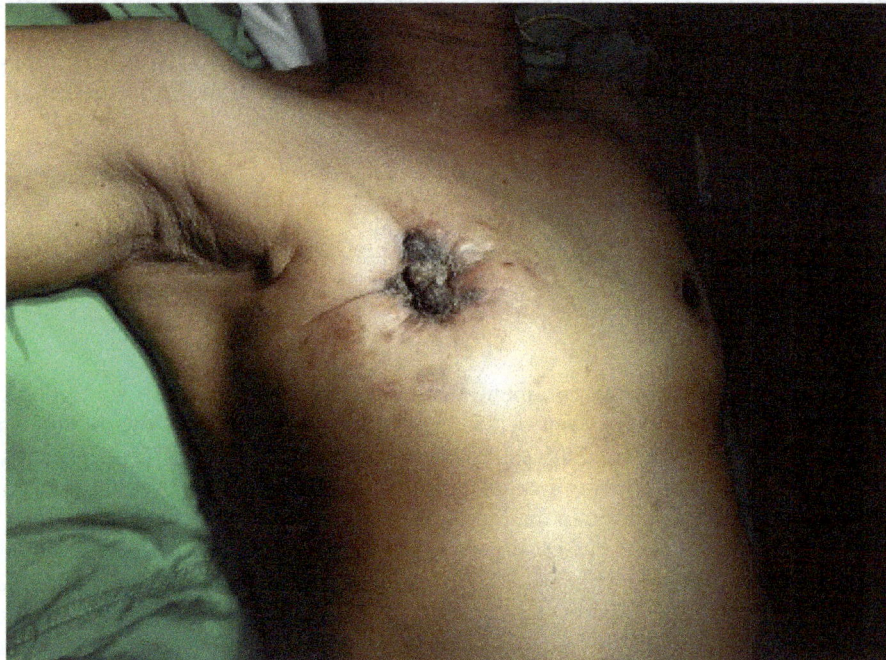

Figure 1. Pre-operative photograph showing a grossly scarred right breast.

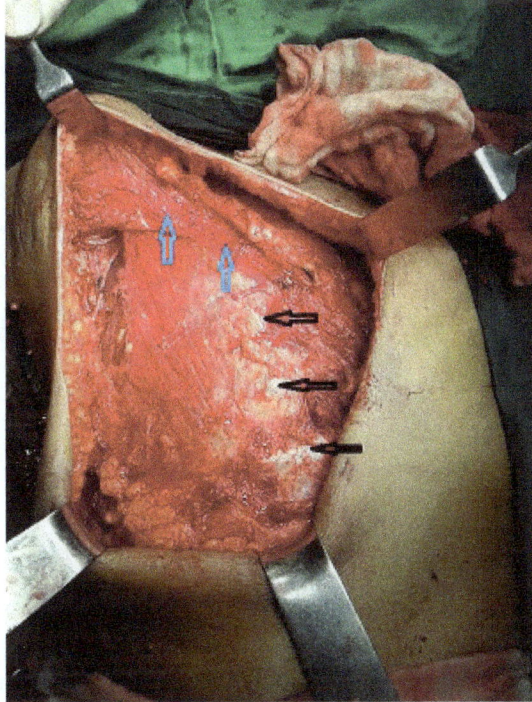

Figure 2. Intraoperative photograph showing exposure of the ribs after removal of amajor portion of the pectoralis major muscle. (exposed ribs marked by black arrows and the cut margin of the pectoralis major is marked by blue arrows).

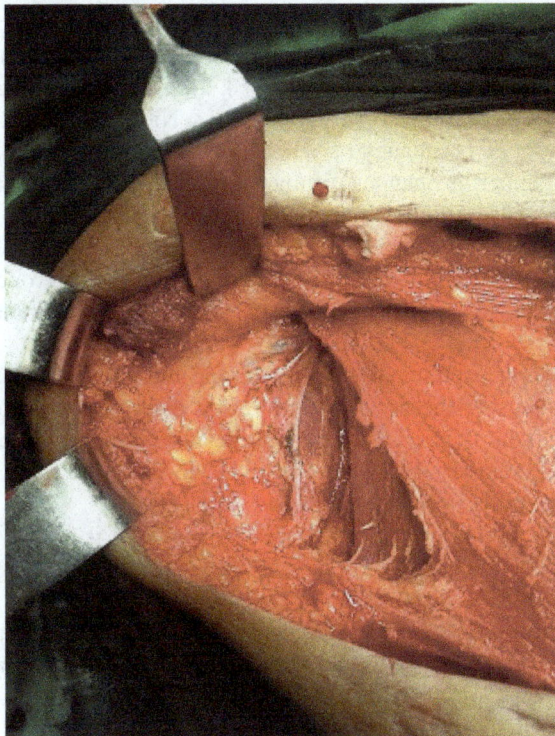

Figure 3. Intraoperative photograph showing the axilla after lymph node clearance.

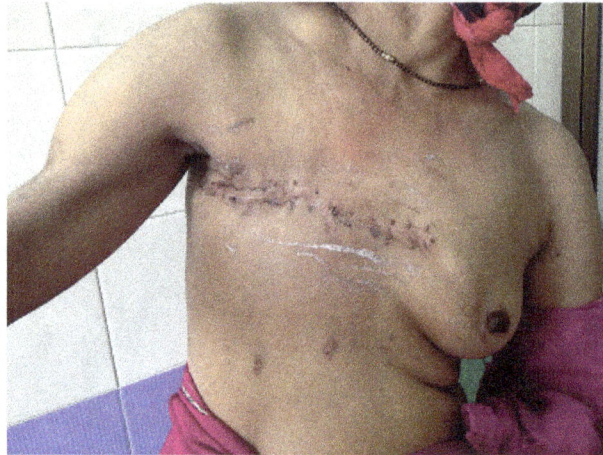

Figure 4. Postoperative state.

3. Discussion

The case presented highlights the fact that fibrocystic disease of breast in middle aged women should be taken seriously. Multiplicity of the cysts, the histology of the cysts removed previously and recurrence of the fibrocystic disease seems to have predisposed to malignant transformation. A detailed analysis of the nature of fibrocystic disease is what is required to determine the chances of malignant transformation. Fibrocystic disease is one of the components of ANDI (Aberrations of Normal Development and involution). Involutional changes in the breast are influenced by the genetic predisposition, socio-cultural factors and hormonal status. Many a times it is extremely difficult to evaluate all issues with an aim to identify those patients who will develop malignancy.

Fibrocystic disease of breast can be divided into non-proliferative and proliferative patterns.

Non proliferative patterns are associated with cystic changes and fibrosis [3]. The lesions are characterised by increase in fibrous stroma associated with dilatation of ducts leading to cysts which may either be single or multiple varying in size ranging from 1 cm to 5 cm [4] [5].

The nature of cyst fluid and lining of the cyst are important factors determining the chances of malignant transformation [3]. Based on nature of breast cyst fluid (BCF), cysts can be divided into two types:

Type I cyst: In this variety the potassium to sodium ratio [K/Na] of the breast cyst fluid is more than 1.5. These women usually have either one pregnancy or are totally nulliparous. They are currently smokers and non coffee drinkers with evidence of apocrine changes. Women with type 1cysts are more prone to malignancy.

Type 2 cyst: These usually have decrease K/Na ratio and have less propensity to develop malignant changes.

Hormonal content or the steroid biochemistry of BCF has also been found to be different in the two types. Increased levels of androsterone-3-α, 17-β-diol glucuronide, dihydroepiandrosterone sulphate (DHEA), oestrogen sulphate, androsterone glucuronide, testosterone and dihydrotestosterone are found in type 1 cysts as compared to type 2 cysts [6].

Type 2 breast cyst fluids have increased levels of progesterone and pregnenolone [6].

The influence of hormonal status of the patients with cystic diseases has also an impact on cyst fluid and breast cancer risk [7]. In women with type 1 cyst, oestrogen levels are high in luteal phase as compared to follicular phase. Whereas in type 2 cysts the DHEA level is higher in follicular phase as compared to luteal phase. Levels are lowest in both types of cysts in post-menopausal state [7].

Number and lining of cysts are also important factors. A Solitary cyst is usually lined by flattened epithelium and is less likely to develop malignant change whereas multiple cysts are usually apocrine in nature and prone to recurrence and malignant changes [4]. This was seen in the case presented.

Type 1 breast cyst fluid and multiplicity have higher chance of malignant changes.

Proliferative pattern of fibrocystic disease is yet another factor which can determine malignant transformation. Epithelial hyperplasia wherein there are more than 2 cell layers can evolve into a spectrum ranging from mild epithelial hyperplasia to atypical hyperplasia eventually leading to malignancy [8]. This was reported by the previous pathologist for the previously excised lumps in the case presented. The histological pattern of epithelial hyperplasia is variable. In a few cases the ducts or the ductules may be filled with orderly cuboidal cells within which small glandular patterns or fenestrations develop. Whereas in other cases proliferating epithelium may project as multiple small papillary excrescences into ductal lumen classically describes as ductal papillomatosis. These changes can be malignant precursors. In few cases, the hyperplastic cells have features resembling Carcinoma in situ. Such lesions can be described as atypical ductal hyperplasia. Both atypical ductal hyperplasia and lobular hyperplasia are associated with increased risk of invasive cancer.

Sclerosing adenosis is another type of fibrocystic disease which is less common than cyst and hyperplasia but whose features closely mimic cancer lesions containing marked intralobular fibrosis and proliferation of ductules and acini [8] [9].

Proliferation of luminal spaces (designated as adenosis) is usually lined by epithelial cells and myoepithelial cells thus yielding masses of small glands within a fibrous stroma. Marked stromal fibrosis may compress and distort proliferating epithelium and is always associated with adenosis. Hence designated as sclerosing adenosis [9].

4. Conclusion

Type 1 breast cyst fluid, multiplicity of cyst and recurrent disease, apocrine metaplasia, atypical ductal hyperplasia and sclerosing adenosis are important determinants for malignant transformation in a patient suffering from fibrocystic disease of breast.

Acknowledgements

We would like to thank the Dean of Dr. D. Y. Patil Medical College, Navi Mumbai, India for allowing us to publish this case report. We would also like to thank Mr. Parth K. Vagholkar for his help in typesetting the manuscripts.

References

[1]   Habo, V., Habor, A., Copotiu, C. and Pantiru, A. (2010) Fibrocystic Breast Disease—Breast Cancer Sequence. *Chirurgia (Bucur)*, **105**, 191-194.

[2]   Vagholkar, K., Dastoor, K. and Gopinathan, I. (2013) Intracystic Papillary Carcinoma in the Male Breast: A Rare Endpoint of a Wide Spectrum. *Case Reports in Oncological Medicine*, 2013, Article ID: 129353.

[3]   Dixon, J.M., Lumsden, A.B. and Miller, W.R. (1985) The relationship of Cyst Type to Risk Factors for Breast Cancer and the Subsequent Development of Breast Cancer in Patients with Breast Cystic Disease. *European Journal of Cancer and Clinical Oncology*, **21**, 1047-1050. http://dx.doi.org/10.1016/0277-5379(85)90289-5

[4]   Naldoni, C., Costantini, M., Dogliotti, L., Bruzzi, P., Bucchi, L., Buzzi, G., Torta, M. and Angeli, A. (1992) Association of Cyst Type with Risk Factors for Breast Cancer and Relapse Rate in Women with Gross Cystic Disease of the Breast. *Cancer Research*, **52**, 1791-1795.

[5]   Dixon, J.M., Scott, W.N. and Miller, W.R. (1985) Natural History of Cystic Disease: The Importance of Cyst Type. *British Journal of Surgery*, **72**, 190-192. http://dx.doi.org/10.1002/bjs.1800720311

[6]   Angeli, A., Dogliott, L., Naldoni, C., Orlandi, F., Puligheddu, B., Caraci, P., Bucchi, L., Torta, M. and Bruzzi, P. (1994) Steroid Biochemistry and Categorization of Breast Cyst Fluid: Relation to Breast Cancer Risk. *The Journal of Steroid Biochemistry and Molecular Biology*, **49**, 333-339. http://dx.doi.org/10.1016/0960-0760(94)90276-3

[7]   Budai, B., Szamel, I., Sulyok, Z., Nemeth, M., Bak, M., Kralovanszky, J., Otto, S., Besznyak, I., Purohit, A., Parish, D.C. and Reed, M.J. (2000) Influence of Hormonal Status of Patients with Cystic Disease on the Composition of Cyst Fluid and Breast Cancer Risk. *Anticancer Research*, **5C**, 3879-3886.

[8]   Celis, J.E., Moreira, J.M., Gromova, I., Cabezon, T., Gromov, P., Shen, T., Timmermans, V. and Rank, F. (2007) Characterization of Breast Precancerous Lesions and Myoepithelial Hyperplasia in Sclerosing Adenosis with Apocrine Metaplasia. *Molecular Oncology*, **1**, 97-119. http://dx.doi.org/10.1016/j.molonc.2007.02.005

[9]   Wells, C.A. and El-Ayat, G.A. (2007) Non Operative Breast Pathology: Apocrine Lesions. *Journal of Clinical Pathology*, **60**, 1313-1320. http://dx.doi.org/10.1136/jcp.2006.040626

18

Serum CK18 as a Predictive Factor of Response to Chemotherapy in Locally Advanced and Metastatic Breast Cancer

Basem Battah[1], Jumana Saleh[1], Marroan Bachour[2], Maher Salamoon[2]*

[1]Faculty of Pharmacy, Damascus University, Damascus, Syria
[2]Al Bairouni University Hospital, Damascus, Damascus, Syria
Email: *maheroncology@yahoo.com

Abstract

Introduction: Breast cancer is the most common cancer in women and the second most frequent cause of cancer death. Several factors affect response to chemotherapy including nodal status, hormonal status and human epidermal growth factor receptor (Her-2). **Aim of Study:** The study is aiming at evaluating M30 antigen in serum of patients with locally advanced and metastatic breast cancer and establishing the relation between M30 level and response to chemotherapy. **Patients and Methods:** The study was performed at Al Bairouni University Hospital and the Faculty of Pharmacy (Damascus-Syria). We have included 60 patients with histologic confirmation of invasive ductal carcinoma of the breast treated with the combination (Docetaxel + Doxorubicin) with M30 levels to be evaluated before treatment and 24 hours after the first and third cycle. **Results:** M30 level increase in serum 24 hours after the 1st cycle correlated with different kinds of response in 39 patients (P value less than 0.03) with better results in those with Estrogen Receptors (ER) positive patients (P value 0.05). There was no correlation between Her-2 status and response (P value 0.3). **Conclusion:** M30 level in serum is a useful predictor marker of response to chemotherapy in both locally advanced and metastatic breast cancer.

Keywords

CK18, Metastatic Breast Cancer, Response

1. Introduction

Breast cancer remains the most common cancer in women and the second most frequent cause of cancer death

---

*Corresponding author.

[1]. There are a number of factors which determine the prognosis of disease and response to treatment. Prognostic factors are those which determine the outcome of disease in the absence of systemic treatment whereas predictive factors predict response to treatment [1]. Estrogen receptor (ER) and progesterone receptor (PR) expressions are the most important and useful predictive factors currently available. ER and PR are intracellular steroid hormone receptors which have received substantial attention since 1986. Measurable amounts of ER and PR are found in about 50% - 85% of patients with breast cancer. The frequency of positivity and the level of ER and PR increase with age, reaching their highest levels in postmenopausal women [2]. Apoptosis (programmed cell death) plays an important role in tissue homeostasis and development. It is regulated by a wide variety of survival signals as well as cellular mechanisms that are in charge of DNA integrity [3]. The apoptosis execution mechanism results in the development of characteristic morphological features such as nucleus and chromatin condensation, cell shrinkage and cytoplasmic blebs. The measure for quantification of apoptosis is the apoptotic index (AI). Many publications have proved that breast cancers with a high apoptosis index (programmed cell death) have a better prognosis compared with the same type of cancer with less or no apoptosis [4].

Although multiple genes are involved in apoptosis, the key mediators of the process are the Caspases. Caspases are Aspartate-specific Cysteine proteases, which cleave their substrates on the carboxyl side of the Aspartate residue and Cytokeratin 18 [5] [6]. Currently at least 14 different Caspases are known to exist, of which two thirds play a role in apoptosis. The Caspases involved in apoptosis can be divided into two main groups, the initiator Caspases (e.g., Caspases 8, 9, and 10) and the downstream effector Caspases (e.g., Caspases 2, 3, 6, and 7). It is the members of the latter group that degrade multiple cell proteins and are responsible for the morphological changes in apoptosis. Caspase 3 is the most widely studied of the effector Caspases. It plays a key role in both the death receptor pathway, initiated by Caspase 8, and the mitochondrial pathway, involving Caspase 9. In addition, several studies have shown that Caspase 3 activation is required for apoptosis induction in response to chemotherapeutic drugs e.g., Taxanes, 5-Fluorouracil, and Doxorubicin [7]-[10]. Cytokeratin 18 (CK 18) is a member of cytoskeletal protein family which is present in epithelial cells [11]. When apoptosis is induced, CK 18 is cleaved from Aspartate amino acids localized at position 238 and 396. Monoclonal antibody M30 recognizes the neoepitope of CK 18 formed after cleavage by Caspases. This newly-formed neoepitope can be regarded as a selective biomarker of apoptosis [12] [13]. Recently, it was reported that serum M30-antigen levels may also be a prognostic marker in some tumor types [14] [15]. In another study, M30-antigen was reported to be associated with the survival in advanced gastric carcinoma patients [16]. Some studies investigated Casepases and their role in breast cancer, some of which studied Caspase levels and expression in breast carcinoma at mRNA level, however, little work has been made to evaluate levels of Caspases in serum of patients under treatment; therefore, the aim of this study is to test the concentration of CK18 level in serum of patients with locally advanced and metastatic breast cancer, then to evaluate the relation between CK18 concentration (fold increase) and response to chemotherapy. In our study, we tried to show the importance of CK18 as a predictive marker of response on chemotherapy in both locally advanced and metastatic breast cancer.

2. Patients and Methods

2.1. Patients

The study is prospective, initiated in September 2012 and included 102 persons (21 disease free patients on follow up, 21 healthy volunteers and 60 patients diagnosed with locally advanced and metastatic invasive ductal carcinoma of the breast). 25 patients presented with hepatic metastasis, 22 with pulmonary metastasis, 3 with bone metastasis and 10 others with locally advanced disease. Age of patients was between 28 and 62 years (51 years in median), good performance status (0, 1 and 2), normal hepatic and renal functions and pathologic confirmation of disease. The study was performed at Breast cancer unit (al Bairouni university hospital) and the faculty of Pharmacy Labs in Damascus (SYRIA). Both locally advanced and metastatic group received the same combination chemotherapy (Docetaxel 75 mg/m² and Doxorubicin 75 mg/m²) repeated every 21 days for 3 cycles then evaluated by CT-Scan and bone scan for those with metastatic disease and by clinical exam for those with locally advanced disease

2.2. Methods

Blood samples were taken from healthy cohort, disease-free then from patients before beginning of treatment, after 24 hours after the first cycle and 24 hours after the completion of the third cycles. Samples were centrifuged and serum was collected and M30 antigen was tested by means of (ELISA). The test measures M30 concentration in serum and CK18 fragments due to K18Asp396 containing Caspase (M30 Apoptosense ELISA) obtained from PEVIVA (Sweden), Kit (ALX-850-270-KI01).

2.3. Biostatistics

Correlation between parameter was assessed by Spearman's test, while Mann-Whitney test was employed to compare between means. To assess the relation between types of response and M30 values after 24 hours of the first chemotherapy, Qui square was used. Statistical significance was assigned to P value less than 0.5.

3. Results

Of the 60 patients included in our study, the disease progressed in 21 patients (35%) with less than 0.5 fold increase in M30 concentration after 24 hours of the first cycle. 10 patients (17%) with M30 concentration fold increase between 0.5 - 0.9 showed stable disease while the remaining 25 patients (42%) showed partial response with M30 fold increase between 1 - 1.9. In the other hand, the 4 complete responders (6%) showed a fold increase between (2-5) 24 hours after the completion of the first cycle as illustrated in **Table 1**.

The mean concentration of M30 was 183 U/L in disease-free patients on follow up versus 182 U/L in healthy volunteers (21 persons each). Concentrations were compared between the two former groups using Mann-Whitney test, showed P value 0.9 with no difference in concentration between the two groups. The test was extended to compare M30 concentration between (healthy and followed-up patients) versus patients before treatment, showed no difference with P value of 0.69.

Interpretation showed a direct correlation between M30 concentration before treatment and 24 hours after the first cycle (P value 0.04), however, M30 increase was not significant after the completion of the third cycle (was not predicting of response) with P value of 0.6. Mean concentration of M30 before treatment, after the first cycle and after the third cycle gives a good indicator of response in both locally advanced and metastatic disease. For example, mean M30 concentration was elevated in patients with metastatic disease (50 patients) compared with those with locally advanced disease (10 patients) as shown in **Table 2**. To evaluate the statistical relation between M-30 fold increase (before and 24 hours after the first cycle) and response to treatment, Chi square was employed showing P value of 0.03.

Among the 60 patients, 35 patients had Estrogen receptors (ER) positive disease (58%), so disease progressed in 8.9% of patients with ER positive disease versus 26% of patients with ER negative disease reflecting a better prognosis in those with ER positive group with P value of 0.05.

Furthermore, M30 concentration at baseline was elevated in Human epidermal growth factor receptor positive patients (Her-2 +) (43 patients) compared with those with Her-2 negative patients with a significant P value of 0.018. However, Her-2 status was not a predictor factor of response (P value 0.3).

Table 1. The relation between M30 concentration and type of response.

Number of patients	M30 fold increase	Type of response	Percentage
21	<0.5	progression	35
10	0.5 - 0.9	Stable	17
25	1 - 1.9	Partial response	42
4	2 - 5	Complete response	6

Table 2. The difference between M30 concentration between locally advanced and metastatic disease.

Type of disease		M30 baseline	M30 after 1st cycle	M30 after 3rd cycle
Locally advanced	Mean	99.66	254.00	194
	Number	10	10	10
	St-deviation	34.32	137.61	127.79
metastatic	Mean	329.20	586.82	317.11
	Number	50	50	50
	St-deviation	298.49	472.59	314.80

4. Discussion

In our study, we measured serum M30 antigen levels in patients with both locally advanced and metastatic breast cancer to reveal the relation between M30 antigen levels and response to chemotherapy protocol (Docetaxel + Doxorubicin). In neoadjuvant and metastatic setting, we do not know which patient will respond better to chemotherapy. Response to chemotherapy is considered a good prognostic factor and may predict a long progression free survival period [17]. Our study showed that M30 antigen elevation especially 24 hours after the first cycle is the most important predictor of response on the short term, and there is a direct proportion between fold increase and degree of clinical and radiologic response.

Death of tumor cells generates detectable protein products in the patient's circulation, which may be used for cancer diagnostics and/or monitoring of therapy efficacy [18]. Apoptosis is a form of regulated cell death that is characterized by specific structural changes, mediated by proteases of the Caspase family [19]. The M30 antibody detects a Caspase-degraded product, CK18-Asp396 (also called M30-antigen), of the important

Cytoskeletal protein called Cytokeratin 18 of epithelial cells. Cytokeratin 18 is expressed by most carcinomas, including those of breast, prostate, lung and colon [13]. It has previously been shown that circulating M30-antigen levels increased in patients with various cancer types and, furthermore, it increased during chemotherapy. For instance, the Docetaxel treatment increased levels of M30-antigen in the serum of breast cancer patients, indicating apoptotic death of tumor cells, while the Cyclophosphamide/Epirubicin/5-fluorouracil treatment led to a heterogeneous response with regard to cell death mode [20]. In preclinical models, studies have shown an increase of apoptotic proteins 1 - 3 days after chemotherapy [21]-[23]. In our study and in a similar way, M30 antigen elevated 24 hours after the first cycle with a serum level decreasing over time to reach a nadir after the 3rd cycle which could be attributed to decrease in tumor volume and consequently apoptotic proteins in responders, however, low level of M30 after the first cycle accompanied with lower levels over time to reveal a chemoresistant cancer cells. This finding may help researchers and clinicians to best tailor the treatment of locally advanced and metastatic breast cancer and to predict the chemoresistant patients from the very beginning. But, if we find low levels after the first cycle, are we able to change chemotherapeutic protocol? It is still a hard question to answer so far, because other factors may affect response to chemotherapy such as ER status, Her-2 status and nodal status.

Regarding chemotherapy, Taxanes induce mitotic catastrophe, characterized by the occurrence of aberrant mitosis followed by cell division. Mitotic catastrophe is not a cell death mode, but will trigger cell death, either by apoptosis or by nonapoptotic mechanisms [24]-[26] and our study is supporting this concept through elevation of M30 in vivo after treatment with Docetaxel in combination with Doxorubicin. Therefore, we can conclude that M30 level in serum could be used as a predictive factor of response in patients with measurable disease breast cancer, however, further studies with other protocols are warranted to tailor our treatment in a better way.

Disclosure

The authors declare no conflict of interest.

References

[1] Burstein, H.J. and Monica, M. (2008) Malignant Tumors of the Breast. In: Devita, V.T., Lawrence, T.S. and Rosenberg, S.A., Eds., *Cancer Principles & Practice of Oncology, Vol.* 2, Williams and Wilkins, Wolters Kluwer Lippincott, 1606-1654.

[2] Shahla, M. (2000) Assessment of Prognostic Factors in Breast Fine-Needle Aspirates. *American Journal of Clinical Pathology*, **113**, S84-S96.

[3] Andrew, G. and Charles, S. (2000) Integrin-Mediated Survival Signals Regulate the Apoptotic Functions of Bax through Its Conformation and Subcellular Localization. *The Journal of Cell Biology*, **149**, 431-445. http://dx.doi.org/10.1083/jcb.149.2.431

[4] Lipponen, P. and Aaltomaa, S. (1994) Apoptosis in Bladder Cancer as Related To Standard Prognostic Factors and Prognosis. *The Journal of Pathology*, **173**, 333-339. http://dx.doi.org/10.1002/path.1711730408

[5] Stennicke, H.R. and Salvesen, G.S. (1998) Properties of the Caspases. *Biochimica et Biophysica Acta*, **1387**, 17-31. http://dx.doi.org/10.1016/S0167-4838(98)00133-2

[6] Thornberry, N.A. and Lazebnik, Y. (1998) Caspases: Enemies within. *Science* (Wash. DC), **281**, 1312-1316.

http://dx.doi.org/10.1126/science.281.5381.1312

[7]   Keane, M.M., Ettenberg, S.A., Nau, M.M., *et al.* (1999) Chemotherapy Augments TRAIL-Induced Apoptosis in Breast
      Cell Lines. *Cancer Research*, **59**, 734-741.

[8]   Bellarosa, D., Ciucci, A., Bullo, A., Nardelli, F., *et al.* (2001) Apoptotic Events in a Human Ovarian Cancer Cell Line
      Exposed to Anthracyclines. *Journal of Pharmacology and Experimental Therapeutics*, **296**, 276-283.

[9]   Kottke, T.J., Blajeski, A.L., Martins, M.L., Mesner, P.W., *et al.* (1999) Comparison of Paclitaxel-, 5-fluoro-2-Deoxy-
      yuridine-, and Epidermal Growth Factor (EGF)-Induced Apoptosis. *The Journal of Biological Chemistry*, **274**, 15927-
      15936. http://dx.doi.org/10.1074/jbc.274.22.15927

[10] Suzuki, A., Kawabata, T. and Kato, M. (1998) Necessity of Interleukin-1β Converting Enzyme Cascade in Tax-
      otere-Initiated Death Signaling. *European Journal of Pharmacology*, **343**, 87-92.
      http://dx.doi.org/10.1016/S0014-2999(97)01520-3

[11] Linder, S. (2007) Cytokeratin Markers Come of Age. *Tumor Biology*, **28**, 189-195.
      http://dx.doi.org/10.1159/000107582

[12] Ueno, T., Toi, M. and Linder, S. (2005) Detection of Epithelial Cell Death in the Body by Cytokeratin 18 Measurement.
      Biomed Pharmacother, **59**, S359-S362. http://dx.doi.org/10.1016/S0753-3322(05)80078-2

[13] Leers, M.P., Kölgen, W., Björklund, V., Bergman, T., *et al.* (1999) Immunocytochemical Detection and Mapping of a
      Cytokeratin 18 Neoepitope Exposed during Early Apoptosis. *The Journal of Pathology*, **187**, 567-572.

[14] de Haas, E.C., di Pietro, A., Simpson, K.L., Meijer, C., *et al.* (2008) Clinical Evaluation of M30 and M65 ELISA Cell
      Death Assays as Circulating Biomarkers in a Drug-Sensitive Tumor, Testicular Cancer. *Neoplasia*, **10**, 1041-1048.

[15] Wu, Y.X., Wang, J.H., Wang, H. and Yang, X.Y. (2003) Study on Expression of Ki-67, Early Apoptotic Protein M30
      in Endometrial Carcinoma and Their Correlation with Prognosis. *Zhonghua Bing Li Xue Za Zhi*, **32**, 314-318.

[16] Yaman, E., Coskun, U., Sancak, B., Buyukberber, S., Ozturk, B. and Benekli, M. (2010) Serum M30 Levels Are Asso-
      ciated with Survival in Advanced Gastric Carcinoma Patients. *International Immunopharmacology*, **10**, 719-722.
      http://dx.doi.org/10.1016/j.intimp.2010.03.013

[17] Scholl, S.M., Beuzeboc, P., Harris, A.L., Pierga, J.Y., Asselain, B., Palangié, T., *et al.* (1998) Is Primary Chemothera-
      py Useful for All Patients with Primary Invasive Breast Cancer? *Recent Results in Cancer Research*, **152**, 217-226.
      http://dx.doi.org/10.1007/978-3-642-45769-2_21

[18] Holdenrieder, S. and Stieber, P. (2004) Apoptotic Markers in Cancer. *Clinical Biochemistry*, **37**, 605-617.
      http://dx.doi.org/10.1016/j.clinbiochem.2004.05.003

[19] Degterev, A. and Yuan, J. (2008) Expansion and Evolution of Cell Death Programmes. *Nature Reviews Molecular Cell
      Biology*, **9**, 378-390. http://dx.doi.org/10.1038/nrm2393

[20] Olofsson, M.H., Ueno, T., Pan, Y., Xu, R., Cai, F., van der Kuip, H., *et al.* (2007) Cytokeratin-18 Is a Useful Serum
      Biomarker for Early Determination of Response of Breast Carcinomas to Chemotherapy. *Clinical Cancer Research*, **13**,
      3198-3206. http://dx.doi.org/10.1158/1078-0432.CCR-07-0009

[21] Meyn, R.E., Stephens, L.C., Hunter, N.R. and Milas, L. (1995) Apoptosis in Murine Tumors Treated with Chemothe-
      rapy Agents. *Anti-Cancer Drugs*, **6**, 443-450. http://dx.doi.org/10.1097/00001813-199506000-00013

[22] Ellis, P.A., Smith, I.E., McCarthy, K., Detre, S., Salter, J. and Dowsett, M. (1997) Preoperative Chemotherapy Induces
      Apoptosis in Early Breast Cancer. *The Lancet*, **349**, 849. http://dx.doi.org/10.1016/S0140-6736(05)61752-7

[23] Green, A.M. and Steinmetz, N.D. (2002) Monitoring Apoptosis in Real Time. *Cancer Journal*, **8**, 82-92.
      http://dx.doi.org/10.1097/00130404-200203000-00002

[24] Morse, D.L., Gray, H., Payne, C.M. and Gillies, R.J. (2005) Docetaxel Induces Cell Death through Mitotic Catastrophe
      in Human Breast Cancer Cells. *Molecular Cancer Therapeutics*, **4**, 1495-1504.
      http://dx.doi.org/10.1158/1535-7163.MCT-05-0130

[25] Jordan, M.A., Wendell, K., Gardiner, S., Derry, W.B., Copp, H. and Wilson, L. (1996) Mitotic Block Induced in HeLa
      Cells by Low Concentrations of Paclitaxel (Taxol) Results in Abnormal Mitotic Exit and Apoptotic Cell Death. *Cancer
      Research*, **56**, 816-825.

[26] Blajeski, A.L., Kottke, T.J. and Kaufmann, S.H. (2001) A Multistep Model for Paclitaxel-Induced Apoptosis in Human
      Breast Cancer Cell Lines. *Experimental Cell Research*, **270**, 277-288.
      http://dx.doi.org/10.1158/1535-7163.MCT-05-0130

19

Metaplastic Carcinoma of the Breast: A Clinical Study of 7 Cases from Balochistan

Abdul Hameed Baloch[1*], Shakeela Daud[2], Jameela Shuja[3], Adeel Ahmad[4], Fateh Ali[3], Mohammad Akram[3], Dost Mohammad Baloch[5], Abdul Majeed Cheema[6], Mohammad Iqbal[7], Jamil Ahmad[1]

[1]Department of Biotechnology and Informatics, BUITEMS, Quetta, Pakistan
[2]Center for Advanced Molecular Biology (CAMB), Lahore, Pakistan
[3]CENAR, Quetta, Pakistan
[4]Institute of Biochemistry and Biotechnology (IBBt), UVAS, Lahore, Pakistan
[5]Lasbela University of Agriculture, Water and Marine Sciences, Balochistan
[6]Institute of Molecular Biology and Biotechnology, The University of Lahore, Pakistan
[7]Bolan Medical College/Hospital (BMC) Quetta
Email: *hameedbaloch77@yahoo.com

Abstract

Metaplastic carcinomas of the breast are rare heterogenous neoplasms characterized by adenocarcinoma with dominant areas of spindle cells, squamous and/or other mesenchymal differentiation, that comprise of <5% of all invasive breast cancers. Our objective in this study was to review the pathological features and clinical outcomes for metaplastic carcinoma of breast in breast cancer patients registered in CENAR (Center for Nuclear Medicines and Radiotherapy), Balochistan. Present study was performed on 7 patients affected with metaplastic carcinoma of breast, who were registered patients in CENAR. Informed consent was taken from the patients and BMI was calculated by measuring the height and weight of the patients. Available clinical history obtained by retrieving the patients file and a copy of biopsy report was also obtained from the file. Metaplastic carcinoma of breast was 4.11% of all 170 breast cancer cases registered in CENAR from 2010-2012. Mean age was 40 years ranging from 25 - 50 years. Four subtypes of metaplastic carcinoma of breast were reported in this study; DCIS component was present in one case and mean tumor size was 6.12 cm ranging from 3.5 - 10 cm. Metaplastic carcinomas of breast are rare heterogenous neoplasm with different characteristics, demographics and tumor biology and accounts for almost >5% of all breast cancer cases.

---

*Corresponding author.

Keywords

Breast Cancer, Metaplastic Carcinoma of Breast, CENAR, Balochistan, BMI, MBC

1. Introduction

Breast tumors arise mostly from glandular epithelium but in some cases glandular epithelium differentiates into non glandular mesenchymal tissue through the process called metaplasia [1]. Metaplastic carcinomas of the breast are rare heterogenous neoplasms characterized by adenocarcinoma with dominant areas of spindle cells, squamous and/or other mesenchymal differentiation [2]-[4]. Metaplastic carcinomas comprises of <5% of all invasive breast cancers [5]-[9], whereas some studies suggest that MBC (Metaplastic Carcinoma of Breast) accounts <1% of all the cases of breast cancer [4] [10]. Another subgroup of metaplastic carcinoma called as carcinosarcoma is the most rare primary malignancies of the breast found in <0.1% of the cases [9]. Metaplastic carcinoma pathologically and clinically differs from typical adenocarcinoma. In metaplastic carcinoma nodal involvement has been shown to be less common compared to typical breast adenocarcinomas, with an incidence ranging from 6% - 26%. In metaplastic carcinoma of breast, hormone receptor expression is uncommon with reported ERPR positivity in 0% - 17% of cases [11]-[13]. Similarly in other studies it has also been shown that most of the MBC cases are triple negative with a worsen prognosis [14]-[20]. MBC presents a different clinical picture as compared to other invasive carcinomas of breast, the mass of the tumor grows rapidly [4] [21] [22]. Despite of a larger palpable mass the axillary lymph nodes less likely be invaded in the patients affected with MBC with a 6% - 26% of the cases [7] [11]-[13] [17] where as in other cases of breast cancer the involvement of axillary lymph nodes is greater than 50% [23].

Present study was performed on 7 patients with metaplastic carcinoma registered in CENAR between 2010-2012. Our aim in this study was to review the pathological features and clinical outcomes for metaplastic carcinoma of breast in patients registered in CENAR.

2. Materials and Methods

This study was conducted in Balochistan University of information Technology, Engineering and Management Sciences, Quetta and Center for Nuclear Medicine and Radiotherapy (CENAR), Quetta. The study was approved by the institutional Review Board of BUITEMS. All the cases of breast cancer affected with MBC type registered in CENAR from 2010-2012 were included. An informed consent was taken from all the patients who took part as volunteers in this study. The clinical features and outcomes of the disease were reviewed by studying the patients file. Body mass index (BMI) was calculated by measuring the height and weight of the patients. All the informations regarding the disease were obtained from the patients files. Following parameters were investigated in this study including patient's ethnicity, age, BMI, histological classification of the cancer, tumor size and grade, involvement of lymph nodes and ERPR and HER2/Neu receptor status by reviewing the pathological reports.

3. Results

Seven cases of metaplastic carcinoma of breast out of 170 breast cancer patients diagnosed between 2010 and 2012 registered in CENAR were reviewed, which was the 4.11% of all breast cancer registered cases in CENAR. All patients were female with mean age at diagnosis of 40 years ranging from 25 - 50 years. BMI of the patients was also calculated by taking their height and weight. There were three patients from Pashtoon ethnic group, two were Afghani, one was Punjabi and one from Hazara ethnic group. Out of seven patients, one was under weight, three were normal, one was overweight and two were obese. Four subtypes of metaplastic carcinoma of breast cancer were recorded in this study including adenosquamous carcinoma, monotonic spindle cell carcinoma, adenocarcinoma with spindle cell metaplasia and metaplastic carcinoma with osteoclast giant cells. All seven cases were diagnosed with IDC, and one case including with DCIS component. The mean tumor size was 6.12 cm ranging from 3.5 - 10 cm. Other pathological and clinical features observed in individual cases were; nuclear pleomorphisms, hyperchromatism, abnormal mitotic figures, tubule formations, come do and cribriforms, fibrocystic changes including epithelial hyperplasia, adenosis, cystically dilated glands, apocrine metaplasia and microcalcification, stromal fibrosis and fibroadrenoma. The features found in the metaplastic carcinoma of breast in the case affected bilaterally were; **Left Breast:** Breast tissue with foreign body giant cell reaction, fat necrosis, chronic inflammation and fibrosis. 14/35 lymph nodes found positive for tumor metastasis. **Right Breast:** Breast tissue with ductal hyperplasia, cystic changes microcalcification and focal fibroadenoma. 6/50 lypmh nodes for tumor metastsis. Clinical features are shown in **Table 1**.

4. Discussion

Metaplastic carcinoma of breast is a rare, uncommon and heterogenous disease consisting of tumors admixed with epithelial and non-epithelial elements and constitute between 0.2 - 5 percent of all breast cancers [24] [25].

In current study we identified 7 breast cancer patients with metaplastic carcinoma which was the 4.11% of all the breast cancer cases registered in CENAR during the period of 2009-2012. Whereas Arce-Grijalval in their study proposed 0.6% cases of metaplastic carcinoma of breast out of all breast cancer cases registered in the Instituto National de Cancerologia from 1995-2005 [26]. Mean age of patients diagnosed with metaplastic carcinoma in our study was 40 years ranging from 25 - 50 years. In their study Arce-Grijalval the mean age of the patients of metaplastic carcinoma was 47.9 years ranging from 24 - 74. But in another study carried out by Brenner R.J. found the median age was 65.5 years ranging from 33 - 87 years and study conducted by Beatty J.D. reported the mean age 55 years ranging from 26 - 80 years [26] [27]. In current study we identified four subtypes of metaplastic carcinoma of breast including adenosquamous carcinoma, monotonic spindle cell carcinoma, adenocarcinoma with spindle cell metaplasia and metplastic carcinoma with osteoclast giant cell. Wargotz *et al.* in their series of studies described five subgroups of metaplastic carcinoma of breast including matrix-producing carcinoma, spindle cell carcinoma, carcinosarcoma, squamous cell carcinoma of ductal origin and metaplastic carcinoma with osteoclast giant cells [7] [11] [12] [28] [29]. Studies suggest that associated ductal carcinoma in situ might be present in 50% of cases [6]. In our study the DCIS component was present in one case which was the 14.23% of all the cases with metaplastic carcinoma of breast. The mean tumor size was 6.12 cm ranging from 3.5 - 10 cm in current study. Most studies suggest a large palpable masses with metaplastic carcinoma of breast [30]. In a study carried out by Kurain and Al-Nafussi presents tumor sizes 2.2 - 10 cm [31]. Park *et al.*, in their study reported mean tumor size 4.2 cm and similarly [32] and Kaufman *et al.*, reported in their study the median tumor size was 4.8cm ranging from 2.5 - 18 cm [22]. whereas smaller tumor sizes have also been reported with metaplastic carcinoma of breast but data are sparse. In a study carried out between 1976 and 1997, the median tumor size was reported 3.4 cm ranging from 0.5 - 0.7 cm [17]. In another study from Nottingham, England the mean tumor size was reported 1.6 cm ranging from 0.7 - 2.4 cm [33].

5. Conclusion

Metaplastic carcinomas of breast are rare heterogenous neoplasm with different characteristics, demographics and tumor biology and accounts for almost >5% of all breast cancer cases.

Table 1. Clinical features of the patients diagnosed with metaplastic carcinoma of breast.

Patient	Ethnicity	Age	BMI	Tumor Size	Tumor Grade	Nodal Status	DCIS	ERPR Status	Laterality
1	Pashtoon	25	17.78	7 cm	III	2/8	-	ERPR+	Left
2	Pashtoon	35	36.7	10 cm	III	3/16	DCIS	ERPR−	Left
3	Pashtoon	40	31.25	6 cm	III	1/8	-	Tripple negative	Left
4	Afghani	50	20.07	9 cm	III	1/20	-	ERPR−	Right
5	Afghani	35	24	3.5 cm	II	14/35 and 6/50	-	ERPR+	Bilateral
6	Panjabi	40	23.17	4 cm	II	3/27	-	ERPR+	Left
7	Hazara	40	29	4 cm	III	4/9	-	ERPR−	Left

Acknowledgements

We thank to all the patients who took part as volunteers in this study, Special thanks to Director CENAR and his team for their kind support.

References

[1]   Brenner, R.J., Turner, R.R., Schiller, V., Arndt, R.D. and Giuliano, A. (1998) Metaplastic Carcinoma of the Breast: Report of Three Cases. *Cancer*, **82**, 1082-1087. http://dx.doi.org/10.1002/(SICI)1097-0142(19980315)82:6<1082::AID-CNCR11>3.0.CO;2-2

[2]   Rauf, F., Kiyani, N. and Bhurgri, Y. (2006) Metaplastic Carcinoma of Breast, an Intriguing Rarity. *Asian Pacific Journal of Cancer Prevention*, **7**, 667-71.

[3]   Pitts, W.C., Rajos, V.A., Gaffey, M.J., Rouse, R.V., Esteban, J., Frierson, H.F., Kempson, R.L. and Weiss, L.M. (1991) Carcinomas with Metaplasia and Sarcomas of the Breast. *American Journal of Clinical Pathology*, **95**, 623-632

[4]   Tavassoli, F.A. (1992) Classification of Metaplstic Carcinomas of the Breast. *Annual Review of Pathology*, **27**, 89-119.

[5]   Rosen, P.P. (1997) Rosen's Breast Pathology. *Lippencott-Raven Philadelphia*, 375-395.

[6]   Elston, C.W. and Ellis, I.O. Vol. 13. The Breast In: Systemic Pathology. 3rd Edition, Churchill Livingstone, Edinburugh, 1998, 323-328.

[7]   Wargotz, E.S. and Norris, H.J. (1990) Metaplastic Carcinomas of the Breast: IV. Squamous Cell Carcinoma of Ductal Origin. *Cancer*, **65**, 272-276. http://dx.doi.org/10.1002/1097-0142(19900115)65:2<272::AID-CNCR2820650215>3.0.CO;2-6

[8]   Oberman, H.A. (1987) Metaplastic Carcinoma of the Breast. *The American Journal of Surgical Pathology*, **11**, 918-929. http://dx.doi.org/10.1097/00000478-198712000-00002

[9]   Feder, J.M., de Paredes, E.S., Hogge, J.P. and Wilken, J.J. (1999) Unusual Breast Lesions: Radiologic-Pathologic Correlation. *Radio Graphics*, **19**, S11-S26. http://dx.doi.org/10.1148/radiographics.19.suppl_1.g99oc07s11

[10] Luini, A., Aguilar, M., Gatti, G., Fasani, R., Brito, J.A., Maisonneuve, P., Vento, A.R. and Viale, G. (2007) Metaplastic Carcinoma of the Breast, an Unusual Disease with Worse Prognosis: The Experience of the European Institute of Oncology and Review of the Literature. *Breast Cancer Research and Treatment*, **101**, 349-353. http://dx.doi.org/10.1007/s10549-006-9301-1

[11] Wargotz, E.S. and Norris, H.J. (1989) Metaplastic Carcinomas of the Breast: I. Matrix-Producing Carcinoma. *Human Pathology*, **20**, 628-635. http://dx.doi.org/10.1016/0046-8177(89)90149-4

[12] Wargotz, E.S. Deos, P.H. and Norris, H.J. (1989) Metaplastic Carcinomas of the Breast: II. Spindle Cell Carcinoma. *Human Pathology*, **20**, 732-740. http://dx.doi.org/10.1016/0046-8177(89)90065-8

[13] Gutman, H., Pollock, R.E., Janjan, N.A. and Johnson, D.A. (1995) Biological Distributions and Therapeutic Implications of Sarcomatoid Metaplasia of Epithelial Carcinoma of the Breast. *Journal of the American College of Surgeons*, **180**, 193-199.

[14] Al Sayed, A.D. El Weshi, A.N., Tulbah, A.M., Rahal, M.M. and Ezzat, A.A. (2006) Metaplastic Carcinoma of the Breast Clinical Presentation, Treatment Results and Prognostic Factors. *Acta Oncologica*, **45**, 188-195. http://dx.doi.org/10.1080/02841860500513235

[15] Tse, G.M., Tan, P.H., Putti, T.C., Lui, P.C.W., Chaiwun, B. and Law, B.K.B. (2006) Metaplastic Carcinoma of the Breast: A Clinicopathological Review. *Journal of Clinical Pathology*, **59**, 1079-1083. http://dx.doi.org/10.1136/jcp.2005.030536

[16] Weigelt, B., Kreike, B. and Reis-Filho, J.A. (2009) Metaplastic Breast Carcinomas Are Basal-Like Breast Cancers: A Genomic Profiling Analysis. *Breast Cancer Research and Treatment*, **117**, 273-280. http://dx.doi.org/10.1007/s10549-008-0197-9

[17] Rayson, D., Adjei, A.A., Suman, V.J., Wold, L.E. and Ingle, J.N. (1999) Metaplastic Breast Cancer: Prognosis and Response to Systemic Therapy. *Annals of Oncology*, **10**, 413-419. http://dx.doi.org/10.1023/A:1008329910362

[18] Bae, S.Y., Lee, S.K., Koo, M.Y., Hur, S.M., Choi, M.Y., Cho, D.H. Kim, S., Choe, J.H., Lee, J.E., Kim, J.H., Kim, J.S., Nam, S.J. and Yang, J.H. (2011) The Prognoses of Metaplastic Breast Cancer Patients Compared to Those of Triple-Negative Breast Cancer Patients. *Breast Cancer Research and Treatment*, **126**, 471-478. http://dx.doi.org/10.1007/s10549-011-1359-8

[19] Jung, S.Y., Kim, H.Y., Nam, B.H., Min, S.Y., Lee, S.J., Park, C., *et al.* (2000) Worse Prognosis of Metaplastic Breast Cancer Patients than Other Patients with Triple-Negative Breast Cancer. *Breast Cancer Research and Treatment*, **120**, 627-637. http://dx.doi.org/10.1007/s10549-010-0780-8

[20] Okada, N., Hasebe, T., Iwasaki, M., Tamura, N., Akashi-Tanaka, S., Hojo, T., *et al.* (2010) Metaplastic Carcinoma of

the Breast. *Human Pathology*, **41**, 960-970. http://dx.doi.org/10.1016/j.humpath.2009.11.013

[21] Kaufman, M.W., Marti, J.R., Gallager, H.S. and Hoehn, J.L. (1984) Carcinoma of the Breast with Pseudosarcomatous Metaplasia. *Cancer*, **53**, 1908-1917. http://dx.doi.org/10.1002/1097-0142(19840501)53:9<1908::AID-CNCR2820530917>3.0.CO;2-F

[22] Chao, T.C., Wang, C.S., Chen, S.C. and Chen, M.F. (1999) Metaplastic Carcinomas of the Breast. *Journal of Surgical Oncology*, **71**, 220-225. http://dx.doi.org/10.1002/(SICI)1096-9098(199908)71:4<220::AID-JSO3>3.0.CO;2-L

[23] Carter, C.L., Allen, C. and Henson, D.E. (1969) Relation of Tumor Size, Lymph Node Status and Survival in 24,740 Breast Cancer Cases. *Cancer*, **63**, 181-187. http://dx.doi.org/10.1002/1097-0142(19890101)63:1<181::AID-CNCR2820630129>3.0.CO;2-H

[24] Smith, D.M., Rongaus, V.A., Wehmann, T.W., Agarwal, P.J. and Classen, G.J. (1996) Metaplastic Breast Carcinoma. *Journal of the American Osteopathic Association*, **96**, 419-421.

[25] Johnson, T.L. and Kini, S.R. (1996) Metaplastic Breast Carcinoma: A Cytohistologic and Clinical Study of 10 Cases. *Diagnostic Cytopathology*, **14**, 226-232. http://dx.doi.org/10.1002/(SICI)1097-0339(199604)14:3<226::AID-DC6>3.0.CO;2-F

[26] Arce-Grijalva, V., Vela-Chávez, T., Pérez-Sánchez, V.M. and Ruvalcaba-Limón, E. (2007) Metaplastic Carcinoma of the Breast: A Clinical and Pathological Study of 40 Cases. *BMC Cancer*, **7**, A6. http://dx.doi.org/10.1186/1471-2407-7-S1-A6

[27] Beatty, J.D., Atwood, M., Tickman, R. and Reiner, M. (2006) Metaplastic Breast Carcinoma-Clinical Significance. *The American Journal of Surgery*, **191**, 657-664. http://dx.doi.org/10.1016/j.amjsurg.2006.01.038

[28] Wargotz, E.S. and Norris, H.J. (1989) Metaplastic Carcinomas of the Breast. *Cancer*, **64**, 1490-1499. http://dx.doi.org/10.1002/1097-0142(19891001)64:7<1490::AID-CNCR2820640722>3.0.CO;2-L

[29] Wargotz, E.S. and Norris, H.J. (1990) Metaplastic Carcinomas of the Breast: V. Metaplastic Carcinoma with Osteoclastic Giant Cells. *Human Pathology*, **21**, 1142-1150. http://dx.doi.org/10.1016/0046-8177(90)90151-T

[30] Gunhan-Bilgen, I., Memiş, A., Üstün, E.E., Zekioglu, O. and Özdemir, N. (2002) Metaplastic Carcinoma of the Breast: Clinical, Mammographic and Sonographic Findings with Histopathologic Correlation. *American Journal of Roentgenology*, **178**, 1421-1425. http://dx.doi.org/10.2214/ajr.178.6.1781421

[31] Kurain, K.M. and Al-Nafussi, A. (2002) Sarcomatoid/Metaplastic Carcinoma of the Breast: A Clinicopathological Study of 12 Cases. *Histopathology*, **40**, 58-64. http://dx.doi.org/10.1046/j.1365-2559.2002.01319.x

[32] Park, J.M, Han, B.K., Moon, W.K., Choe, Y.H., Ahn, S.H. and Gong, G. (2000) Metaplastic Carcinoma of the Breast: Mammographic and Sonographic Findings. *Journal of Clinical Ultrasound*, **28**, 179-186. http://dx.doi.org/10.1002/(SICI)1097-0096(200005)28:4<179::AID-JCU5>3.0.CO;2-Y

[33] Denley, H., Pinder, S.E., Tan, P.H., Sim, C.S., Brown, R., Barker, T., Gearty, J., Elston, C.W. and Ellis, I.O. (2000) Metaplastic Carcinoma Arising within Complex Sclerosing Lesions: A Report of Five Cases. *Histopathology*, **36**, 203-209. http://dx.doi.org/10.1046/j.1365-2559.2000.00849.x

20

GP88 (Progranulin) Confers Fulvestrant (Faslodex, ICI 182,780) Resistance to Human Breast Cancer Cells

Wisit Tangkeangsirisin[1,2], Ginette Serrero[1,3]*

[1]A&G Pharmaceutical Inc., Columbia, USA
[2]Present Address: Department of Biopharmacy, Faculty of Pharmacy, Silpakorn University, Nakhon Pathom, Thailand
[3]Program in Oncology, Greenebaum Cancer Center of the University of Maryland, Baltimore, USA
Email: *gserrero@agpharma.com

Abstract

The 88 kDa glycoprotein known as GP88, Progranulin or PC cell derived growth factor is an autocrine growth factor with a unique cysteine rich motif that is over expressed in breast cancer whereas it is negative in normal mammary epithelial cells. It has been shown to play a major role in estrogen independence, tamoxifen resistance and tumorigenesis of breast cancer cells. In the present study, we investigated the effect of GP88 overexpression on the response of the human breast cancer MCF-7 cells to the pure estrogen receptor antagonist fulvestrant (ICI 182,780). While fulvestrant effectively inhibited cell proliferation of empty vector transfected cells, it had no inhibitory effect on the proliferation of GP88 overexpressing breast cancer cells. Mouse xenograft experiments in athymic ovariectomized nude mice showed that GP88 over expressing cells were fulvestrant resistant *in vivo* in contrast to low GP88 expressing cells. We show that the ability of fulvestrant to induce apoptosis determined by measuring cleavage of poly (ADP-ribose) polymerase was inhibited by GP88. Anti-apoptotic activity of GP88 was associated with sustained expression of bcl-2 and bcl-x_L after fulvestrant treatment. In contrast, fulvestrant was still able to inhibit the ability of estrogen to stimulate ERE-luciferase reporter gene activity as well as vEGF expression in GP88 over expressing MCF-7 cells similarly to control MCF-7 cells. Collectively, our data suggest that GP88 prevents apoptosis induced by faslodex and contributes to antiestrogen resistance in human breast cancer.

Keywords

Progranulin (GP88), Fulvestrant, Faslodex, Breast Cancer, Anti-Estrogen Resistance

---

*Corresponding author.

1. Introduction

Anti-estrogen therapy is the treatment of choice in all stages of estrogen receptor positive (ER$^+$) breast cancer [1]. These agents target either estrogen binding, interaction with its receptor or estrogen synthesis. They include Selective Estrogen Receptor Modulator (SERM) such as tamoxifen and its derivatives, Selective Estrogen Receptor down-regulators (SERD) such as faslodex (fulvestrant or ICI 182, 780) and aromatase inhibitors such as letrozole or anastrozole. Tamoxifen is the first developed antiestrogen that acts by inhibiting the binding of estrogen to its receptor [2]. It has been the most commonly prescribed drug for breast cancer, and is currently used for the treatment of advanced disease as well as adjuvant therapy after surgery for early breast cancer [3]. Fulvestrant (faslodex, ICI 182,780) is a steroidal estrogen receptor (ER) pure antagonist that acts by binding with high affinity to the ER and down-regulating ER expression [4] [5]. It was developed as an alternative anti-estrogen therapy due to the unfavorable agonistic effect of tamoxifen in the endometrium [6]. Unlike tamoxifen, the conformation fulvestrant-ER complex inhibits the activation function of ER, disrupts dimerization and nuclear translocation of the complex and results in ER degradation. Fulvestrant is well-tolerated and produces good response rates when used in patients who develop tamoxifen resistance. In fact, clinical studies have suggested fulvestrant as a second line antiestrogen [7] [8]. Although these agents are effective and show promising clinical results, resistance to these agents can also be observed after a period of treatment [9] [10]. More than half of the patients, who failed previous treatment with tamoxifen, still do not respond to fulvestrant [8] [11]. There have been several mechanisms of action to explain anti-estrogen resistance. Among them, one possible mechanism of anti-estrogen therapy resistance in ER$^+$ tumors [3] [12] has been the constitutive overexpression of autocrine growth/survival factors, and/or the upregulation of growth factor receptor by tumor cells [13] [14]. Such increased autocrine or paracrine growth factor signaling network may bypass the need for ER-mediated growthstimulation in human breast cancer cells, thus rendering anti-estrogen therapy ineffective. For example, clinical studies have reported a decreased efficacy of tamoxifen for tumors overexpressing c-erbB2 (6) and EGFR [15]-[18]. In addition to inhibiting the growth promoting effect of estrogen, anti-estrogen have also been shown to induce programmed-cell death in breast cancer cell lines and in clinical samples [19]-[24]. Failure to undergo apoptosis in response to anti-estrogen would also confer drug resistance [25] Therefore, increase in growth factor signaling that mediates both proliferation signals and anti-apoptotic signals may induce resistance to anti-estrogen therapy.

GP88 is the 88 kDa cysteine-rich glycoprotein autocrine growth factor originally purified from the highly tumorigenic mouse teratoma PC cells by applying a biological screen to mine for drivers of tumorigenesis [26]. GP88, (also known as granulin/epithelin precursor, progranulin, acrogranin or PC-cell derived growth factor) is the largest member of the granulin-epithelin family of growth modulators characterized by 71/2 granulin repeats containing a unique double cysteine rich motif [27]. This protein has been found to have pleiotropic functions in normal and diseased human tissues. In particular, GP88 has been found to be overexpressed in many cancers whereas it is not expressed in the normal tissue counterparts [26]-[28]. GP88 stimulates proliferation, survival and metastasis in several cancer cell types via activation of multiple pathways that include MAP kinase and P-I-3 kinase pathways, FAK kinase [27]. In human breast cancer cells, GP88 expression was stimulated by estradiol in a time- and dose-dependent fashion in estrogen receptor positive cells [29]. In these cells, GP88 was shown to mediate the mitogenic activity of estrogen by stimulating cyclin D1 expression [29]. Inhibition of GP88 expression in estrogen receptor negative MDA-MB-468 cells by antisense transfection led to a complete inhibition of tumorigenesis in nude mice [30].

Overexpression of the autocrine growth factor GP88 in ER$^+$ breast cancer cells leads to tamoxifen resistance in vitro and *in vivo* while the cells remained ER$^+$ [31]. In addition, we have shown that GP88 confers resistance to the aromatase inhibitor letrozole in aromatase overexpressing cells MCF7-CA and AC1 cells while estrogen receptor expression remained unchanged [32]. Naturally letrozole resistant cells LTLT and AC1LTR cells overexpressed GP88 whereas inhibition of GP88 by SiRNA restored letrozole responsiveness [32]. Pathological studies with paraffin embedded breast cancer biopsies have shown positive GP88 tissue expression in 60% of ductal carcinoma *in situ* (DCIS) and 80% of invasive ductal carcinoma (IDC) whereas normal mammary epithelium and benign tumors were GP88 negative [33] In IDC, GP88 expression correlated with parameters of poor prognosis such as tumor grade, proliferation index and p53 expression. Recent studies investigating the correlations of GP88 tumor tissue expression in ER$^+$ IDC with clinical outcomes showed that patients with high GP88 tumor expression (GP88 3+) were associated with a 4-fold increase in recurrence and mortality when compared to patients with low or no GP88 tissue expression [34]. Increased levels of circulating GP88 were found in breast cancer patients when compared to healthy subjects [35].

Because of the role of GP88 on breast cancer cells and since GP88 confers resistance to a SERM (tamoxifen) and to an aromatase inhibitor (letrozole), it would be interesting to examine the effect of GP88 on anti-estrogen compound with a different mode of action such as the SERD faslodex. The present study focused on investigating the effect of GP88 on the faslodex responsiveness of breast cancer cells in vitro and *in vivo*.

2. Material and Methods

2.1. Materials

17β-Estradiol (E2) was purchased from Calbiochem (San Diego, CA). G418, Taq polymerase and Superscript II were obtained from Gibco BRL (Gaithersburg, MD). Fulvestrant was purchased from Tocris (Ellisville, MO). Oligonucleotide primers used in the RT-PCR were synthesized by the Biopolymer Core Laboratory of the University of Maryland (Baltimore, MD). Placebo and fulvestrant time-release pellets were manufactured at Innovative Research of America (Sarasota, FL). Enhanced chemiluminescence kit was obtained from Pierce (Rockford, IL). Mouse anti-poly (ADP-ribose) polymerase antibody (anti-PARP) was purchased from Oncogene Research (Boston, MA).

2.2. Cell Lines

MCF-7 cell line was originally obtained from the American Type Culture Collection (Manassas, VA). GP88 overexpressing MCF-7 cells and empty vector MCF-7 control cells were developed in our laboratory as previously described [30] [31]. These cells were cultured in DMEM/F12 supplemented with 5% FBS and 50 μg/ml gentamicin (Sigma) and 400 μg/ml G418 (Gibco).

2.3. Proliferation Assay

Proliferation assay was performed in 6-well tissue culture plates (Costar, Cambridge, MA). 5×10^4 cells were plated in phenol red-free α-MEM (PFMEM) supplemented with 5% charcoal extracted fetal bovine serum (CHX-FBS). Cells were treated with either 1 nM E2 alone or in combination with 10 nM fulvestrant. Control cells were treated with vehicle alone (0.01% DMSO). Medium was changed at day 4. Cell numbers were determined with a hemocytometer. Each time point was performed in triplicate.

2.4. *In Vivo* Tumorigenesis Assay

All animal studies were approved by the Institutional Animal Care and Use Committee of the University of Maryland, Baltimore. Control and GP88 overexpressing MCF-7 cells (5×10^6 cells per site) were injected subcutaneously in two sites into six-week-old ovariectomized athymic female nude mice (National Cancer Institute, Frederick, MD). E2 pellets (1.7 mg, 60 day release) were implanted subcutaneously in the back, one day before inoculating the cells. The animals received fulvestrant pellets (2.5 mg, 60-day release) or placebo pellets (Innovative Research of America, Sarasota, FL), ten days after the cell inoculation, when the tumors were visible. The width (W) and length (L) of individual tumors were measured using a caliper. Average tumor volume was calculated with the widely used formula: Tumor volume = $(W^2 \times L) \times 0.5$.

2.5. Determination of mRNA Expression for bcl-2, bcl-x_L, bax and VEGF by RT-PCR

Total RNA was isolated with Trizol reagent (Gibco) and was reverse transcribed into single strand cDNA by Superscript II (Gibco). A total of 30 - 35 PCR cycles depending on the gene amplified was performed, followed by electrophoresis on 1% agarose gel. Specific primers for glyceraldehyde 3-phosphate dehydrogenase (GAPDH) for bcl-2 and for V-EGF have been previously described [31] [36] .Other specific primers used here were:

for bax: forward primer 5' GAGCAGATCATGAAGACAGGGG 3', reverse primer 5' CTCCAGCAAGGCCCAGCGTC 3';

for bcl-x_L: forward primer 5' CAGTGAGTGAGCAGGTGTTTTGG 3', reverse primer 5' GTTCCACAAAAGTATCCCAGCCG 3';

2.6. Western Blot Analysis of PARP Cleavage

Cells were seeded at a density of 7×10^5 cells in 60-mm dish in DMEM/F12 supplemented with 5% FBS. After 24 hours, medium was changed to serum-free phenol red-free DMEM/F12 supplemented with vehicle or purified GP88 (400 ng/ml) for another 24 hours. Cells were treated with either vehicle only or factors under investigation for 24 hours. Cell lysates were prepared as described before [31]. 100 μg of protein from eachsample was used for immunoblotting. Intact and cleaved forms of PARP were detected using a mouse monoclonal anti-PARP antibody. The band intensity of PARP cleaved form was determined by densitometric analysis and normalized to the β-actin.

2.7. Statistical Analysis

All experiments were conducted in triplicates and repeated at least twice. Data were analyzed by Student t test for mean comparison and statistical significance. The values are reported as mean ± standard error.

3. Results

3.1. GP88 Overexpression Prevent Growth Inhibitory Effect of Fulvestrant

The effect of increasing concentrations of fulvestrant on the proliferation of MCF-7 EV cells and GP88 over expressing cells was first examined by thymidine incorporation assay. Fulvestrant inhibited proliferation of control MCF-7 EV cells in a dose-dependent fashion. Concentrations as low as 0.2 nM, inhibited by 90% thymidine incorporation in MCF-7 EV cells. At similar dose, thymidine incorporation into DNA of GP88 overexpressing cells had been inhibited by only 20%. Even at concentration of 2 nM of fulvestrant, inhibition did not exceed 40% (**Figure 1(a)**). This dose had no effect on the DNA synthesis of GP88 overexpressing cells. Long-term proliferation assay showed that fulvestrant inhibited the proliferative effect of estradiol (E2) in MCF-7 EV cells whereas the proliferation of GP88 overexpressing cells was mostly unchanged (**Figure 1(b)**). As shown in **Table 1**, the mean doubling time of MCF-7 EV cells treated with E2 and fulvestrant was significantly higher than in cells treated with E2 alone ($p < 0.05$). On the other hand, the mean doubling time of GP88 overexpressing cells treated with fulvestrant and E2 was similar to the one of cells treated with E2 only, indicating that fulvestrant did not inhibit the growth of cells overexpressing GP88 ($p < 0.05$).

3.2. GP88 Overexpression Results in Fulvestrant Resistance *in Vivo*

Since fulvestrant failed to inhibit the proliferation of GP88 overexpressing cells *in vitro*, its effect on tumorigenesis of ER$^+$ breast cancer cells expressing or not GP88 was then examined in mouse xenografts. Control and GP88 overexpressing MCF-7 cells were injected into female nude mice one day after they had been implanted with E2 pellets, as described in the method section. Ten days later, when the tumors were visible, the mice were randomized and segregated into experimental groups that received either placebo or fulvestrant pellets. The groups were then monitored for an additional 45 days. Tumor size was determined with a caliper and tumor volume determined as described in the method section. As shown in **Figure 2**, fulvestrant significantly inhibited MCF-7 EV tumor growth as evidenced by a 35% inhibition of tumor incidence and a 70% inhibition of mean tumor volume when compared to mice treated with E2 only ($p < 0.05$), in agreement with the reported inhibitory effect of fulvestrant in MCF-7 tumor growth. In contrast, GP88 overexpressing cells formed larger tumors in mice with or without fulvestrant without any change in tumor incidence (100%) or tumor growth. Monitoring of tumor volume was performed over 45 days after start of treatment (**Figure 2**). In the agreement with our previous experiments [31], it is clear that GP88 overexpression in breast cancer cells promotes antiestrogen resistance.

3.3. Fulvestrant Inhibits Estrogen Responsive Element Activity in MCF-7EV and O4 Cells

It is well established that fulvestrant acts as a pure estrogen receptor antagonist by inhibiting the formation of E2-ER complexes and its subsequent binding to estrogen responsive element (ERE) within the promoter [7]. Since fulvestrant did not show growth inhibitory effect on GP88 overexpressing MCF-7 cells, we examined the effect of fulvestrant on ERE responsiveness to E2 in these cells when compared to control cells. As shown in **Figure 3**, E2 stimulated ERE-luciferase activity in both MCF-7 EV and O4 cells by 4.4 and 3.9-fold, respectively when compared to the untreated cells. Fulvestrant treatment resulted in a 95% inhibition of E2 mediated effect on ERE-luciferase in both cells ($p < 0.05$, compared to untreated groups). These data suggest that fulvestrant still acts as an E2 antagonist of in both cells. Therefore, GP88 overexpression in MCF-7 cells does not change the genomic

Table 1. Effect of estrogen and fulvestrant on doubling time in breast cancer cell lines.

	Doubling Time (h)		
	Control	E2	E2 + Fulvestrant
MCF-7EV	61.8 ± 1.0	$37.9 \pm 1.0^*$	$64.6 \pm 0.9^*$
O4	42.1 ± 0.7	$37.3 \pm 1.6^*$	39.7 ± 1.1
O7	47.4 ± 1.3	$42.6 \pm 2.2^*$	47.4 ± 1.3

$p < 0.05$ compared to control group. The proliferation of Two GP88 overexpressing MCF-7 cell lines and the empty vector transfected control MCF-7 cell line was examined as described in the material and Methods section. Doubling times in each culture conditions were determined from the growth curves of **Figure 1**.

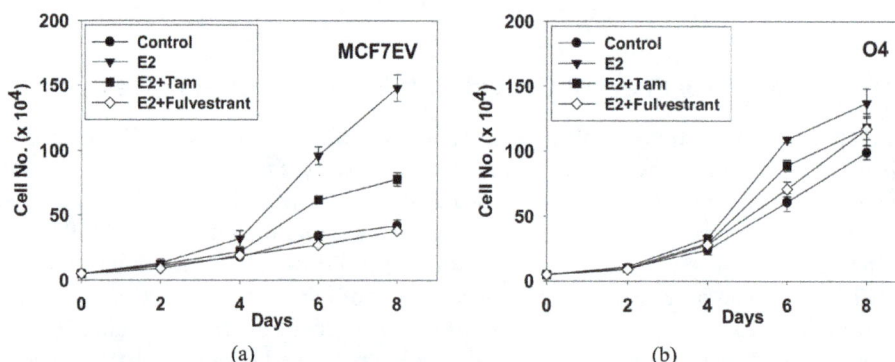

(a)   (b)

Figure 1. Effect of E2 and fulvestrant on Cell proliferation of MCF-7EV, and GP88 overexpressing cells O4 cells. Long-term growth of MCF-7EV and O4 cells in estrogen–depleted medium. Cells (5×10^4 cells) were cultivated in phenol red-free DMEM/F12 containing 5% charcoal-stripped FBS supplemented with vehicle (●), with 1 nM17β-estradiol (E2) alone (○) or in combination with 1 μM tamoxifen (▼) or 10 nM ICI 182,780 (▽). Cell number was counted using hemocytometer. Experiments were performed in triplicates.

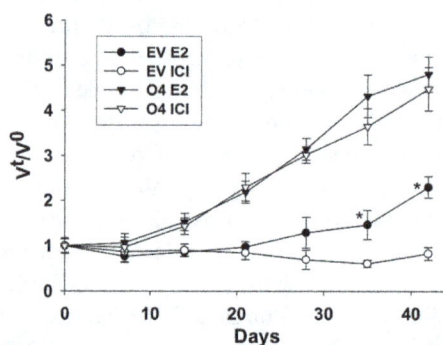

Figure 2. *In vivo* fulvestrant resistance of MCF-7 EV and O4 cells. Exponentially growing MCF-7 EV or O4 cells (5×10^6 cells/site) were subcutaneously inoculated into the lower abdominal area of ovariectomized athymic nude mice supplemented with E2 pellets. Ten days after cell inoculation, fulvestrant pellets were implanted. Tumor growth was monitored and tumor volume was calculated as described in the method section. Results shown here were plotted as the mean tumor volume at each time point (V^t) over the mean tumor volume at day fulvestrant pellet implanted (V^0). Bar; SE.

response to fulvestrant.

3.4. GP88 Prevents Apoptosis Induced by Fulvestrant

It has been documented that fulvestrant, similarly to tamoxifen, induces apoptosis of MCF-7 cells [22]. We determined whether GP88 blocked the apoptotic effect of fulvestrant by using PARP cleavage assay. As shown in

Figure 4, incubation with fulvestrant induced PARP cleavage in MCF-7 EV cells. GP88 treatment inhibited PARP cleavage induced by fulvestrant in MCF-7 EV cells (>80% inhibition suggesting that GP88 inhibited fulvestrant-induced apoptosis as one possible mechanism of fulvestrant resistance.

3.5. Failure of Fulvestrant to Downregulate Bcl-2 in GP88 Overexpressing Cells

Bcl-2 is a key regulator for apoptosis in many cell types. Previous reports have suggested that bcl-2 expression was downregulated by fulvestrant treatment leading to activation of apoptosis in MCF-7 cells [22] [37]. Bcl-2 expression was examined in MCF-7 EV and O4 cells treated or not with fulvestrant. Fulvestrant induced the down-regulation of bcl-2 transcript in MCF-7 EV cells in a dose dependent manner (**Figure 5**). In contrast, fulvestrant failed to downregulate bcl-2 in O4 cells even at the highest dose tested (10 nM). Fulvestrant (10 nM) also downregulated the mRNA expression of bcl-x_L an homolog of bcl-2 in MCF-7EV cells by 72%. The reduction of bcl-x_L mRNA expression was not observed in O4 cells treated with the same fulvestrant concentration. Bax expression was slightly but not significantly decreased in both cells at all fulvestrant doses tested. These results indicate that fulvestrant-induced apoptosis can be prevented by GP88 overexpression by preventing down regulation of bcl-2, and possibly bcl-x_L, mRNA expression.

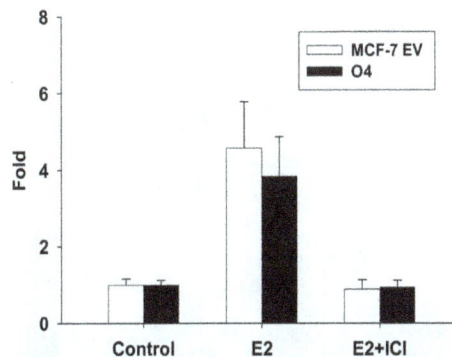

Figure 3. Effect of E2 and fulvestrant on ERE-luciferase reporter gene activity in MCF-7 EV and O4 cells. Cells were cotransfected with pGL2-ERE-luciferase and β-galactosidase reporter gene constructs. E2 (1 nM) and/or fulvestrant (ICI, 10 nM) were added after transfection. Cell lysates were collected 36 hours later for measuring luciferase activity as described in the method section. The values were normalized to the values of b-galactosidase activity used as internal control to determine transfection efficiency. The data are presented in folds of activation above the control untreated cells.

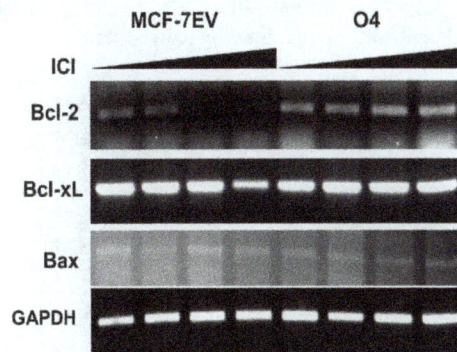

Figure 4. GP88 prevents down regulation of fulvestrant-induced bcl-2 expression. Bcl-2, Bcl-x_L and Bax mRNA expression were determined by semi-quantitative RT-PCR of total RNA samples isolated from MCF-7 EV and O4 cells cultivated in estrogen-depleted medium and treated for 24 h with increasing concentrations of fulvestrant (0.1, 1, and 10 nM) as described in the method section. GAPDH mRNA expression was used as internal control for loading. PCR products were resolved by agarose gel electrophoresis and visualized by ethidium bromide staining.

3.6. Fulvestrant Effect on V-EGF Expression in GP88 Overexpressing Cells

It is known that VEGF expression in MCF-7 cells is stimulated by E2 and inhibited by tamoxifen and fulvestrant. We have also shown previously that GP88 stimulated VEGF expression in MCF-7 cells ([36]). We examined here the effect of fulvestrant on VEGF expression in GP88 overexpressing cells and in MCF-7 control cells. As shown in **Figure 6**, fulvestrant inhibited E2 effect on VEGF expression in both MCF-7 EV and O4 cells.

4. Discussion

We have shown previously that GP88 overexpression in MCF-7 cells conferred estrogen independence and tamoxifen resistance both in vitro and *in vivo* [31] [36]. The present study demonstrates that GP88 also confers fulvestrant resistance to MCF-7 cells both in vitro and *in vivo*. We show here that fulvestrant was ineffective in inhibiting the long-term proliferation of MCF-7 cells that overexpressed GP88 in contrast to what was observed with MCF-7 control cells. More interestingly, fulvestrant failed to inhibit tumor formation of GP88 overexpressing cells injected in nude mice. No change in tumor volume as well as tumor incidence was observed in mice

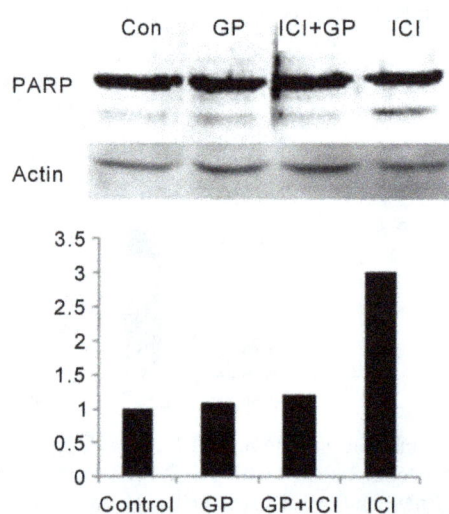

Figure 5. GP88 prevents PARP cleavage and inhibits apoptosis induced by fulvestrant in MCF-7 EV cells. MCF-7 EV cells were cultivated in estrogen-depleted medium and treated with 10 nM fulvestrant (ICI), 1 nM E2 or 400 ng/ml GP88 for 48 hours. Cell lysates were prepared in RIPA buffer containing 6 M urea for the western blot analysis. The level of PARP cleavage was determined by the presence of 85 kDa band (upper panel). Level of α-actin was determined as internal control for equal loading (lower panel).

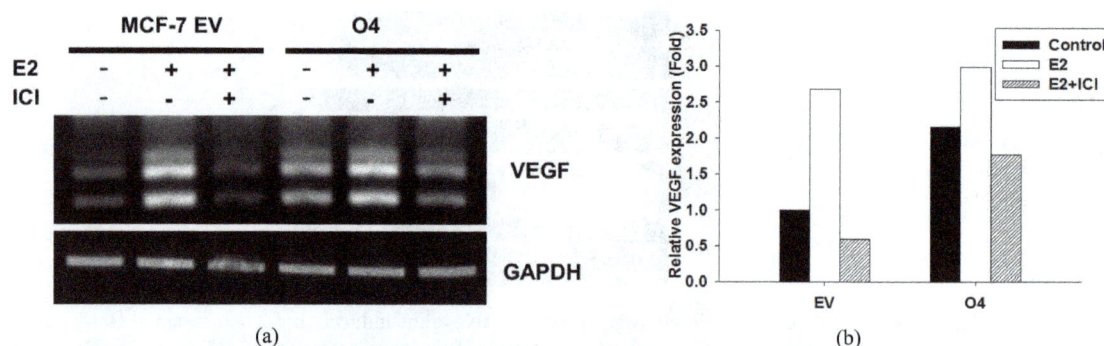

Figure 6. Effect of fulvestrant and E2 on VEGF expression in MCF-7EV and O4 cells. Cells were treated as described previously and incubated with 1 nM E2 or 10 nM fulvestrant (ICI) for 5 days. RNA samples were collected. VEGF mRNA expression was compared using RT-PCR. (a) RT-PCR products of VEGF in MCF-7EV and O4 cells. (b) Relative expression of VEGF. VEGF expression was normalized with GAPDH and compared with MCF-7 EV cells treated with vehicle only

injected with O4 cells treated with fulvestrant when compared to mice that received placebo pellets in contrast to what was observed with mice injected with control MCF-7EV cells. It is interesting to note that fulvestrant-resistant MCF-7 variants, isolated by cultivating MCF-7 cells in the continuous presence of fulvestrant displayed a 10-fold increase in GP88 expression as measured by quantitative EIA (data not shown). These data would confirm the close correlation between GP88 expression and resistance to fulvestrant in MCF-7 cells.

In addition to preventing fulvestrant inhibition of cell proliferation, we show here that GP88 prevented apoptosis induced by fulvestrant. This was observed with GP88 added exogenously as well as in GP88 overexpressing cells. GP88 overexpression as well as GP88 added exogenously prevented PARP cleavage induced by fulvestrant and also sustained bcl-2 and bcl-x_L expression during fulvestrant treatment. We have reported previously that GP88 inhibited tamoxifen apoptotic effect in MCF-7 cells by preventing tamoxifen induced bcl-2 down regulation [31]. Both tamoxifen and fulvestrant induce apoptosis in human breast cancer cells although fulvestrant is more effective than tamoxifen on inducing apoptosis in MCF-7 cells [22] [24].

In MCF-7 cells, fulvestrant, similarly to tamoxifen, induced apoptosis via down regulation of bcl-2 [20]-[24]. In addition, fulvestrant can downregulate bcl-x_L unlike tamoxifen [20]. This data could explain that fulvestrant has a more potent effect than tamoxifen in stimulating apoptosis. However, the role of bax in fulvestrant treatment remains unclear. While it has been reported that fulvestrant induced bax expression [22], other reports, in agreement with our results, showed that bax expression remained unchanged [24].

Even though, GP88 could inhibit the effect of fulvestrant on cell proliferation and apoptosis, we show here that fulvestrant was still able to inhibit the stimulation by estradiol of ERE-luciferase reporter gene activity in GP88 overexpressing cells as well as in MCF-7 control cells. Moreover, fulvestrant maintained its ability to inhibit the expression of the angiogenic factor V-EGF in GP88 over expressing cells as well as in MCF-7 control cells. Both data are in agreement with the fact that ER expression in GP88 over expressing cells remained unchanged compared to MCF-7 control cells [29]. These later results are different from the ones obtained with tamoxifen that not only failed to inhibit VEGF expression in GP88 over expressing cells but also cooperated with GP88 to stimulate VEGF expression [31] [33]. This effect is in agreement with the fact that tamoxifen has been reported as having a weak agonistic effect on VEGF expression [38]. This data is in the agreement with the results from in vitro and *in vivo* growth study that fulvestrant has no stimulatory effect in GP88 over expressing cells. The results suggested that even though fulvestrant is more effective than tamoxifen, both agents could not counteract the mitogenic effect of GP88. This is unlikely with fulvestrant, since no known agonist effect has been reported yet. Moreover, fulvestrant has been shown to have anti-angiogenic effect in human umbilical vein endothelial cells by inducing apoptosis and preventing the formation of tube-structure in matrigel [39]. Although Progranulin (GP88) has been reported to enhance growth of vascular cells [40], it is possible that the inhibitory effect of fulvestrant may overcome the proliferative effect of GP88 on vessel growth. Our *in vivo* experiments have shown that fulvestrant did not promote the growth of GP88 overexpressing tumors in nude mice. In contrast, tamoxifen treatment had resulted in a two-fold increase in tumor growth of GP88 overexpressing cells when compared to mice treated with placebo pellets [31]. Since this effect was observed *in vivo* and not *in vivo*, we had hypothesized that it could be due to the increased angiogenesis observed *in vivo* with tamoxifen and GP88. Based on this, it is possible that no stimulatory effect of fulvestrant on O4 tumor growth was observed because the inhibitory effect of fulvestrant on vessel growth may have neutralized the proliferative effect of GP88. This data would suggest that in ER$^+$ breast tumors that overexpress GP88, fulvestrant would be a better choice of therapy than tamoxifen.

Resistance to anti-estrogen therapies has been observed in cells over expressing other growth factor pathways. GP88 overexpression of several growth factors or growth factor receptors has been found to be associated with tamoxifen resistance, especially in MCF-7 cells [5]. Her-2 receptor overexpression promotes tamoxifen resistance in MCF-7 [28]. However, in this case, the resistance corresponded to a decreased ability of tamoxifen to inhibit tumor growth *in vivo* rather than a complete loss of tamoxifen response. Enhanced Epidermal Growth Factor Signaling was found in faslodex (fulvestrant resistant) MCF-7 cells [17]. It has been shown that tamoxifen resistance and fulvestrant resistance occurred when fibroblast growth factor (FGF) was overexpressed in MCF-7 cells [13]. Taken together, these results suggest that estrogen independent pathways induced by growth factors may overcome the suppression of estrogen dependent pathway by antiestrogens, allowing cells to grow in estrogen independent condition and abolishing the response to antiestrogen treatment. However, whether GP88 overexpression leads to the resistance to aromatase inhibitor remains to be investigated.

ER and PR status is a good predictor of response to endocrine therapy [41] [42]. Several groups have proposed other additional negative predictors such as kallikrein 10, VEGF, prostate specific antigen, Fas ligand/Fas ratio [42]

[43].

Combined VEGF and TP53 status has been found to predict poor response to tamoxifen therapy in estrogen receptor positive advanced breast cancer [44]. In addition, positive association between expression of transforming growth factor alpha was observed in endocrine unresponsive tumors [45]. Concerning GP88 expression in clinical samples, we have reported that GP88 was expressed in 80% of invasive ductal carcinoma in correlation with poor prognosis such as tumor grade, p53 expression and Ki67 [33] [34]. GP88 expression was found both in ER positive as well as ER negative tumors [33] suggesting that GP88 may play a role in both types of tumors. Since GP88 has been found associated with both tamoxifen resistance and fulvestrant resistance, it would be interesting to hypothesize that its expression may serve as a predictive marker of anti-estrogen response. Clinical studies are necessary to investigate this hypothesis in detail.

References

[1]   Howell, A. (2001) Future Use of Selective Estrogen Receptor Modulators and Aromatase Inhibitors. *Clinical Cancer Research*, **7**, 4402s-4410s; Discussion 11s-12s.

[2]   Cole, M.P., Jones, C.T. and Todd, I.D. (1971) A New Anti-Oestrogenic Agent in Late Breast Cancer. An Early Clinical Appraisal of ICI46474. *British Journal of Cancer*, **25**, 270-275. http://dx.doi.org/10.1038/bjc.1971.33

[3]   Clarke, R., Skaar, T.C., Bouker, K.B., Davis, N., Lee, Y.R., Welch, J.N. and Leonessa, F. (2001) Molecular and Pharmacological Aspects of Antiestrogen Resistance. *The Journal of Steroid Biochemistry and Molecular Biology*, **76**, 71-84.

[4]   Hu, X.F., Veroni, M., De Luise, M., Wakeling, A., Sutherland, R., Watts, C.K. and Zalcberg, J.R. (1993) Circumvention of Tamoxifen Resistance by the Pure Anti-Estrogen ICI 182,780. *International Journal of Cancer*, **55**, 873-876. http://dx.doi.org/10.1002/ijc.2910550529

[5]   Morris, C. and Wakeling, A. (2002) Fulvestrant ("Faslodex")—A New Treatment Option for Patients Progressing on Prior Endocrine Therapy. *Endocrine-Related Cancer*, **9**, 267-276. http://dx.doi.org/10.1677/erc.0.0090267

[6]   Kellen, J.A. (2001) Raloxifene: Another Selective Estrogen Modulator. *In Vivo*, **15**, 459-460.

[7]   Howell, A., DeFriend, D.J., Robertson, J.F., Blamey, R.W., Anderson, L., Anderson, E., Sutcliffe, F.A. and Walton, P. (1996) Pharmacokinetics, Pharmacological and Anti-Tumour Effects of the Specific Anti-Oestrogen ICI 182780 in Women with Advanced Breast Cancer. *British Journal of Cancer*, **74**, 300-308. http://dx.doi.org/10.1038/bjc.1996.357

[8]   Howell, A., Robertson, J.F., Quaresma, Albano. J., Aschermannova, A., Mauriac, L., Kleeberg, U.R., Vergote, I., Erikstein, B., Webster, A. and Morris, C. (2002) Fulvestrant, formerly ICI 182,780, Is as Effective as Anastrozole in Postmenopausal Women with Advanced Breast Cancer Progressing after Prior Endocrine Treatment. *Journal of Clinical Oncology*, **20**, 3396-3403. http://dx.doi.org/10.1200/JCO.2002.10.057

[9]   Johnston, S.R. (1997) Acquired Tamoxifen Resistance in Human Breast Cancer-Potential Mechanisms and Clinical Implications. *Anticancer Drugs*, **8**, 911-930. http://dx.doi.org/10.1097/00001813-199711000-00002

[10]   Foekens, J.A., Peters, H.A., Grebenchtchikov, N., Look, M.P., Meijer-van Gelder, M.E., Geurts-Moespot, A., van der Kwast, T.H., Sweep, C.G. and Klijn, J.G. (2001) High Tumor Levels of Vascular Endothelial Growth Factor Predict Poor Response to Systemic Therapy in Advanced Breast Cancer. *Cancer Research*, **61**, 5407-5414.

[11]   Osborne, C.K., Pippen, J., Jones, S.E., Parker, L.M., Ellis, M., Come, S., Gertler, S.Z., May, J.T., Burton, G., Dimery, I., Webster, A., Morris, C., Elledge, R. and Buzdar, A. (2002) Double-Blind, Randomized Trial Comparing the Efficacy and Tolerability of Fulvestrant versus Anastrozole in Postmenopausal Women with Advanced Breast Cancer Progressing on Prior Endocrine Therapy: Results of a North American Trial. *Journal of Clinical Oncology*, **20**, 3386-3395. http://dx.doi.org/10.1200/JCO.2002.10.058

[12]   Johnston, S.R., Saccani-Jotti, G., Smith, I.E., Salter, J., Newby, J., Coppen, M., Ebbs, S.R. and Dowsett, M. (1995) Changes in Estrogen Receptor, Progesterone Receptor, and pS2 Expression in Tamoxifen-Resistant Human Breast Cancer. *Cancer Research*, **55**, 3331-3338.

[13]   McLeskey, S.W., Zhang, L., El-Ashry, D., Trock, B.J., Lopez, C.A., Kharbanda, S., Tobias, C.A., Lorant, L.A., Hannum, R.S., Dickson, R.B. and Kern, F.G. (1998) Tamoxifen-Resistant Fibroblast Growth Factor-Transfected MCF-7 Cells Are Cross-Resistant *in Vivo* to the Antiestrogen ICI 182,780 and Two Aromatase Inhibitors. *Clinical Cancer Research*, **4**, 697-711.

[14]   Nicholson, R.I., Staka, C., Boyns, F., Hutcheson, I.R. and Gee, J.M.W. (2004) Growth-Factor Driven Mechanisms Associated with Resistance to Estrogen Deprivation in Breast Cancer: New Opportunities for Therapy. *Endocrine-Related Cancer*, **11**, 623-641. http://dx.doi.org/10.1677/erc.1.00778

[15]   Carlomagno, C., Perrone, F., Gallo, C., De Laurentiis, M., Lauria, R., Morabito, A., Pettinato, G., Panico, L., D'Antonio, A., Bianco, A.R. and De Placido, S. (1996) c-erb B2 Overexpression Decreases the Benefit of Adjuvant

Tamoxifen in Early-Stage Breast Cancer without Axillary Lymph Node Metastases. *Journal of Clinical Oncology*, **14**, 2702-2708.

[16] Pietras, R.J., Arboleda, J., Reese, D.M., Wongvipat, N., Pegram, M.D., Ramos, L., Gorman, C.M., Parker, M.G., Sliwkowski, M.X. and Slamon, D.J. (1995) HER-2 Tyrosine Kinase Pathway Targets Estrogen Receptor and Promotes Hormone-Independent Growth in Human Breast Cancer Cells. *Oncogene*, **10**, 2435-2446.

[17] McClelland, R.A., Barrow, D., Madden, T.A., Dutkowski, C.M., Pamment, J., Knowlden, J.M., Gee, J.M. and Nicholson, R.I. (2001) Enhanced Epidermal Growth Factor Receptor Signaling in MCF7 Breast Cancer Cells after Long-Term Culture in the Presence of the Pure Antiestrogen ICI 182,780 (Faslodex). *Endocrinology*, **142**, 2776-2788.

[18] Okubo, S., Kurebayashi, J., Otsuki, T., Yamamoto, Y., Tanaka, K. and Sonoo, H. (2004) Additive Antitumour Effect of the Epidermal Growth Factor Receptor Tyrosine Kinase Inhibitor Gefitinib (Iressa, ZD1839) and the Antioestrogen Fulvestrant (Faslodex, ICI 182,780) in Breast Cancer Cells. *British Journal of Cancer*, **90**, 236-244. http://dx.doi.org/10.1038/sj.bjc.6601504

[19] Cameron, D.A., Keen, J.C., Dixon, J.M., Bellamy, C., Hanby, A., Anderson, T.J. and Miller, W.R. (2000) Effective Tamoxifen Therapy of Breast Cancer Involves Both Antiproliferative and Pro-Apoptotic Changes. *European Journal of Cancer*, **36**, 845-851. http://dx.doi.org/10.1016/S0959-8049(00)00013-7

[20] Zhang, G.J., Kimijima, I., Onda, M., Kanno, M., Sato, H., Watanabe, T., Tsuchiya, A., Abe, R. and Takenoshita, S. (1999) Tamoxifen-Induced Apoptosis in Breast Cancer Cells Relates to Down-Regulation of Bcl-2, but Not Bax and bcl-X(L), without Alteration of p53 Protein Levels. *Clinical Cancer Research*, **5**, 2971-2977.

[21] Kang, Y., Cortina, R. and Perry, R.R. (1996) Role of c-myc in Tamoxifen-Induced Apoptosis Estrogen-Independent Breast Cancer Cells. *Journal of the National Cancer Institute*, **88**, 279-284. http://dx.doi.org/10.1093/jnci/88.5.279

[22] Diel, P., Smolnikar, K. and Michna, H. (1999) The Pure Antiestrogen ICI 182780 Is More Effective in the Induction of Apoptosis and Down Regulation of BCL-2 than Tamoxifen in MCF-7 Cells. *Breast Cancer Research and Treatment*, **58**, 87-97. http://dx.doi.org/10.1023/A:1006338123126

[23] Lim, K.B., Ng, C.Y., Ong, C.K., Ong, C.S., Tran, E., Nguyen, T.T., Chan, G.M. and Huynh, H. (2001) Induction of Apoptosis in Mammary Gland by a Pure Anti-Estrogen ICI 182780. *Breast Cancer Research and Treatment*, **68**, 127-138. http://dx.doi.org/10.1023/A:1011929222555

[24] Somaï, S., Chaouat, M., Jacob, D., Perrot, J.Y., Rostène, W., Forgez, P. and Gompel, A. (2003) Antiestrogens Are Pro-Apoptotic in Normal Human Breast Epithelial Cells. *International Journal of Cancer*, **105**, 607-612. http://dx.doi.org/10.1002/ijc.11147

[25] Clarke, R., Liu, M.C., Bouker, K.B., Gu, Z., Lee, R.Y., Zhu, Y., Skaar, T.C., Gomez, B., O'Brien, K., Wang, Y. and Hilakivi-Clarke, L.A. (2003) Antiestrogen Resistance in Breast Cancer and the Role of Estrogen Receptor Signaling. *Oncogene*, **22**, 7316-7339. http://dx.doi.org/10.1038/sj.onc.1206937

[26] Bateman, A. and Bennett, H.P. (1998) Granulins: The Structure and Function of an Emerging Family of Growth Factors. *Journal of Endocrinology*, **158**, 145-151. http://dx.doi.org/10.1677/joe.0.1580145

[27] Serrero, G. (2003) Autocrine Growth Factor Revisited: PC-Cell-Derived Growth Factor (Progranulin), a Critical Player in Breast Cancer Tumorigenesis. *Biochemical and Biophysical Research Communications*, **308**, 409-413. http://dx.doi.org/10.1016/S0006-291X(03)01452-9

[28] Halper, J. (2010) Growth Factors as Active Participants in Carcinogenesis: A Perspective. *Veterinary Pathology*, **47**, 77-97. http://dx.doi.org/10.1177/0300985809352981

[29] Lu, R. and Serrero, G. (2001) Mediation of Estrogen Mitogenic Effect in Human Breast Cancer MCF-7 cells by PC-Cell-Derived Growth Factor (PCDGF/Granulin Precursor). *Proceedings of the National Academy of Sciences of the United States of America*, **98**, 142-147. http://dx.doi.org/10.1073/pnas.98.1.142

[30] Lu, R. and Serrero, G. (2000) Inhibition of PCDGF Expression by Antisense cDNA Transfection Inhibits Tumorigenicity of the Human Breast Carcinoma Cell Line MDA-MB-486. *Proceedings of the National Academy of Sciences of the United States of America*, **97**, 3993-3998.

[31] Tangkeangsirisin, W., Hayashi, J. and Serrero, G. (2004) PC Cell-Derived Growth Factor Mediates Tamoxifen Resistance and Promotes Tumor Growth of Human Breast Cancer Cells. *Cancer Research*, **64**, 1737-1743. http://dx.doi.org/10.1158/0008-5472.CAN-03-2364

[32] Abrhale, T., Brodie, A., Sabnis, G., Macedo, L., Tian, C., Yue, B. and Serrero, G. (2011) GP88 (PC-Cell Derived Growth Factor, Progranulin) Stimulates Proliferation and Confers Letrozole Resistance to Aromatase Overexpressing Breast Cancer Cells. *BMC Cancer*, **11**, 231. http://dx.doi.org/10.1186/1471-2407-11-231

[33] Serrero, G. and Ioffe, O. (2003) Expression of the PC-Cell Derived Growth Factor in benign and Malignant Human Breast Epithelium. *Human Pathology*, **34**, 1148-1154. http://dx.doi.org/10.1016/S0046-8177(03)00425-8

[34] Serrero, G., Hawkins, D.M., Yue, B., Ioffe, O., Bejarano, P., Phillips, J.T., Head, J.F., Elliott, R.L., Tkaczuk, K.R., Godwin, A.K., Weaver, J.E. and Kim, W. (2012) Progranulin (GP88) Tumor Tissue Expression Is Associated with In-

creased Risk of Recurrence in Breast Cancer Patients Diagnosed with Estrogen Receptor Positive Invasive Ductal Carcinoma. *Breast Cancer Research*, **14**, R26-R35. http://dx.doi.org/10.1186/bcr3111

[35] Tkaczuk, K.R., Yue, B., Zhan, M., Tait, N., Yarlagadda, L., Dai, H. and Serrero, G. (2011) Increased Circulating Level of the Survival Factor GP88 (Progranulin) in the Serum of Breast Cancer Patients When Compared to Healthy Subjects. *Breast Cancer Basic and Clinical Research*, **5**, 155-162.

[36] Tangkeangsirisin, W. and Serrero, G. (2004) PC Cell-Derived Growth Factor (PCDGF/GP88, Progranulin) Stimulates Migration, Invasiveness and VEGF Expression in Breast Cancer Cells. *Carcinogenesis*, **25**, 1587-1592. http://dx.doi.org/10.1093/carcin/bgh171

[37] Lilling, G., Hacohen, H., Nordenberg, J., Livnat, T., Rotter, V. and Sidi, Y. (2000) Differential Sensitivity of MCF-7 and LCC2 Cells, to Multiple Growth Inhibitory Agents: Possible Relation to High bcl-2/Bax Ratio? *Cancer Letters*, **161**, 27-34. http://dx.doi.org/10.1016/S0304-3835(00)00579-6

[38] Takei, H., Lee, E.S. and Jordan, V.C. (2002) *In Vitro* Regulation of Vascular Endothelial Growth Factor by Estrogens and Antiestrogens in Estrogen-Receptor Positive Breast Cancer. *Breast Cancer*, **9**, 39-42. http://dx.doi.org/10.1007/BF02967545

[39] Soares, R., Guo, S., Russo, J. and Schmitt, F. (2003) Role of the Estrogen Antagonist ICI 182,780 in Vessel Assembly and Apoptosis of Endothelial Cells. *Ultrastructural Pathology*, **27**, 33-39. http://dx.doi.org/10.1080/01913120309946

[40] He, Z., Ong, C.H., Halper, J. and Bateman, A. (2003) Progranulin Is a Mediator of the Wound Response. *Nature Medicine*, **9**, 225-229. http://dx.doi.org/10.1038/nm816

[41] Elledge, R.M., Green, S., Pugh, R., Allred, D.C., Clark, G.M., Hill, J., Ravdin, P., Martino, S. and Osborne, C.K. (2000) Estrogen Receptor (ER) and Progesterone Receptor (PgR), by Ligand-Binding Assay Compared with ER, PgR and pS2, by Immuno-Histochemistry in Predicting Response to Tamoxifen in Metastatic Breast Cancer: A Southwest Oncology Group Study. *International Journal of Cancer*, **89**, 111-117.

[42] Osborne, C.K., Yochmowitz, M.G., Knight 3rd, W.A. and McGuire, W.L. (1980) The Value of Estrogen and Progesterone Receptors in the Treatment of Breast Cancer. *Cancer*, **46**, 2884-2888.

[43] Luo, L.Y., Diamandis, E.P., Look, M.P., Soosaipillai, A.P. and Foekens, J.A. (2002) Higher Expression of Human Kallikrein 10 in Breast Cancer Tissue Predicts Tamoxifen Resistance. *British Journal of Cancer*, **86**, 1790-1796. http://dx.doi.org/10.1038/sj.bjc.6600323

[44] Berns, E.M., Klijn, J.G., Look, M.P., Grebenchtchikov, N., Vossen, R., Peters, H., Geurts-Moespot, A., Portengen, H., van Staveren, I.L., Meijer-van Gelder, M.E., Bakker, B., Sweep, F.C. and Foekens, J.A. (2003) Combined Vascular Endothelial Growth Factor and *TP53* Status Predicts Poor Response to Tamoxifen Therapy in Estrogen Receptor-Positive Advanced Breast Cancer. *Clinical Cancer Research*, **9**, 1253-1258.

[45] Nicholson, R.I., McClelland, R.A., Gee, J.M., Manning, D.L., Cannon, P., Robertson, J.F., Ellis, I.O. and Blamey, R.W. (1994) Transforming Growth Factor-Alpha and Endocrine Sensitivity in Breast Cancer. *Cancer Research*, **54**, 1684-1689.

21

Failure to Engage in Breast Screening and Risk Assessment Results in More Advanced Stage at Diagnosis

Alison Johnston, Sharon Curran, Michael Sugrue*

Breast Centre North West, Letterkenny Hospital, Donegal Clinical Research Academy, Donegal, Ireland
Email: *michael.sugrue@hse.ie

Abstract

Background: Although well established, population based screening and family risk assessment for breast cancer have come under increasing scrutiny. The concept of over diagnosis is increasingly cited in cancer publications. This study assessed the impact of failure to screen or risk assess patients attending with a new diagnosis of breast cancer. Methods: A retrospective review was undertaken of 200 consecutive patients diagnosed with breast cancer between January 2010 and September 2012 at Letterkenny Hospital. Appropriate screening was defined as biennial in those aged 50 - 66 and in those 40 - 49 with moderate/high family history risk (NICE criteria or IBIS criteria). Patient demographics, screening history, diagnosis date and stage (TNM) were documented. Patients with previous breast cancer were not included (n = 17). Results: 200 consecutive patients, whose mean age was 61 (range 28 - 99), were studied. 112/200 (56%) met no criteria for screening or family history assessment, and 88/200 (44%) met criteria for either screening (in 56) or family history assessment (in 32). 61/88 (69.3%) meeting criteria did not have a mammogram or risk assessment. The stage of breast cancer was significantly earlier in those screened appropriately, with early stage cancer in n = 111/139 (79.9 %) and late in n = 28/139 (20.1%), compared with 38/61 (62.3%) and 23/61 (37.7%) in those failing to be screened appropriately (p = 0.01 χ^2 df1). Conclusion: Failure to engage in breast screening and risk assessment resulted in more advanced stage at diagnosis.

Keywords

Breast Cancer, Breast Cancer Detection, Breast Screening, Breast Outcomes

---

*Corresponding author.

1. Introduction

Over the last decade, there has been significant global reduction in mortality in breast cancer [1]. Early detection of breast cancer optimizes outcomes and survival [2]-[5]. This is facilitated by appropriate breast screening and triage of women of increased risks [6]. While it is universally accepted that breast screening increases breast cancer survival, recent heated discussions question whether it reduces breast cancer mortality [7]-[9]. It has even been suggested that breast screening be abandoned [10]. The concept of over diagnosis and harm of screening and risk assessment has been highlighted [11] [12]. Current international guidelines suggest that women with a moderate or greater family history breast cancer risk should have a mammogram from the age of 40. Those between 50 and 65 should be enrolled in breast screening [13]-[15].

The uptake rates of utilization of existing screening programs are influenced by socioeconomic factors, ease of access, advertising and public awareness. However, not all studies show a positive relationship between familial breast cancer risk and mammographic uptake [16] [17]. There has been a lack of published data assessing enrolment and uptake of breast screening and risk assessment in patients with a known family history risk and or those of breast screening age who should have undergone breast screening [18]. Some countries, such as Ireland and Estonia, have higher breast cancer mortality than the European on average. This is a multifactorial issue with many potential explanations including public awareness, organization and access to services as well as treatments employed. Understanding the stage of presentation of breast cancer may identify opportunities to improve outcome [1]. It is clear, however, that tumor size at presentation predicts long term survival [19].

This study assessed uptake of breast screening and compliance with risk assessment in patients, either with a familial breast cancer history or those meeting screening age criteria in patients presenting with a new index breast cancer.

2. Methods

An ethically approved retrospective review of 200 consecutive newly diagnosed breast cancer patients, presenting to the Symptomatic Breast Unit of Letterkenny Hospital between January 2010 and September 2012, was undertaken. Patients with a known previous diagnosis of breast cancer were excluded from the study (n = 17). Letterkenny Hospital is a designated provider of multidisciplinary breast cancer care under the Irish National Cancer Control Program (NCCP, 2007), working as a satellite centre of its parent cancer centre at University College Hospital Galway [20]. Breast screening in Ireland commenced in 2000 in Dublin and spread nationally throughout the country having arrived in the North West (where this study took place) in October 2009 [13]. Open access or family doctor referral for non-screening mammography is not available for asymptomatic women.

The cohort was divided into one of two groups; the appropriately screened group or the inappropriately screened group. Appropriate screening for the study was defined as biennial in those of breast screening age (50 - 65 years old) [13]. Biennial mammography was considered optimal in those aged 40 - 49 who met 2006 NICE criteria for a moderate family history risk or had an IBIS (Tyrer-Cuzick) 10 yr risk > 3% or a lifetime risk ≥ 17% [15] [21]. Appropriate screening and assessment was deemed to have occurred if a mammogram had been performed within 2 years of diagnosis. Low-risk patients outside breast screening age were also deemed to have been appropriately screened with no previous mammogram performed.

Inappropriate screening and assessment was deemed to have occurred if a mammogram had not been performed within 2 years of diagnosis in those of breast screening age and /or having a moderate or high family history risk.

Patient demographics, date of diagnosis, stage and previous visits to a breast clinic were documented. TNM staging was used to classify stage at presentation [22]. Those stages 0 - 2 were deemed to be early stage and those stages 3 - 4 late stages. A second clinically focused staging system was also used classifying stage as localised, loco-regional or distant. Localised was T0-3 N0 M0; loco-regional was T0-3 N1-3 M0 or T4 N any M0 and distant was T any N any M1 [2]. Data was retrospectively extracted from prospectively entered medical records and hospital databases. Patients were not contacted to determine a reason for non screening to avoid creating anxiety or distress.

Breast cancers detected through the National Screening Programme were not included in this study as they are processed through a standalone breast screening service. In the study period we estimate that 11,822 women were screened with Breast Screening in the Northwest and 137 cancers detected on what would have been a preliminary round of screening for most patients [23]. Data was expressed as mean and standard deviation for normally distributed data and medians and inter quartile range for non-normal data. Chi square test or Student's T-test was used as appropriate for categorical and continuous variables. Data was considered significantly different if p-value was <0.05.

3. Results

200 patients, mean age 61.4 ± 15.4 years (range 28 - 99), all female, were studied. The age distribution is shown in **Figure 1**. 172/200 patients were symptomatic when diagnosed and 28/200 asymptomatic. Of the 28, 12 were incidentally identified during unrelated body imaging, 12 detected by surveillance screening for family history and 4 by other modalities. The dominant symptom at presentation is shown in **Table 1**.

139/200 (69.5%) patients were appropriately screened and 61/200 (30.5%) inappropriately screened. Of the 200 patients, 112 (56%) met no screening or family history risk assessment indication. 88/200 met criteria for mammography: 56/88 met age criteria for breast screening, 21 purely because of family history and 11 met both criteria. Of the 32 family history cohort 29 had a moderate family history risk and 3 were high risk. Of those meeting the screening and risk assessment criteria, only 27/88 (30.7%) were assessed appropriately with mammography. Of the 61 failing to meet screening targets 19 (31.1%) were in the family history risk group and 42 (68.9%) were in the breast screening group. Of those with a family history 13/32 (40.6%) were appropriately screened and 14/56 (25%) in the breast screening age group. 36/61 (59.0%) never had a mammogram while the

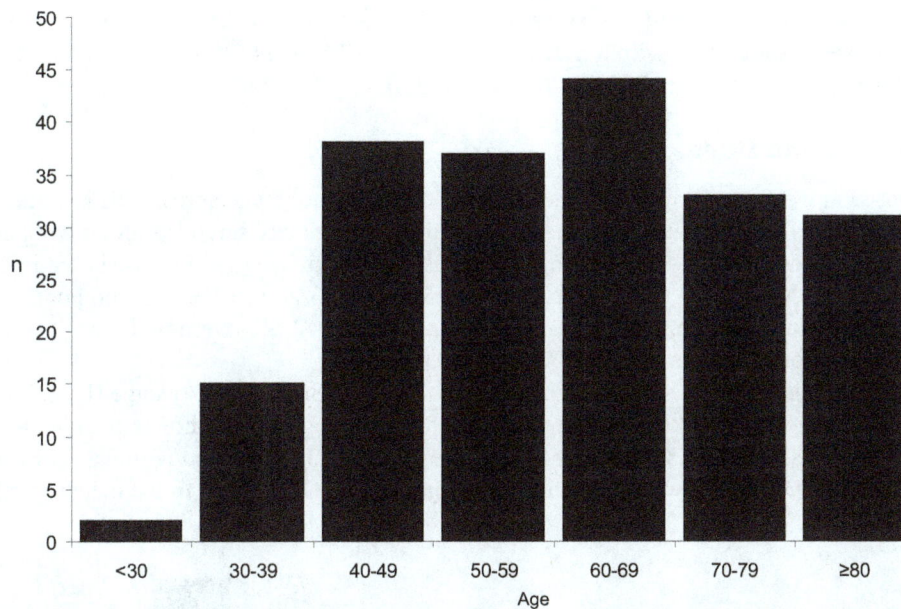

Figure 1. Age distribution of breast cancer (n = 200).

Table 1. Dominant symptom at presentation (n = 172).

Dominant symptom	n
Breast lump	125
Mastalgia	17
Nipple retraction	9
Skin and nipple changes	8
Fungating breast lesion	6
Nipple discharge	4
Altered breast sensation	3

remaining 25/61 (41%) had a mammogram performed more than 2 years pre-diagnosis. The previous mammogram was performed on average 9 ± 7.8 years prior to diagnosis. 26/61 had attended a specialist breast clinic previously, before 2008. Failure to follow up these women was due to both system factors n = 24 and patient factors n = 2. System failures to review patients occurred within the family history service in n = 12 and within the asymptomatic National breast screening services in n = 12.

In patients with increased family risk, the mean 10 year and lifetime IBIS risk was 7.2% ± 5.0% (range 2.7 - 29.1) and 18.9% ± 10.5% (range 6.4 - 61.4) respectively. The BCRA 1 and 2 risks were low for this sub group, at 1.2% ± 3.6% (range 0 - 17.1) and 0.5% ± 1.1% (range 0 - 5.8) respectively. 24 patients in total met NICE criteria for secondary care referral to family history clinics and only one for tertiary care referral to genetic services.

88 of the 200 (44%) had previously attended the breast unit; their first attendance was a median of 84 months prior to the date of diagnosis (range 2 - 408). No cancer was considered a missed diagnosis. Interval cancers were detected in 18 (9%) (≤24 months), 11 of these being ≤12 months. One had a delay of 10 months from initial presentation to final diagnosis. Interval cancers were detected a mean of 10.6 ± 4.7 months (range 2 - 20) after the last mammogram. The pathology of the interval cancers were invasive ductal n = 11, DCIS n = 4 and lobular n = 3.

Of the 82/200 (41%) who had had a previous mammogram, the interval between the last mammogram and the current diagnostic mammogram was on average 58.4 months ± 61.3 (range 1 month to 312 months). The number of years from previous mammogram to diagnosis is shown in **Figure 2**. The cancers were mammography occult in 4/200, three in the appropriately screened group and one in the inappropriately screened group. Mammograms were not performed in three patients, due to tumour ulceration in two and immobility in one.

The appropriateness of screening and risk assessment within each age bracket is shown in **Figure 3**. The appropriate group (n = 139) were older with a mean age of 63.4 ± 17.5 years (28 - 99) compared to the inappropriately screened group (n = 61) 56.7 ± 7.2 (42 - 66) (p = <0.01).

Tumour Pathology and Stage

DCIS was diagnosed in n = 21 and invasive tumours in n = 179. Tumour stage across all 200 patients is show in **Table 2**. Overall T3 and T4 tumour occurred in 14.4% of the appropriately screened group compared to 24.6% of those inappropriately screened (p = 0.08). The mean invasive tumour size (n = 179) is shown in **Table 3**.

107/200 (53.5%) were N0, 54/200 (27%) N1, 17/200 (8.5%) N2, 13/200 (6.5%) N3 and nodal status was unknown in 9/200 (4.5%). In the appropriately screened group 59/139 (42.5%) were nodal positive and in the inappropriately screened group this was 34/61 (55.7%) (p = 0.08 χ^2 df1).

21/200 (10.5%) were diagnosed at stage 0, 41/200 (20.5%) stage I, 86/200 (43%) stage II, 28/200 (14%) stage III and 24/200 (12%) stage IV. TNM stage of presentation for the two groups is shown in **Table 4**. In the appropriately screened group 81/139 (58.3%) had local disease, 45/139 (32.4%) loco/regional disease and 12/139 (8.6%) distant disease. 1/139 (0.7%) was not completely staged due to CT phobia. In the inappropriately screened

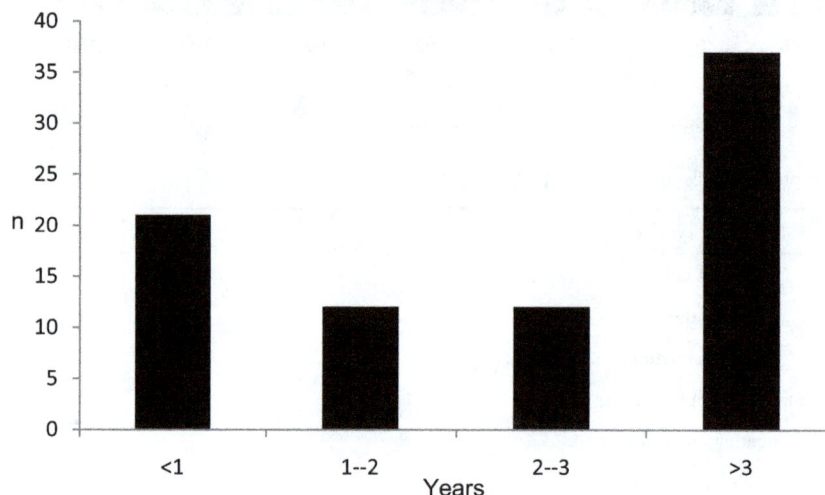

Figure 2. Years from previous mammogram to diagnosis (n = 82).

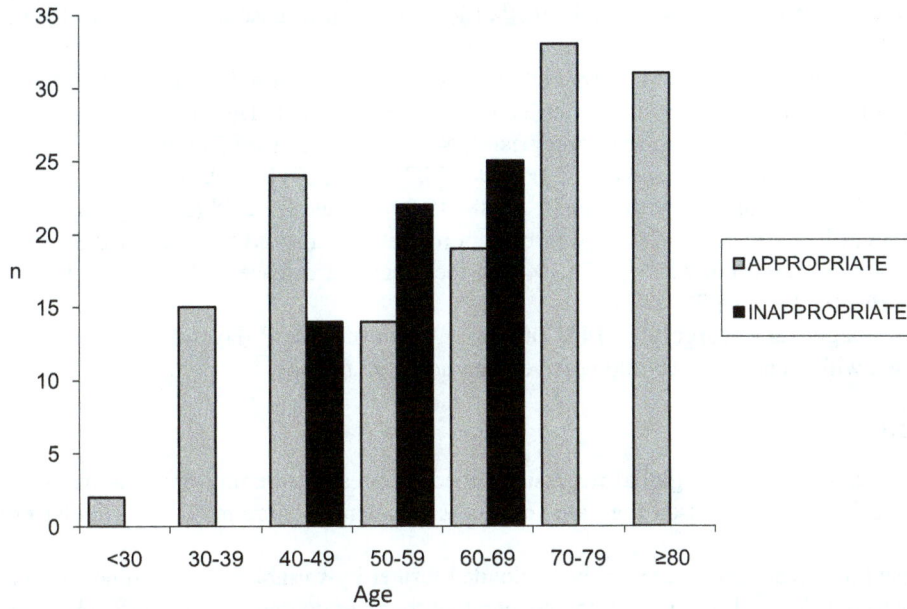

Figure 3. Appropriateness of screening and risk assessment according to age (n = 200).

Table 2. Tumour stage across all 200 patients.

Tumour stage	Appropriately screened (n = 139)		Inappropriately screened (n = 61)	
	n	%	n	%
Tis	13	9.3	8	13.1
T1	41	29.5	15	24.6
T2	65	46.8	23	37.7
T3	14	10.1	8	13.1
T4	6	4.3	7	11.5

(p = 0.25).

Table 3. Invasive tumour size (mm) (n = 179).

Stage (TNM)*	All invasive tumours n = 179	Appropriately screened n = 126	Inappropriately screened n = 53
Early	n = 128	n = 98	n = 30
	24.1 ± 14.1 (0.8 - 105)	24.5 ± 15.3 (0.8 - 105)	22.6 ± 9.9 (5.5 - 40)
Late	n = 51	n = 28	n = 23
	54.8 ± 32.6 (11 - 150)	58.1 ± 34.9 (11 - 150)	50.9 ± 29.9 (11.6 - 120)

*TNM stages 1 - 2 were deemed to be early stage and stages 3 - 4 late stage.

Table 4. TNM stage of breast cancer at presentation.

Stage (TNM)*	All		Appropriately screened		Inappropriately screened	
	n=200		n = 139		n = 61	
	n	%	n	%	n	%
Early	149	74.5	111	79.9	38	62.3
Late	51	25.5	28	20.1	23	37.7

p-value 0.01 χ^2 df = 1. *TNM stages 0 - 2 were deemed to be early stage and stages 3 - 4 late stage.

group 27/61 (44.3%) had local disease, 22/61 (36.1%) loco/regional disease and 12/61 (19.6%) distant disease (p-value 0.05 χ^2 df = 2).

In those meeting screening criteria (n = 88), DCIS was diagnosed in n = 14 and invasive tumours in n = 74. Tumour stages for those meeting screening criteria are shown in **Figure 4**. The mean invasive tumour size (mm) in n = 74 was 32.1 ± 24.6 (5 - 120). In the appropriately screened group (n = 21) this was 25.0 ± 22.1 (5 - 105) and in the inappropriately screened group (n = 53) 34.9 ± 25.2 (5.5 - 120) (p = 0.1).

14 of the 88 (15.9%) were stage 0 at diagnosis, 17/88 (19.3 %) stage I, 32/88 (36.4%) stage II, 12/88 (13.6%) stage III and 13/88 (14.8%) stage IV. 74.1% of those appropriately screened had localised disease versus 44.2% in those inappropriately screened. 22.2% v 36.1% had loco/regional disease and 3.7% v 19.7% distant disease respectively (p-value 0.02 χ^2 df = 2).

The time from diagnosis to surgery in 143/200 was a mean of 13 ± 8 days (1 - 50) with a median of 12. 41/200 was treated without surgery; 16/200 received neo-adjuvant therapy.

4. Discussion

Optimizing breast cancer care is a global necessity, aided by breast screening and risk assessment. Recently, however, there has been doubt cast on the value of risk assessment programmes, in particular breast screening [10] [24].

The optimal path in breast cancer care has been clouded further by variability in outcomes from different countries and healthcare services. More recently the concepts of the over diagnosis have seriously questioned the actual benefits of breast screening and risk assessment programmes.

Heated discussion has arisen in relation to the provision of balanced outcome reporting and balanced messages, to enable informed choices, for women attending breast risk assessment and screening [25]. This study has identified that failure to enrol in breast risk assessment and breast screening results in significantly later stage of breast cancer presentation.

Breast screening has developed at different times in different countries. Scandinavia, USA and the United Kingdom developed formal screening programmes between 1990 and 2006. In Ireland the Breast Check programme rolled out to the entire country in 2009. The last region for this programme to be enrolled was in Donegal in the North West of Ireland, the site of the study. Ireland has a designated regionalised breast cancer programme with 8 designated units of which Letterkenny Hospital is the provider for a population of 160,000 in the North West; a relatively remote geographic area and one of Ireland's poorest from a socioeconomic viewpoint. The region does not have GP access mammography and mammography can only be organized through attendance at a Symptomatic Breast Unit or through the breast screening service between the ages of 50 and 64.

Patients entering the Breast Screening Programme were not included in this study. The enrolment rate for breast screening in Ireland is falling and now approaches 71.4% in line with other recruitments internationally. Of particular concern of those aged 50 - 54, invited for a first screening, 49.6% in the West region accepted the offer [23]. The average lifetime risk of breast cancer is between 10% and 12.3% and the 10-year risk of invasive breast cancer at the ages of 40, 50 and 60 years are 1.5%, 2.3%, and 3.5% respectively [26].

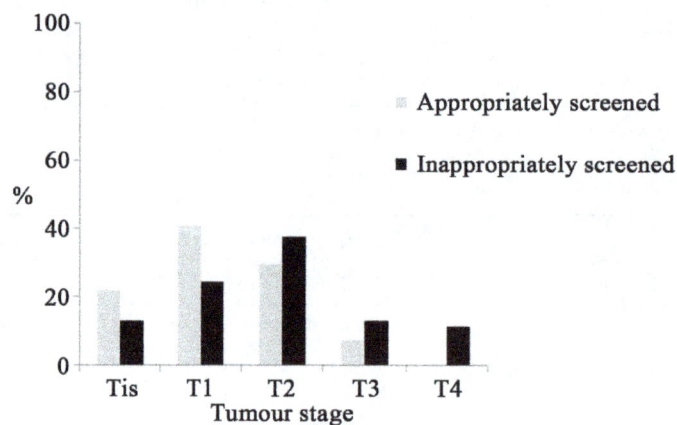

Figure 4. Tumour stages in those meeting screening criteria (n = 88).

In our study the dominant symptom was a lump leading to the patients' presentation. 44% of our study population met criteria for breast screening, under international guidelines moderate to high risk patients should be screened [27]-[30]. Madlensky and colleagues (2005) have shown that moderate risk women have undertaken mammography in 47% of cases compared to 82% in high risk and 35% among the population risk [16].

There are many factors involved in failure to undertake mammography. These are patient and system related. Some are related to poor literacy, fatalistic fears and external decision making pressures [31]. Anxiety and stress also play a role [32]. New strategies to reduce the late presentation of breast cancer are considered important. Devi and colleagues [4] were able to reduce the prevalence of Stage III and Stage IV breast cancers from 60% to 35% by educating health staff on the theoretical and practical aspects of breast cancer and by strengthening public awareness programs and referral system for positive cases. Similarly in Singapore, Chang and colleagues found that up to 20% of patients were still presenting with Stage III and Stage IV breast cancer [33]. Surprisingly the stage and tumour size at presentation in this study was quite late with a mean invasive tumour size of 32 mm versus 35 mm, and a significant over representation of stage III and IV and regional and metastatic disease in those failing to be risk assessed and screened.

Tabár and colleagues suggested that there was a 63% reduction in mortality in those screened and more recently Paap *et al.* found a 58% reduction [34] [35]. Multiple individual studies, randomised controlled trials, meta-analysis and systematic review of the literature have challenged this. The Marmot report suggests there is a 20% reduction in mortality [11]. Pace and Keating suggests that this is 15% for women in their 40s and 32% for women in their 60s. They have suggested that 19% of cancers diagnosed during the 10 year period would have become clinically apparent without screening and feel that this represents over diagnosis [26]. Others feel that over diagnosis is less of a problem at 0.7% in 40 to 49 years old [36]. Many studies have looked at delays, usually in the peri-operative period. A key National performance indicator [37] is that surgery occurs in over 90% of patients within 4 weeks of diagnosis, unless having neoadjuvant treatment. There were no significant peri-operative delays; the median time to surgery was 12 days. It has been suggested that a delay of more than 6 months may affect outcome [38]. Others are showing that peri-operative delays had no impact on survival [39].

Patients presenting in this series were direct referrals to the Breast Unit and all but one of the patients were diagnosed on their visit following triple assessment. This compares with more economically challenged countries such as Mexico where 7.9 clinic visits were required before diagnosis [40].

Patient factors relating to failure to attend were not analysed and it is a limitation of the study. It was decided, despite ethical approval for this study, that it may have created an element of retrospective anxiety as to question the women as to why they had not attended for screening. A system problem with failure to recall patients before 2008 in 12 patients was deduced from auditing medical records; however at that time clear international guidelines were not as well developed in risk assessment. Currently the unit uses computerized and manual NICE guidelines for risk assessment [27] [41] [42].

International variation occurs in outcome from breast cancer across Europe, United States and other health areas. Stage has been felt to be one of the most dominant predictors of outcome [2] [3] [28] [43]-[45]. It is important to differentiate between adherences to mammography as a random or guideline event. In conclusion this study has identified that failure to risk assess and perform mammography in line with International current guidelines will result in delayed presentation of breast cancer. New strategies for risk assessment and screening in moderate risk patients need to be developed. Newer options in breast imaging may improve detection and outcome, but have not yet been validated [46] [47].

This study identified that women who failed to attend appropriate screening and risk assessment would have more advanced breast cancer. A public health review of enrolment and risk assessment process needs to be undertaken in the region.

References

[1]   De Angelis, R., Sant, M., Coleman, M.P., *et al.* (2014) Cancer Survival in Europe 1999-2007 by Country and Age: Results of EUROCARE-5—A Population-Based Study. *The Lancet Oncology*, **15**, 23-34. http://dx.doi.org/10.1016/S1470-2045(13)70546-1

[2]   Barburin, A., Aareleid, T., Padrik, P., *et al.* (2014) Time Trends in Population-Based Cancer Survival in Estonia: Analysis by Age and Stage. *Acta Oncologica*, **53**, 226-234. http://dx.doi.org/10.3109/0284186X.2013.806992

[3]   Richards, M.A. (2009) The Size of the Prize for Earlier Diagnosis of Cancer in England. *British Journal of Cancer*, **101**, S125-S129. http://dx.doi.org/10.1038/sj.bjc.6605402

[4] Devi, B.C., Tang, T.S. and Corbex, M. (2007) Reducing by Half the Percentage of Late-Stage Presentation for Breast and Cervix Cancer over 4 Years: A Pilot Study of Clinical Downstaging in Sarawak, Malaysia. *Annals of Oncology*, **18**, 1172-1176. http://dx.doi.org/10.1093/annonc/mdm105

[5] Friedman, L.C., Kalidas, M., Elledge, R., *et al.* (2006) Medical and Psychosocial Predictors of Delay in Seeking Medical Consultation for Breast Symptoms in Women in a Public Sector Setting. *Journal of Behavioral Medicine*, **29**, 327-334. http://dx.doi.org/10.1007/s10865-006-9059-2

[6] Mathis, K., Hoskin, T., Boughey, J., *et al.* (2010) Palpable Presentation of Breast Cancer Persists in the Era of Screening Mammography. *Journal of American College of Surgeons*, **210**, 314-318. http://dx.doi.org/10.1016/j.jamcollsurg.2009.12.003

[7] Miller, A., Wall, C., Baines, C., *et al.* (2014) Twenty Five Year Follow-Up for Breast Cancer Incidence and Mortality of the Canadian National Breast Screening Study: Randomised Screening Trial. *British Medical Journal*, **348**, g366-g366.

[8] Bleyer, A. and Welch, H.G. (2012) Effect of Three Decades of Screening Mammography on Breast-Cancer Incidence. *The New England Journal of Medicine*, **367**, 1998-2005. http://dx.doi.org/10.1056/NEJMoa1206809

[9] Tabár, L., Vitak, B., Chen, T.H., *et al.* (2011) Swedish Two-County Trial: Impact of Mammographic Screening on Breast Cancer Mortality during 3 Decades. *Radiology*, **260**, 658-663. http://dx.doi.org/10.1148/radiol.11110469

[10] Biller-Andorno, N. and Juni, P. (2014) Abolishing Mammography Screening Programs? A View from the Swiss Medical Board. *The New England Journal of Medicine*, **370**, 1965-1967. http://dx.doi.org/10.1056/NEJMp1401875

[11] Marmot, M. (2013) Sorting through the Arguments on Breast Screening. *JAMA*, **309**, 2553-2554. http://dx.doi.org/10.1001/jama.2013.6822

[12] McCartney, M. (2014) A Trial to Extend Breast Cancer Screening May Be Unethical. *British Medical Journal*, **349**, g5105. http://dx.doi.org/10.1136/bmj.g5105

[13] National Cancer Screening Service (NCSS) (2000) Breast Check—The National Breast Screening Programme. http://www.breastcheck.ie/

[14] Armstrong, A. and Evans, G. (2014) Management of Women at High Risk of Breast Cancer. *British Medical Journal*, **348**, g2756. http://dx.doi.org/10.1136/bmj.g2756

[15] National Institute for Health and Clinical Excellence (2006) Quick Reference Guide. Clinical Guideline 41. Familial Breast Cancer: The Classification and Care of Women at Risk of Familial Breast Cancer in Primary, Secondary and Tertiary Care. NICE, London.

[16] Madlensky, L., Vierkant, R., Vachon, C.M., Pankratz, V.S., Cerhan, J.R., Vadaparampil, S.T. and Sellers, T.A. (2005) Preventive Health Behaviors and Familial Breast Cancer. *Cancer Epidemiology, Biomarkers & Prevention*, **14**, 2340-2345. http://dx.doi.org/10.1158/1055-9965.EPI-05-0254

[17] Price, M.A., Butow, P.N., Charles, M., Bullen, T., Meiser, B., McKinley, J.M., *et al.* (2010) Predictors of Breast Cancer Screening Behavior in Women with a Strong Family History of the Disease. *Breast Cancer Research and Treatment*, **124**, 509-519. http://dx.doi.org/10.1007/s10549-010-0868-1

[18] Samphao, S., Wheeler, A.J., Rafferty, E., Michaelson, J.S., Specht, M.C., Gadd, M.A., *et al.* (2009) Diagnosis of Breast Cancer in Women Age 40 and Younger: Delays in Diagnosis Result from Underuse of Genetic Testing and Breast Imaging. *American Journal of Surgery*, **198**, 538-543. http://dx.doi.org/10.1016/j.amjsurg.2009.06.010

[19] Narod, S., Valentini, A., Nofech-Mozes, S., Sun, P. and Hanna, W. (2012) Tumour Characteristics among Women with Very Low-Risk Breast Cancer. *Breast Cancer Research and Treatment*, **134**, 1241-1246. http://dx.doi.org/10.1007/s10549-012-2065-x

[20] Health Service Executive. Galway University Hospitals Cancer Centre—Annual Report 2012. http://www.wnwhg.ie/sites/default/files/publications/cancer-centre-annual-report-2012.pdf

[21] IBIS Breast Cancer Risk Evaluation Tool. V6 2004. http://www.ems-trials.org/riskevaluator/

[22] AJCC (American Joint Committee on Cancer) (2010) Cancer Staging Manual. 7th Edition, Edge, S.B., Byrd, D.R., Compton, C.C., *et al.*, Eds., Springer-Verlag, New York.

[23] National Cancer Screening Service (2014) Breast Check—Programme Report 2012-2013. Health Service Executive, Dublin. http://www.breastcheck.ie/sites/default/files/bcheck/documents/bc_pr_2013.pdf

[24] Smith, R. (2014) Counterpoint: Overdiagnosis in Breast Cancer Screening. *Journal of the American College of Radiology*, **11**, 648-652. http://dx.doi.org/10.1016/j.jacr.2014.03.011

[25] Hersch, J., Barratt, A., Jansen, J., Irwig, L., McGeechan, K., Jacklyn, G., *et al.* (2015) Use of a Decision Aid Including Information on Overdetection to Support Informed Choice about Breast Cancer Screening: A Randomised Controlled Trial. *The Lancet*, Published Online18 February 2015.

[26] Pace, L. and Keating, N. (2014) A Systematic Assessment of Benefits and Risks to Guide Breast Cancer Screening

Decisions. *JAMA*, **311**, 1327-1335. http://dx.doi.org/10.1001/jama.2014.1398

[27] National Institute for Health and Clinical Excellence (2013) Familial Breast Cancer: Classification and Care of People at Risk of Familial Breast Cancer and Management of Breast Cancer and Related Risks in People with a Family History of Breast Cancer. CG164. http://guidance.nice.org.uk/CG164/Guidance

[28] Møller, H., Sandin, F., Bray, F., Klint, Å., Linklater, K.M., Purushotham, A., *et al.* (2010) Breast Cancer Survival in England, Norway and Sweden: A Population-Based Comparison. *International Journal of Cancer*, **127**, 2630-2638. http://dx.doi.org/10.1002/ijc.25264

[29] Anderson, E., Berg, J., Black, R., Bradshaw, N., Campbell, J., Carnaghan, H., *et al.* (2008) Prospective Surveillance of Women with a Family History of Breast Cancer: Auditing the Risk Threshold. *British Journal of Cancer*, **98**, 840-844. http://dx.doi.org/10.1038/sj.bjc.6604155

[30] Gui, G., Hogben, R., Walsh, G., A'Hern, R. and Eeles, R. (2001) The Incidence of Breast Cancer from Screening Women According to Predicted Family History Risk: Does Annual Clinical Examination Add to Mammography? *European Journal of Cancer*, **37**, 1668-1673. http://dx.doi.org/10.1016/S0959-8049(01)00207-6

[31] Taib, N., Yip, C. and Low, W. (2014) A Grounded Explanation of Why Women Present with Advanced Breast Cancer. *World Journal of Surgery*, **38**, 1676-1684. http://dx.doi.org/10.1007/s00268-013-2339-4

[32] Schwartz, M., Taylor, K., Wilard, K., Siegel, J.E., Lamdan, R.M. and Moran, K. (1999) Distress, Personality and Mammography Utilization among Women with a Family History of Breast Cancer. *Health Psychology*, **18**, 327-332. http://dx.doi.org/10.1037/0278-6133.18.4.327

[33] Chang, G., Chan, C. and Hartman, M. (2011) A Commentary on Delayed Presentation of Breast Cancer in Singapore. *Asian Pacific Journal of Cancer Prevention*, **12**, 1635-1639.

[34] Tabár, L., Vitak, B., Chen, H., Yen, M.F., Duffy, S.W. and Smith, R.A. (2001) Beyond Randomized Controlled Trials. *Cancer*, **91**, 1724-1731. http://dx.doi.org/10.1002/1097-0142(20010501)91:9<1724::AID-CNCR1190>3.0.CO;2-V

[35] Paap, E., Verbeek, A., Botterweck, A., *et al.* (2014) Breast Cancer Screening Halves the Risk of Breast Cancer Deaths: A Case-Referent Study. *The Breast*, **23**, 439-444. http://dx.doi.org/10.1016/j.breast.2014.03.002

[36] Gunsoy, N., Garcia-Closas, M. and Moss, S. (2012) Modelling the Overdiagnosis of Breast Cancer Due to Mammography Screening in Women Aged 40 to 49 in the United Kingdom. *Breast Cancer Research*, **14**, R152. http://dx.doi.org/10.1186/bcr3365

[37] HSE, NCCP Symptomatic Breast Disease. Key Performance Indicators: 3 Year Report 2010-2012. http://www.hse.ie/eng/services/list/5/cancer/pubs/intelligence/NCCP%20KPI%20report%20symptomatic%20breast%20disease%202010%20-%202013.pdf

[38] Love, R., Duc, N., Baumann, L., Thi Hoang Anh, P., Van To, T., Qian, Z. and Havighurst, T.C. (2004) Duration of Signs and Survival in Premenopausal Women with Breast Cancer. *Breast Cancer Research and Treatment*, **86**, 117-124. http://dx.doi.org/10.1023/B:BREA.0000032980.55245.c3

[39] Brazda, A., Estroff, J., Euhus, D., Leitch, A.M., Huth, J., Andrews, V., *et al.* (2010) Delays in Time to Treatment and Survival Impact in Breast Cancer. *Annals of Surgical Oncology*, **17**, S291-S296. http://dx.doi.org/10.1245/s10434-010-1250-6

[40] Bright, K., Barghash, M., Donach, M., de la Barrera, M.G., Schneider, R.J. and Formenti, S.C. (2011) The Role of Health System Factors in Delaying Final Diagnosis and Treatment of Breast Cancer in Mexico City, Mexico. *The Breast*, **20**, S54-S59. http://dx.doi.org/10.1016/j.breast.2011.02.012

[41] Gorman, A., Sugrue, M., Ahmed, Z. and Johnston, A. (2014) An Evaluation of FaHRAS Computer Programmes' Utility in Family History Triage of Breast Cancer. *Advances in Breast Cancer Research*, **3**, 17-21. http://dx.doi.org/10.4236/abcr.2014.32004

[42] Thomas, J., Sugrue, M., Curran, S., Furey, M. and Sugrue, R. (2013) Are Family Doctors Compliant with Breast Family History Guidelines? *Advances in Breast Cancer Research*, **2**, 149-153. http://dx.doi.org/10.4236/abcr.2013.24024

[43] Olesen, F., Hansen, R. and Vedsted, P. (2009) Delay in Diagnosis: The Experience in Denmark. *British Journal of Cancer*, **101**, S5-S8. http://dx.doi.org/10.1038/sj.bjc.6605383

[44] Woods, L., Rachet, B., O'Connell, D., Lawrence, G., Tracey, E., Willmore, A. and Coleman, M.P. (2009) Large Difference in Patterns of Breast Cancer Survival between Australia and England: A Comparative Study Using Cancer Registry Data. *International Journal of Cancer*, **124**, 2391-2399. http://dx.doi.org/10.1002/ijc.24233

[45] Sant, M., Allemani, C., Capocaccia, R., Hakulinen, T., Aareleid, T., Coebergh, J.W., *et al.* (2003) Stage at Diagnosis Is a Key Explanation of Differences in Breast Cancer Survival across Europe. *International Journal of Cancer*, **106**, 416-422. http://dx.doi.org/10.1002/ijc.11226

[46] Kopans, D. (2014) A New Era in Mammography Screening. *Radiology*, **271**, 629-631. http://dx.doi.org/10.1148/radiol.14140177

[47] Skaane, P., Bandos, A., Eben, E., Jebsen, I.N., Krager, M., Haakenaasen, U., *et al.* (2014) Two-View Digital Breast Tomosynthesis Screening with Synthetically Reconstructed Projection Images: Comparison with Digital Breast Tomosynthesis with Full-Field Digital Mammographic Images. *Radiology*, **271**, 655-663. http://dx.doi.org/10.1148/radiol.13131391

22

Unusual Case of Bilateral Breast Cancer: A Pure Encapsulated Papillary Breast Tumor of the Right Breast and a Contralateral Invasive Ductal Carcinoma

Alberto Testori[1], Valentina Errico[1], Edoardo Bottoni[1], Emanuele Voulaz[1], Stefano Meroni[2], Roberto Travaglini[1], Marco Alloisio[1]

[1]General and Thoracic Surgery, IRCCS Humanitas Research Hospital, Via Manzoni, Rozzano (Milan), Italy
[2]Breast Imaging Division, European Institute of Oncology, Via Ripamonti, Milan, Italy
Email: stefano.meroni@ieo.it

Abstract

Background: Intracystic papillary breast cancer is a very rare tumor that occurs most frequently in elderly postmenopausal women. Aim: In this article we presented a case of a 66-year-old woman who underwent excisional biopsy due to a right breast mass. Case presentation: Histological examination revealed the "pure" encapsulated papillary breast carcinoma without coexisting *in situ* neoplasm and/or invasive carcinoma. This is a rare lesion of the breast that can clinically mimic breast benign mass with only local or regionally aggressive course. Conclusion: In order to avoid misdiagnosis, both the clinician and the breast radiologist should have the possibility of diagnosing this tumor. Intracystic papillary carcinoma of the breast associated with lymph node metastasis has rarely been reported, but the sentinel lymph node biopsy may be prudent in such cases, despite the non aggressive behavior.

Keywords

Encapsulated Papillary Breast Carcinoma, Intracystic Papillary Breast Carcinoma, Lymph Node Breast Metastases

1. Introduction

Intracystic papillary breast cancer is a ductal carcinoma of papillary variety surrounded by a fibrous capsule that develops in a cystic space. It occurs most frequently in elderly postmenopausal women.

It is a rare clinicopathological entity, and its *in situ* or invasive character is difficult to establish, particularly on biopsy. Surgery and breast conservation are treatment options, depending on the size of the tumor. This tumor may be multifocal and can be as a "pure" form or associated with *in situ* neoplasms or invasive carcinomas. Lymph node exploration is currently debated. Although rare and despite being a large and bulky tumor, invasive papillary cancer has an excellent prognosis [1] due to a high-grade hormonal response and uncommon axillary node metastases. The prognosis is favorable also for women presenting with axillary metastases [2].

The aim of this article is to present a case of unexpected bilateral breast cancer and to make breast radiologists and surgeons aware of the spread of the axillary tumor.

2. Clinical Summary

We report a case of a 66-year-old female presenting with a painless mass in the upper inner quadrant of the right breast.

On physical examination the breast surgeon appreciated a rather firm palpable lump without any evidence of dermal invasion and no suspicious axillary lymph nodes. A round, high-density mass without microcalcifications, with well-defined margins and 15 mm in diameter was found in the right breast on a mammography (**Figure 1**). An ultrasound examination revealed one well-delimited oval mass with a slightly heterogeneous echostructure. The nodule featured cystic collections in hypoechoic solid parts containing millimetric cystic regions. There was no acoustic shadowing; a slight acoustic enhancement behind the mass was noticed instead and there were no sonographic signs of adjacent tissue invasion (**Figure 2**). No suspicious axillary lymph nodes were found on ultrasound examination. The breast ecographic findings did not raise any suspicion of malignancy: the radiological work-up was rather suggestive of a benign etiology such as pseudoangiomatous stromal hyperplasia (PASH), fibroadenoma, intraductal papilloma, or complex cyst. In contrast, rare malignant tumors including medullary or mucinous carcinoma were considered as well. The serum CEA and CA15-3 levels were within normal range. A fine needle aspiration cytology (FNAC) under ultrasound guidance of the nodule was performed and revealed a C3 diagnosis, most likely a benign lesion. Lumpectomy was performed in another medical center; no surgical margin was positive for malignancy.

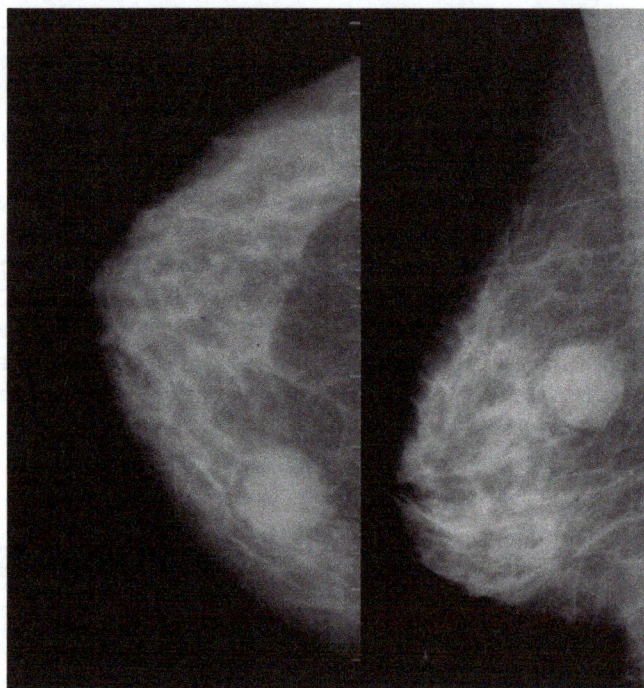

Figure 1. Mediolateral oblique and craniocaudal mammograms of the right breast showing a high opacity round mass without microcalcification and with well-defined margins in the upper inner quadrant.

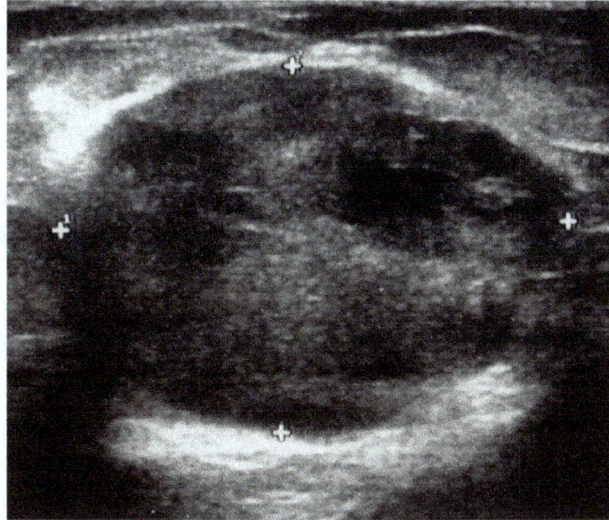

Figure 2. Ultrasound imaging demonstrating a round mass with well-defined margins and a slight acoustic enhancement behind the mass. Multiple areas of hypoechogenicity are detectable, revealing cystic areas.

Microscopic evaluation revealed a "pure" encapsulated papillary breast carcinoma without coexisting *in situ* neoplasm (ER 90%, PgR 90%, Ki67 30% Her2 negative).

The patient was referred to our institution for sentinel lymph node biopsy. Sentinel lymph node metastasis was detected in the right axilla using SNOLL (Sentinel Node and Occult Lesion Localization) procedure. We performed a lymph node dissection of the right axilla. Due to axillary tumor spread, the patient underwent breast MRI (Magnetic Resonance Imaging), which showed a small suspicious nodule in the left breast undetected with the traditionally triplet diagnostics (physical examination, mammography and ultrasound).

At the breast MR imaging, the suspicious nodule showed an ill-defined mass without a cystic component, characterized by hypointensity at axial T2-weighted image, hypointensity at the T1-weighted imaging findings and hyperintensity after administration of gadolinium-based contrasting agent. This finding represented the vascularized stroma.

The dynamic enhancement pattern is typically the type III washout pattern in the solid portion.

So we performed a left quadrantectomy with sentinel node biopsy using SNOLL procedure without a subsequent axillary dissection. In the left breast, the final diagnosis was invasive ductal carcinoma not otherwise specified, G2 (ER 90%, PgR 75%, Ki67 10% Her2 negative), with isolated tumor cells in one lymph node.

According to the biological characteristics of ductal breast cancer, we proposed radiation therapy on both breasts and hormone therapy.

An annual mammography and a six month breast ultrasound with senological examination were scheduled, considering the malignant nature of the lesion in a right breast. After two years of follow-up, we found no recurrence.

3. Discussion

The aim of this article is to highlight an uncommon case of encapsulated papillary breast cancer with an atypical clinical presentation [1] [3]-[6]. Imaging is crucial for the identification of the lesion and local staging, guiding tissue diagnosis, and follow-up while the final diagnosis still relies on the interventional approach (biopsy or surgery). Considering the radiological features of the right breast mass (rounded shape, well-defined margins, heterogeneous echostructure, absence of acoustic shadowing, absence of microcalcifications and an expansive rather than infiltrative growth pattern) the diagnosis of a benign or probably benign lesion could be erroneously made.

Differentiation between benign and malignant papillary lesions may be difficult on FNAC (as in our case), because FNAC targets the centre whereas invasion is at the periphery, as well as the trucut biopsy of the lesion. Despite the fact that these tumors are invasive or *in situ* neoplasms, encapsulated papillary breast carcinomas rarely metastasize, and when they do, they must be considered as indistinguishable from general mammary carcinomas.

Based on the available clinical data [3]-[6], little is known about encapsulated papillary breast cancer with positive axillary lymph node [2]. Axillary dissection is rare because nodal metastases are poor in this group of patients, however sentinel node biopsy may be warranted. Our case indicates that some papillary breast cancers can widely spread and sentinel lymph node biopsy may be a prudent way to evaluate axillary involvement in these patients. It is difficult to make a correct preoperative evaluation in such cases but, in our opinion, the sentinel lymph node biopsy is a reasonable option. Since encapsulated papillary breast carcinomas rarely metastasize, when we found metastases in the sentinel node, we decided to reassess the initial diagnosis by subjecting the patient to a breast MRI with contrasting agents. Interestingly, using MRI to detect an eventual another breast cancer in a right breast, we found an otherwise occult contralateral breast cancer not detected with traditional diagnostic triplet (physical examination, mammography and ultrasound).

Invasive papillary carcinoma often has a favorable prognosis than ductal carcinoma. In a recent study [7], the majority of invasive papillary carcinoma patients were positive for ER and PgR and negative for Her2 (as in our case), low-grade and slow growing cancer. The incidences of local recurrence, distant metastasis, and cancer related death were relatively low to that previously reported [6]-[8]. Surgical resection remains the cornerstone of treatment with an undefined role for radiation therapy and chemotherapy in the neoadjuvant, adjuvant, and metastatic management [6]-[8]. The aim of this article is to present a case report of encapsulated breast cancer with axillary node metastasis tumor and to make the clinician and the radiologist aware of the possible axillary tumor spread of these tumors. The second aim of this report is to raise the radiologist awareness towards ultrasound abnormalities in breast nodules and to evaluate accurately the axillary node in case of breast lesion with atypical clinical and radiological presentations.

4. Conclusion

In conclusion, we demonstrate a case of invasive papillary carcinoma of the breast with omolateral axillary tumor spread, rare by definition and an undetected tumor on the left side. Recommendation from this case report is to have a great attention on benign diagnosis. Make an adequate follow-up also for benign lesions as pseudoangiomatous stromal hyperplasia (PASH), fibroadenoma, intraductal papilloma, or complex cyst to evaluate a possible variation, and perform MRI in all doubt or uncommon cases.

Disclosure Statement

This research was not supported by any organization and none of the authors has a financial relationship that would represent a conflict of interest. The informed consent was obtained by the patient.

References

[1]   Rakha, E.A., Gandhi, N., Climent, F., van Deurzen, C.H., Haider, S.A., Dunk, L., Lee, A.H., Macmillan, D. and Ellis, I.O. (2011) Encapsulated Papillary Carcinoma of the Breast: An Invasive Tumor with Excellent Prognosis. *American Journal of Surgical Pathology*, **35**, 1093-1103. http://dx.doi.org/10.1097/PAS.0b013e31821b3f65

[2]   Mulligan, A.M. and O'Malley, F.P. (2007) Metastatic Potential of Encapsulated (Intracystic) Papillary Carcinoma of the Breast: A Report of 2 Cases with Axillary Lymph Node Micrometastases. *International Journal of Surgical Pathology*, **15**, 143-147. http://dx.doi.org/10.1177/1066896906299119

[3]   Rodríguez, M.C., Secades, A.L. and Angulo, J.M. (2010) Best Cases from the AFIP: Intracystic Papillary Carcinoma of the Breast. *Radiographics*, **30**, 2021-2027. http://dx.doi.org/10.1148/rg.307105003

[4]   Dogan, B.E., Whitman, G.J., Middleton, L.P. and Phelps, M. (2003) Intracystic Papillary Carcinoma of the Breast. *American Journal of Roentgenology*, **181**, 186. http://dx.doi.org/10.2214/ajr.181.1.1810186

[5]   Akagi, T., Kinoshita, T., Shien, T., Hojo, T., Akashi-Tanaka, S. and Murata, Y. (2009) Clinical and Pathological Features of Intracystic Papillary Carcinoma of the Breast. *Surgery Today*, **39**, 5-8. http://dx.doi.org/10.1007/s00595-008-3792-9

[6]   Grabowski, J., Salzstein, S.L., Sadler, G.R. and Blair, S. (2008) Intracystic Papillary Carcinoma: A Review of 917 Cases. *Cancer*, **113**, 916-920. http://dx.doi.org/10.1002/cncr.23723

[7]   Liu, Z.Y., Liu, N., Wang, Y.H., Yang, C.C., Zhang, J., Ly, S.H. and Niu, Y. (2013) Clinicopathologic Characteristics and Molecular Subtypes of Invasive Papillary Carcinoma of the Breast: A Large Case Study. *Journal of Cancer Re-*

search and Clinical Oncology, **139**, 77-84. http://dx.doi.org/10.1007/s00432-012-1302-3

[8] Solorzano, C.C., Middleton, L.P., Hunt, K.K., Mirza, N., Meric, F., Kuerer, H.M., Ross, M.I., Ames, F.C., Feig, B.W., Pollock, R.E., Singletary, S.E. and Babiera, G. (2002) Treatment and Outcome of Patients with Intracystic Papillary Carcinoma of the Breast. *The American Journal of Surgery*, **184**, 364-368. http://dx.doi.org/10.1016/S0002-9610(02)00941-8

23

The Centricity Score: A Novel Measurement to Aid in Conservative Breast Cancer Surgery

Ryan Sugrue, Katherine McGowan, Cillian McNamara, Michael Sugrue*

Department of Breast Surgery and Radiology Letterkenny and Donegal Clinical Research Academy, National University of Ireland, Galway, Ireland
Email: *michael.sugrue@hse.ie

Abstract

Introduction: This study describes an intra-operative scoring system to advise the surgeon of the centricity of the tumour in the excised specimen. Methods: Spatial estimations were prospectively made in 10 consecutive patients undergoing wide local excision (WLE) using Bioptics intra-operative digital specimen imaging. The centricity score was defined as 100 − (ICD/SD × 100), where ICD is the inter-centre distance between the specimen's centre and the tumour's centre. Results: 10 patients with invasive breast cancer (T1b to T4a), mean age 56 years (range 44 - 71) were studied. The mean tumour and specimen diameter was 24 mm ± 10 (range 12 - 48) and 101 mm ± 22 (range 64 - 140). The mean centricity score was 86 ± 9 (range 65 - 95). Conclusion: This study successfully describes an intraoperative radiological spatial scoring system for patients undergoing WLE. Tumours were well centered in specimens with an overall score of 86/100. The centricity score could be used to guide excision and potentially set benchmarks for conservative breast surgery.

Keywords

Breast Cancer, Wide Local Excision, Positive Margins, Re-Excision Rates, Specimen Radiography

1. Introduction

The majority of patients diagnosed with breast cancer now opt for breast conserving surgery [1]. While wide local excision (WLE) may reduce morbidity and promote excellent cosmesis [2], there is a risk of re-operation for positive margins. This is associated with additional physical and psychological consequences for the patient and financial costs to the health service.

From a surgical perspective, ideally the tumour should be as close to the centre of the excised specimen and

---

*Corresponding author.

out of this concept the centricity score developed. Fundamentally the more central the tumour is in the excision specimen the higher the score. The higher the score the better, indicating the tumour should be more eqi-distant from the margin and theoretically reduce risk of margin involvement. Margin status is the primary determinant of local recurrence after breast conserving therapy (BCT) [3] and the rate of re-excision [4].

From a patient perspective, it is important to achieve an excellent cosmetic effect. This is essentially obtained by avoiding excessive excision. The larger the volume excised the worse the cosmetic outcome [5], This balance between a good oncological outcome and an appropriate cosmetic effect reflects the "success" of a WLE and also forms the basis for The Centricity Score.

Rates of re-excision vary internationally with an average of 25%, ranging from 10% - 54% [1] [6] and therefore remain a major challenge in health care delivery. Although re-excision rates cannot themselves be used as a quality measure in breast cancer care delivery, multiple operations are undesirable [1] and wide variations that exist indicate a potential gap in quality of care [7]. This potential shortfall in patient care is not helped by scarcity of aids to assist a surgeon in performing complete tumour excision at the index operation.

This study assesses the feasibility of measuring the centricity of breast cancer in the surgical specimen during wide local excision.

2. Materials and Methods

A prospective study was undertaken in 2012 in Letterkenny Hospital, Donegal, Ireland—a regional designated provider of breast cancer care—to measure the centricity score in a sample of 10 consecutive patients undergoing WLE. Letterkenny Hospital is a satellite centre with its parent cancer centre at University College Hospital Galway (UCHG) under the Irish National Cancer Control Program designation.

The centricity score was defined by the formulae; $100 - (ICD/SD \times 100)$, where ICD is the inter-centre distance between the breast specimen's centre and the tumour's centre. The specimen diameter (SD) is measured along the long axis of the specimen. Both values are calculated in millimeters using the intra-operative specimen X-ray of the excised breast specimen (**Figure 1**). Specimens were orientated with a standard specimen marking system, with three clips superior, two clips anterior and one clip medial. Margins were considered positive if tumour was at the inked surface or close, if within 2 mm [7]. A score of 100 would be considered a perfect score indicating the tumour was the exact centre of the excised breast specimen ("bull's-eye"). As the specimen diameter increases there will be a reduction in the centricity score. Tumour and specimen measurements were obtained both radiologically and pathologically and included mass, width, length and depth. The tumour distance to nearest margin was also calculated. Perpendicular margin assessment was used where the tumour was close to the margin; otherwise macroscopic measurement was used [8].

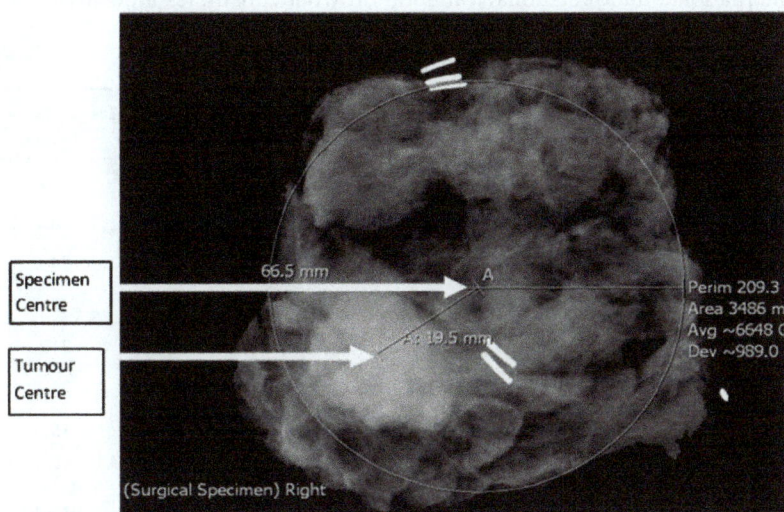

Figure 1. Specimen X-ray with marking clips demonstrating Centricity Score Cal- culation. The ICD is 19.5 mm between the Specimen and Tumour Centres (SC and TC) [CS = 100 − (19.5 mm/66.5 mm × 100)] = 70.7

Patient demographics and histology were recorded. Patients with primary DCIS or mammographically occult cancers were not included. Data was expressed as mean, standard deviation and range. Specimen radiographs were performed using Bioptics® intra-operative digital specimen imaging. One standard non-compressed AP view was obtained following a standard specimen orientation by a single consultant surgeon and operating theatre staff, guided by written protocols. The specimens were carefully placed by the attending surgeon on the positioning plate with a protocol for orientation in the AP plane. Specimen X-rays were taken in the OR and were available in 3 minutes. Lateral views were done but were not used in the calculation of the centricity score. Images were then analyzed and recorded with Agfa IMPAX 6.4 radiological imaging. The study was approved by the hospital ethics committee.

3. Results

10 consecutive patients, mean age was 56 years (range 44 - 71), with a mean BMI of 25 (range 22 - 26) with invasive ductal breast cancer were studied. All patients were symptomatic and 9/10 had palpable lesions, 1/10 had a non-palpable cancer and underwent wire guided localization prior to excision. All patients had invasive cancer, ductal in 9 and lobular in 1. The mean tumour diameter was 24 mm (range 12 to 48 mm) and grade 1 in 1/10, grade 2 in 5/10 and grade 3 in 4/10. 8/10 were ER/PR positive and 2 were HER2 positive. There was associated ductal carcinoma in situ (DCIS) in 4/10 and one had an extensive intra-duct component. Lymphovascular invasion (LVI) was present in 5. There was associated ductal carcinoma in situ (DCIS) in 4/10. The margins were clear, and none were close, either radiologically on the specimen X-ray or on histology in all patients. No patient underwent re-excision. The mean specimen weight was 129 g ± 8.5 g (range 29 - 240 g). The mean centricity score was 86 ± 9 (65.3 - 94.5). All other parameters are shown in **Table 1**. The nearest radiological margin was 15 mm and the furthest 24 mm.

4. Discussion

This study describes a novel method of recording the spatial intra-operative location of a breast cancer's relative position within the excised specimen in patients undergoing conservative breast surgery. This is one of the first studies to describe an objective radiological assessment of tumour location in wide local excision specimens.

This method is founded on two important principles. Firstly, understanding the importance of achieving a "clear margin" histologically free of any residual tumour whilst avoiding excessive resection. The strongest predictor of local recurrence remains that of surgical margin status [3] [9] [10]. Despite this, there is currently no consensus regarding the definition of a negative margin [4] [11]. Secondly, there is a surprisingly large variation in positive margins and re-excision rates [1] [6]. Re-excision rates themselves are not a true quality indicator as there is a large international interpretational variation on what constitutes a positive margin and need for re-op-

Table 1. Spatial Analysis and Centricity Score in patients undergoing WLE.

Patient N = 10	Specimen Max Diameter (mm)	Tumour Max Diameter (mm)	Intercentric Distance (mm)	Margin Distance (mm)	Centricity Score
Patient 1	64	22	6.3	15.2	90.2
Patient 2	92.4	16.9	12.5	24.2	86.5
Patient 3	110.1	19.3	6.1	24.5	94.5
Patient 4	100.4	14.5	34.8	15.3	65.3
Patient 5	121.6	31.5	22.6	21.8	81.4
Patient 6	111.2	24.9	13.2	23.1	88.1
Patient 7	78	12.1	5.4	15.9	93.1
Patient 8	140.1	48.3	13.7	16.1	90.2
Patient 9	103.7	24.5	8.2	17.4	92.1
Patient 10	90.4	23.9	16	18.2	82.3
Mean ± SD	101 ± 22	24 ± 10	14 ± 9	19 ± 4	86 ± 9

eration. Some surgeons will aim for a macroscopic margin of 1 cm, whilst others aim for a 2 cm margin [11]. More so, some surgeons value and perform intra-operative specimen radiography; others use intra-operative ultrasound (US). This variation in surgical philosophy suggests that the technique of breast wide local excision, although a relatively simple surgical procedure, may not achieve the planning and analysis it deserves both from a pre-operative work-up and intra-operative approach. Essentially, there is a need to raise surgical awareness for the importance of centrally locating the tumour in the excised specimen. There are conflicting views in the surgical literature regarding whether consultant surgeons obtain superior results than trainees, either supervised or unsupervised [12].

While outcome determination in itself is not an exact science even with the use of objective analysis tools, quality of life is important after breast cancer surgery and may reflect the operative approach [13]. To suggest that there can be a standard approach to an individual patient's breast cancer would be naive. Confounders include patient breast size, breast density, need for localization, type of tumour histology, presence of DCIS and the position within the breast.

Since its introduction over 50 years ago breast surgical specimen radiography has been a controversial area. Some authors favour the technique, while others argue that it does not correlate with a positive/negative histological margin [14]-[16], or in DCIS the mammographic appearance of calcification often does not reflect the extent of the cancer on the final histology. To counter these limitations and enhance the value of specimen radiography, a number of modifications have been suggested: notably, two-dimensional views, compression, use of grids and fluid immersion [17]. The specimens in this study were uncompressed to avoid distortion [17] [18] and the centricity score used refers to one plane (antero-posterior) only. As far back as 1990, Aitkin [19] has advocated two-dimensional specimen radiology to enhance the spatial perception of the tumour in the specimen. The centricity score used in this only looks at one plane. The lateral view on specimen X-ray in general does not provide as much useful information as the AP view. It is generally accepted that the radial rather than the anterior and posterior margins are keys to outcome. Many intra-operative aids have been suggested including pre-operative radio-isotope guided seeds, Quantum-Dot Molecular Probe, radiofrequency spectroscopy with the Margin Probe [20]-[25].

There are definite specific limitations to the centricity score. Patients undergoing neo-adjuvant therapy, where tumour regression occurs may result in inability to radiologically localize the tumour. Such patients were not included in this pilot study. More so, peripherally placed tumours will not and should not be in the centre of the excised specimen and hence the centricity score described here is not useful for this subgroup of patients.

The centricity score will also be unhelpful in radiological occult tumors. Patients with lobular cancer often fall into this category, as will patients with DCIS. Patients with DCIS even when visible on mammogram, will have more extensive disease than that predicted on the mammogram.

While this surgery was undertaken by a single consultant in this study, it has been suggested that residents' performance in completely excising tumour may not be inferior to consultant [12]. It is unclear from the literature whether high volume surgeons have lower re-excision rates, with some studies in favour [26] and some against [6].

Whilst margin indexes have been reported in pathological margin assessment, existing radiology systems do not provide robust intra-operative measurement [27] [28]. The margin indexes previously reported are histologically based and look at edge rather than centre of tumour, the margin index has failed external validation as a predictive tool for margin involvement [28]. The uniqueness of the centricity score lies in the fact that it can be easily calculated intra-operatively. This ease of access and instant feedback creates a new market in breast surgery. The centricity score provides the very important ability to predict a potential positive margin [29] [30] and could potentially focus the mind of the surgeon. More so, by incorporating the specimen diameter into the centricity score formula, it's an attempt to regulate excessive excisions as a large specimen will result in a reduced need for re-excision but have adverse cosmetic and outcome measures for the patient [31]. Recent consensus guidelines on WLE margins produced by the American Society of Clinical Oncology, American Society for Radiation Oncology, and Society of Surgical Oncology indicating that no ink on tumour is now considered an adequate margin will also help reduce re-excision [32].

This study only describes the measurements and spatial analysis and in itself does not provide a validation of the score. Internal and external validation would be required before wider use could be advocated. It can, in its current format, provide a semi-objective analysis of a surgeon's ability to centrally locate an excised tumour within a specimen. We now routinely undertake the centricity score, calculated by the surgical team using manual mapping on the digital radiology system. This analysis can provide a standardized means of comparison between surgeons. This may aid in resident training and in the future offer a potential tool to reduce some of the excess variability in conservative breast surgery.

Conflict of Interest Statement

The Authors declare that there is no conflict of interests.

Funding Source

None.

Ethical Approval

The study was approved by the hospital ethics committee.

References

[1]   Jeevan, R., Cromwell, D.A., Trivella, M., *et al.* (2012) Reoperation Rates after Breast Conserving Surgery for Breast Cancer among Women in England: Retrospective Study of Hospital Episode Statistics. *BMJ*, **345**, e4505. http://dx.doi.org/10.1136/bmj.e4505

[2]   Fisher, B., Anderson, S., Bryant, J., *et al.* (2012) Twenty-Year Follow-Up of a Randomized Trial Comparing Total Mastectomy, Lumpectomy, and Lumpectomy Plus Irradiation for the Treatment of Invasive Breast Cancer. *NEJM*, **347**, 1233-1241. http://dx.doi.org/10.1056/NEJMoa022152

[3]   Park, C.C., Mitsumori, M., Nixon, A., *et al.* (2000) Outcome at 8 Years after Breast-Conserving Surgery and Radiation Therapy for Invasive Breast Cancer: Influence of Margin Status and Systemic Therapy on Local Recurrence. *Journal of Clinical Oncology*, **18**, 1668-1675.

[4]   Morrow, M., Harris, J.R. and Schnitt, S.J. (2012) Surgical Margins in Lumpectomy for Breast Cancer-Bigger Is Not Better. *NEJM*, **367**, 79-82. http://dx.doi.org/10.1056/NEJMsb1202521

[5]   Olivotto, I.A., Rose, M.A., Osteen, R.T., *et al.* (1989) Late Cosmetic Outcome after Conservative Surgery and Radiotherapy: Analysis of Causes of Cosmetic Failure. *International Journal of Radiation Oncology*Biology*Physics*, **17**, 747-753. http://dx.doi.org/10.1016/0360-3016(89)90061-8

[6]   McCahill, L.E., Single, R.M., Aiello Bowles, E.J., *et al.* (2012) Variability in Re-Excision Following Breast Conservation Surgery. *JAMA*, **307**, 467-475. http://dx.doi.org/10.1001/jama.2012.43

[7]   Morrow, M., Katz, S.J. (2012) The Challenge of Developing Quality Measures for Breast Cancer Surgery. *JAMA*, **307**, 509-510. http://dx.doi.org/10.1001/jama.2012.74

[8]   Moo, T.A., Choi, L., Culpepper, C., Olcese, C., Heerdt, A., Sclafani, L., *et al.* (2014) Impact of Margin Assessment Method on Positive Margin Rate and Total Volume Excised. *Annals of Surgical Oncology*, **21**, 86-92. http://dx.doi.org/10.1245/s10434-013-3257-2

[9]   Bedwinek, J.M., Perez, C.A., Kramer, S., *et al.* (1980) Irradiation as the Primary Management of Stage I and II Adenocarcinoma of the Breast. *Cancer Clinical Trials*, **3**, 11-18.

[10] Singletary, S.E. (2002) Surgical Margins in Patients with Early-Stage Breast Cancer Treated with Breast Conservation Therapy. *The American Journal of Surgery*, **184**, 383-393. http://dx.doi.org/10.1016/S0002-9610(02)01012-7

[11] Blair, S.L., Thompson, K., Rococco, J., Malcarne, V., Beitsch, P.D. and Ollila, D.W. (2009) Attaining Negative Margins in Breast-Conservation Operations: Is There a Consensus among Breast Surgeons? *Journal of the American College of Surgeons*, **209**, 608-613. http://dx.doi.org/10.1016/j.jamcollsurg.2009.07.026

[12] Aguilar, B., Sheikh, F., Pockaj, B., Wasif, N. and Gray, R. (2011) The Effect of Junior Residents on Surgical Quality: A Study of Surgical Outcomes in Breast Surgery. *The American Journal of Surgery*, **202**, 654-657. http://dx.doi.org/10.1016/j.amjsurg.2011.05.018

[13] Sugrue, R., MacGregor, G., Sugrue, M., Curran, S. and Murphy, L. (2013) An Evaluation of Patient Reported Outcomes Following Breast Reconstruction Utilizing Breast Q. *The Breast*, **22**, 158-161. http://dx.doi.org/10.1016/j.breast.2012.12.001

[14] Britton, P.D., Sonoda, A.K., Yamamoto, B., Koo, B., Soh, E. and Goud, A. (2011) Breast Surgical Specimen Radiographs: How Reliable Are They? *European Journal of Radiology*, **79**, 245-249. http://dx.doi.org/10.1016/j.ejrad.2010.02.012

[15] Graham, R.A., Homer, M.J., Katz, J., Rothschild, J., Safaii, H. and Supran, S. (2012) The Pancake Phenomenon Contributes to the Inaccuracy of Margin Assessment in patients with Breast Cancer. *The American Journal of Surgery*, **184**, 89-93. http://dx.doi.org/10.1016/S0002-9610(02)00902-9

[16] Bimston, D.N., Bebb, G.G. and Wagman, L.D. (2000) Is Specimen Mammography Beneficial? *Archives of Surgery*, **135**, 1083-1086. http://dx.doi.org/10.1001/archsurg.135.9.1083

[17] Chilcote, W.A., Davis, G.A., Suchy, P. and Paushter, D.M. (1988) Breast Specimen Radiography: Evaluation of a Compression Device. *Radiology*, **168**, 425-427. http://dx.doi.org/10.1148/radiology.168.2.3393660

[18] Clingan, R., Griffin, M., Phillips, J., Coberly, W. and Jennings, W. (2003) Potential Margin Distortion in Breast Tissue by Specimen Mammography. *Archives of Surgery*, **138**, 1371-1374. http://dx.doi.org/10.1001/archsurg.138.12.1371

[19] Aitkin, R.J., Going, J.J. and Chetty, U. (1990) Assessment of Surgical Excision during Breast Conservation Surgery by Intraoperative Two-Dimensional Specimen Radiology. *British Journal of Surgery*, **77**, 322-323. http://dx.doi.org/10.1007/s00268-012-1577-1

[20] Bernardi, S., Bertozzi, S., Londero, A.P., Gentile, G., Giacomuzzi, F. and Carbone, A. (2012) Incidence and Risk Factors of the Intraoperative Localization Failure of Nonpalpable Breast Lesions by Radio-Guided Occult Lesion Localization: A Retrospective Analysis of 579 Cases. *World Journal of Surgery*, **36**, 1915-1921. http://dx.doi.org/10.1007/s00268-012-1577-1

[21] Cox, E.C., Furman, B., Stowell, N., Ebert, M., Clark, J., Dupont, E., *et al.* (2003) Radioactive Seed Localization Breast Biopsy and Lumpectomy: Can Specimen Radiographs Be Eliminated? *Annals of Surgical Oncology*, **10**, 1039-1047. http://dx.doi.org/10.1245/ASO.2003.03.050

[22] Allweis, T.M., Kaufman, Z., Lelcuk, S., Pappo, I., Karni, T., Schneebaum, S., *et al.* (2008) A Prospective, Randomized, Controlled, Multicenter Study of a Real-Time, Intraoperative Probe for Positive Margin Detection in Breast-Conserving Surgery. *The American Journal of Surgery*, **196**, 483-489. http://dx.doi.org/10.1016/j.amjsurg.2008.06.024

[23] Feldman, S.M. (2013) Editorial-Surgical Margins in Breast Conservation. *International Journal of Surgical Oncology*, **2013**, Article ID: 136387. http://dx.doi.org/10.1155/2013/136387

[24] Murphy, J.O., Moo, T.A., King, T.A., Van Zee, K.J., Villegas, K.A., Stempel, M., *et al.* (2013) Radioactive Seed Localization Compared to Wire Localization in Breast-Conserving Surgery: Initial 6-Month Experience. *Annals of Surgical Oncology*, **20**, 4121-4127. http://dx.doi.org/10.1245/s10434-013-3166-4

[25] Ramos, M., Diaz, J.C., Ramos, T., Ruano, R., Aparicio, M., Sancho, M., *et al.* (2012) Ultrasound-Guided Excision Combined with Intraoperative Assessment of Gross Macscopic Margins Decreases the Rate of Reoperations for Non-Palpable Invasive Breast Cancer. *The Breast*, **22**, 520-524. http://dx.doi.org/10.1016/j.breast.2012.10.006

[26] Cancela, M., Comber, H. and Sharp, L. (2013) Hospital and Surgeon Caseload Are Associated with Risk of Re-Operation Following Breast-Conserving Surgery. *Breast Cancer Research and Treatment*, **140**, 535-544. http://dx.doi.org/10.1007/s10549-013-2652-5

[27] Margenthaler, J.A., Gao, F. and Klimberg, V.S. (2010) Margin Index: A New Method for Prediction of Residual Disease after Breast-Conserving Surgery. *Annals of Surgical Oncology*, **17**, 2696-2701. http://dx.doi.org/10.1111/j.1524-4741.2012.01249.x

[28] Bolger, J.C., Solon, J.G., Power, C. and Hill, A.D. (2012) Analysis of Margin Index as a Method for Predicting Residual Disease after Breast-Conserving Surgery in a European Cancer Center. *Annals of Surgical Oncology*, **19**, 207-211.

[29] Atalay, C. and Irkkan, C. (2012) Predictive Factors for Residual Disease in Re-Excision Specimens after Breast-Conserving Surgery. *The Breast Journal*, **18**, 339-344. http://dx.doi.org/10.1111/j.1524-4741.2012.01249.x

[30] Waljee, J.F., Hu, E.S., Newman, L.A. and Alderman, A.K. (2008) Predictors of Re-Excision among Woman Undergoing Breast-Conserving Surgery for Cancer. *Annals of Surgical Oncology*, **15**, 1297-1303. http://dx.doi.org/10.1245/s10434-007-9777-x

[31] Krekel, N.M., Haloua, M.H., Cardozo, A.M.L., de Wit, R.H., Bosch, A.M., de Widt-Levert, L.M., *et al.* (2013) Intraoperative Ultrasound Guidance for Palpable Breast Cancer Excision (COBALT Trial): A Multicentre, Randomised Controlled Trial. *The Lancet Oncology*, **14**, 48-54. http://dx.doi.org/10.1016/S1470-2045(12)70527-2

[32] Moran, M.S., Schnitt, S.J., Giuliano, A.E., Harris, J.R., Khan, S.A., Horton, J., *et al.* (2014) Society of Surgical Oncology-American Society for Radiation Oncology Consensus Guideline on Margins for Breast-Conserving Surgery with Whole-Breast Irradiation in Stages I and II Invasive Breast Cancer. *Journal of Clinical Oncology*, **32**, 1507-1515. http://dx.doi.org/10.1200/JCO.2013.53.3935

24

Snai-1 and Epithelial-Mesenchymal Transition-Related Protein Immunoexpression in Canine Mammary Carcinomas

Breno S. Salgado[1*], Rafael M. Rocha[3], Fernando A. Soares[3], Fátima Gärtner[4], Noeme S. Rocha[1,2]

[1]Departamento de Patologia, Faculdade de Medicina de Botucatu, Universidade Estadual Paulista (UNESP), Botucatu, Brazil
[2]Laboratório de Patologia Investigativa e Comparada, Departamento de Clínica Veterinária, Faculdade de Medicina Veterinária e Zootecnia, Universidade Estadual Paulista (UNESP), Botucatu, Brazil
[3]Departamento de Anatomia Patológica, Hospital A. C. Camargo, Fundação Antônio Prudente, São Paulo, Brazil
[4]Institute of Pathology and Molecular Immunology (IPATIMUP), Oporto, Portugal
Email: [*]brenosalgado@globo.com

Abstract

Epithelial-mesenchymal transition (EMT) is defined as switching of polarized epithelial cells to a migratory fibroblastoid phenotype. EMT is known to be involved in the progression and metastasis of various cancers in humans, but this specific process is still little explored in the veterinary literature. The aim of this research was to evaluate the expression of EMT-related proteins in canine mammary carcinomas (CMCs). The expression of six EMT-related proteins in 94 CMCs of female dogs was evaluated by immunohistochemistry using a tissue array method. Additionally, clinicopathological characteristics were compared with the expression of EMT-related proteins. Loss of epithelial protein and/or acquisition of the expression of mesenchymal proteins were observed in CMCs. Loss of epithelial protein and/or acquisition of the expression of mesenchymal proteins were observed, particularly in tumors with evidence of stromal invasion; however, significance was only observed between the S100A4 and vascular invasion. In addition, Snai-1 nuclear immunoexpression was significantly related to E-cadherin loss. In conclusion, loss of epithelial proteins and/or the acquisition of mesenchymal proteins are associated with EMT and may have an important role in the evaluation of CMC patients. The unique immunoexpression pattern of Snai-1 could help to distinguish between an adenoma and a non-metastatic carcinoma and seems to be related

---

[*]Corresponding author.

to conversion of myoepithelial cells to a complete mesenchymal-like phenotype. Loss of E-cadherin and cytokeratin and change of immunoexpression pattern of Snai-1, N-cadherin, S100A4 and MMP-2 indicate the occurrence of EMT in canine mammary carcinomas and should result in an en bloc resection or a close follow-up.

Keywords

EMT, S100A4, Keratin, Mammary Tumors, Dog

1. Introduction

Mammary gland tumors are the most common neoplasms of the female dog and represent a remarkably heterogeneous group in terms of morphology and biological behavior [1]. Consequently, the identification of reliable prognostic factors is very important in order to assess the individual risk and evaluate the clinical outcome. The prognosis of advanced mammary carcinoma patients is most likely related to the degree of metastatic spread. Although the process of cancer metastasis appears to be regulated by a variety of gene products, little is known about the molecular aspects of progression of canine mammary carcinoma (CMC) cells.

Recently, the conversion of epithelial cells to migratory fibroblastoid cells—known as epithelial-mesenchymal transition (EMT)—was suggested to be involved in metastasis. Such event is crucial during gastrulation and neural crest formation in embryogenesis [2], but has been suggested to be also involved in inflammation and neo-plastic progression. During EMT, cells lose epithelial polarity and acquire a spindle-shaped, highly motile mesenchymallike phenotype. Moreover, this transition involves loss or redistribution of tight- and adherence-junction proteins and a switch to mesenchymal gene expression which confers upon cells the ability to pass through the basement membrane [3]. This phenomenon is reactivated during the progression of numerous cancers and was demonstrated to be associated with poor histological differentiation, local invasiveness and distant metastasis [4] [5].

Different studies regarding expression of EMT-related proteins in canine mammary neoplasms were performed; however, none of them focused on the specific event of EMT and its implication in the diagnosis and prognosis of any canine tumor type. In the present study we therefore evaluated the expression of 6 established human breast cancer EMT markers (Snai-1, E-cadherin, N-cadherin, MMP-2, S100A4, and cytokeratin) in canine mammary carcinomas and compared their expression with different pathological parameters.

2. Materials and Methods

2.1. Tissue Samples

Consecutively collected, surgically resected 94 CMC tissue specimens were obtained from female dogs which underwent mastectomy at the São Paulo State University's Veterinary Hospital, Botucatu, Brazil, between March 2009 and September 2010. All patients had the tumor specimens surgically removed by radical mastectomy and none of them had received preoperative chemotherapy or radiotherapy. Tissue samples from these neoplasms were formalin-fixed and paraffin-embedded. For routine microscopic examination, 4 μm thick sections were obtained and stained with hematoxylin and eosin with subsequent evaluation under light microscopy.

2.2. Histologic Evaluation

Three independent pathologists were responsible for the evaluation of tissues and diagnosis of the neoplasms, according to the World Health Organization criteria for canine mammary tumors [6]. Malignant epithelial neoplasms were graded histologically in accordance with the Nottingham scoring system for mammary cancer [7], based on the assessment of three morphological features: tubule formation, nuclear pleomorphism and mitotic counts. Each of these features was scored on a scale of 1 - 3 to indicate whether it was present in slight, moderate or marked degree, giving a putative total of 3 - 9 points. Grade was allocated by an arbitrary division of the total points as follows: grade I (well differentiated), 3, 4 or 5 points; grade II (moderately differentiated), 6 or 7 points; and grade III (poorly differentiated), 8 or 9 points. Cases of mammary carcinomas were assessed for mode of growth (expansive vs. infiltrative), presence of intratumoral necrosis, stromal and vascular invasion.

Additionally, lesions were classified according to standard diagnostic criteria provided by the World Health Organization [6] and classified using the Nottingham grading system for mammary neoplasms [7]. Presence of vascular invasion, invasion depth, mode of growth, and presence of intratumoral necrotic tissue were also evaluated. Tissue samples were arrayed for performing subsequent analysis.

2.3. Immunohistochemistry

Firstly, 3 μm thick histologic sections were obtained, deparaffinized, and rehydrated. Immunohistochemistry was performed by using a polymeric labeling detection system (Novolink Polymer Detection System, Novocastra Laboratories, Newcastle, UK). Antigen retrieval was carried out by heat treatment in 10 mM citrate buffer pH 6.0 for all primary antibodies except for N-cadherin, for which the antigen retrieval was carried by heating the slides in a water bath using a Tris EDTA buffer pH 9.0. **Table 1** summarizes the used primary antibodies and staining procedures adopted for each antibody in this study and their immunoexpression patterns in nonneoplastic and CMC tissues. After cooling (20 minutes at room temperature), the sections were immersed for 30 minutes in a solution of 3% hydrogen peroxide diluted in methanol in order to block endogenous peroxidase activity. All slides were then incubated with a protein block reagent (Novocastra Laboratories, Newcastle, UK) for 10 minutes and subsequently overnight incubated at 4°C with the specific primary antibodies. Then, the slides were immersed with the detection systems following the manufacturer's instructions. Subsequently, 3,3' diaminobenzidine tetrahydrochloride (DAB) was used as chromogen in order to allow the visualization of antigen-antibody reaction. Then, slides were counterstained using Harris's hematoxylin, dehydrated, and mounted for evaluation and light microscopy.

For immunollabeling evaluation, S100A4 was considered as positive when more than 10% of neoplastic cells revealed nuclear staining. N-cadherin was considered as positive when membranous immunostaining was observed in luminal neoplastic cells. On the other hand, E-cadherin was considered as negative when loss of membranous staining was observed in such cells. For cytokeratin tumor cells were considered as negative when loss of membranous/cytoplasmic staining was observed. For MMP-2, neoplastic cells were considered as positive when cytoplasmic/membranous staining was observed. The assessment of Snai-1 expression in canine mammary tissues was based on detectable immunoreactivity in nuclear region and on a semiquantitative analysis using the following scoring system: 0, no staining; 1+, nuclear staining in 1% to 25% of neoplastic cells; 2+, nuclear staining in 26% to 50% of neoplastic cells; and 3+: nuclear staining in more than 50% of neoplastic cells, as previously described (Hung *et al.*, 2009).

2.4. Statistical Analysis

Differences in EMT-related proteins expression were compared using Fisher's exact test or Pearson's X^2 test for qualitative variables and using Student's t-test or analysis of variance for continuous variables. Survival curves were estimated using Kaplan-Meier product-limit method, and the significance of differences between survival curves was determined using the log rank text. Multivariate analysis was performed by Cox proportional hazards regression modeling. All statistical tests were two sided, and statistical significance was accepted at the $P < 0.05$ level. All analyses were performed using the Prism GraphPad software version 5.0 (San Diego, CA).

Table 1. Antibodies used, dilution, and expression patterns.

Antibody	Dilution	Source	Clone	Manufacturer	Expression pattern
Snai-1	1:500	Rabbit	Polyclonal	LifeSpan Biosciences	Nuclear
S100A4	1:1200	Rabbit	Polyclonal	Abcam	Nuclear
MMP-2	1:100	Mouse	4D3	Abcam	Cytoplasmic
E-Cadherin	1:100	Mouse	NCL-E-cad	Novocastra	Cytoplasmic/membrane
N-Cadherin	1:50	Mouse	6G11	Dako	Cytoplasmic/membrane
Cytokeratin	1:500	Mouse	AE1/AE3	Dako	Cytoplasmic

*MMP-2: matrix metalloproteinase 2.

3. Results

3.1. Snai-1 Immunoexpression Patterns in Canine Mammary Tissues

Snai-1 nuclear positive immunostaining was not observed in normal or hyperplastic mammary tissue adjacent to tumor areas and from female dogs that never developed mammary tumors. Dysplastic areas revealed only single positive cells. In mixed benign tumors, Snai-1 nuclear expression was observed in fibroblastoid cells, myoepithelial cells, and cells under chondroid/osteoid differentiation. In simple carcinomas, Snai-1 expression was observed in luminal cells (**Figure 1**), infiltrating cells of the invasive front and stromal cells, with absence of nuclear expression in myoepithelial cells. In complex carcinomas and carcinomas in mixed tumors, Snai-1 expression was observed in carcinomatous luminal cells, myoepithelial cells and cells under chondroid/osteoid differentiation (**Figure 2**). No or rare Snai-1 positive immunoreactivity (+) was observed in normal, hyperplastic, or dysplastic mammary tissue. A similar pattern was observed in mammary adenomas and within the benign luminal component of carcinomas in mixed tumors. On the other hand, high expression of Snai-1 was detected in mammary carcinomas. The results regarding the Snai-1 immunoexpression quantification are summarized in **Table 2**.

No relation with invasion depth, presence of intratumoral necrosis, vascular invasion, tumor mode of growth, HER-2 and hormone receptor status were statistically found.

3.2. Relation between Immunoexpression of EMT-Related Proteins and Pathologic Parameters

Epithelial protein loss frequencies were 25.53% (28/94) for cytokeratin and 38.29% (36/94) for E-cadherin, and aberrant mesenchymal protein expression frequencies were 59.57% (56/94) for N-cadherin, 36.17% (34/94) for matrix metalloproteinase 2, and 10.63% (10/94) for S100A4. Additionaly, 59.57% (56/94) highly expressed Snai-1. **Figure 2** shows a representative immunohistochemical result.

Expression loss of the epithelial protein E-cadherin was found to be significantly related to high nuclear expression of Snai-1 ($P = 0.045$). Novel mesenchymal protein expression of S100A4 was found to be related to vascular invasion ($P = 0.001$). Although in our study the number of Snai-1-highly-expressing cases increased with the occurrence of stromal invasion, a statistical significant correlation was not evident. Additionally, no relation between EMT related proteins immunoexpression and invasion depth, presence of intratumoral necrosis, vascular invasion, and tumor mode of growth was statistically found except for S100A4 and vascular invasion.

3.3. EMT-Related Protein Expression and Survival Analysis

Overall patient survival rates were determined using the log rank test with respect to expression of the six proteins. In terms of the epithelial proteins, cytokeratin loss ($P = 0.02$) (**Figure 3(a)**) was found to be significantly associated with a poor outcome. For mesenchymal proteins, the nuclear expression S100A4 ($P = 0.02$) (**Figure 3(d)**) was found to be significantly associated with an unfavorable prognosis. However, no significant difference in patient outcome was found with respect to E-cadherin loss (**Figure 3(b)**), N-cadherin expression (**Figure 3(c)**), Snai-1 expression (**Figure 3(e)**), or MMP-2 (**Figure 3(f)**) in the cases herein studied. Multivariate analysis was performed to determine relations between markers but no statistical significance was observed.

4. Discussion

Many recent studies have demonstrated the importance of EMT in various tumor types and humans [2]-[4] and, less extensively, in dogs [8] [9]. An important aspect of EMT is the loss of epithelial protein markers, *i.e.* cytokeratins and E-cadherin. E-cadherin is required for the formation of stable adherens junctions and, thus, for the maintenance of an epithelial phenotype [10]. Loss of epithelial proteins such as E-cadherin is a hallmark of metastatic carcinoma and, furthermore, proteomic analysis in breast cancer has revealed that circulating mammary tumor cells or those found in micrometastases reveal evidence of mesenchymal [10]. We observed both loss in the important epithelial proteins E-cadherin and cytokeratin expression. Loss in cytokeratin expression revealed to be related to overall survival ($P = 0.02$; risk four times higher than in dogs that did express cytokeratin) in dogs with CMCs and demonstrated to be an independent predictive factor in multivariate analysis. This feature is quite interesting since in cancer keratins are used as prognostic indicators in tumors and/or peripheral blood and several studies have provided evidence for active keratin involvement in cancer cell invasion and metastasis [11].

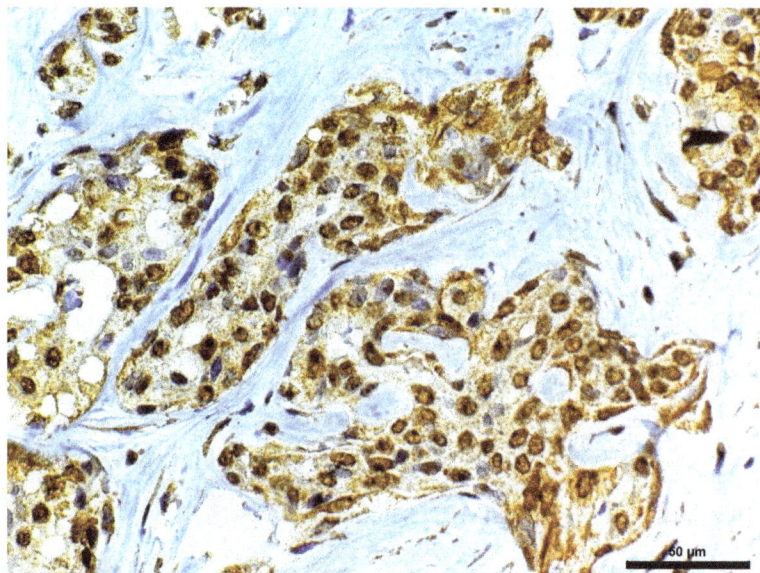

Figure 1. Nuclear Snai-1 expression in mammary luminal cells (DAB immunohistochemistry, Harris hematoxylin counterstain; bar = 50 μm).

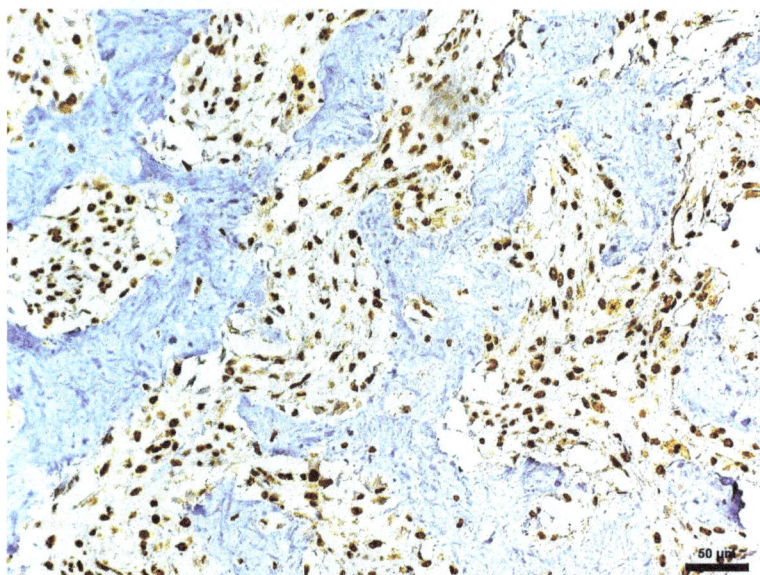

Figure 2. Nuclear Snai-1 expression in neoplastic cells under chondroid metaplasia/differentiation (DAB immunohistochemistry, Harris hematoxylin counterstain; bar = 50 μm).

Table 2. Snai-1 expression in luminal cells from mammary tissues and their relation to histological classification.

		Snai-1 expression in luminal cells		
Histological diagnosis	*Number of samples*	*−/+*	*++*	*+++*
Lipid-rich carcinoma	1	1	0	0
Carcinoma arising in mixed tumor	9	2	5	2
Complex carcinoma	34	7	19	8
Tubulopapillary carcinoma	34	18	15	8
Solid carcinoma	9	1	4	4

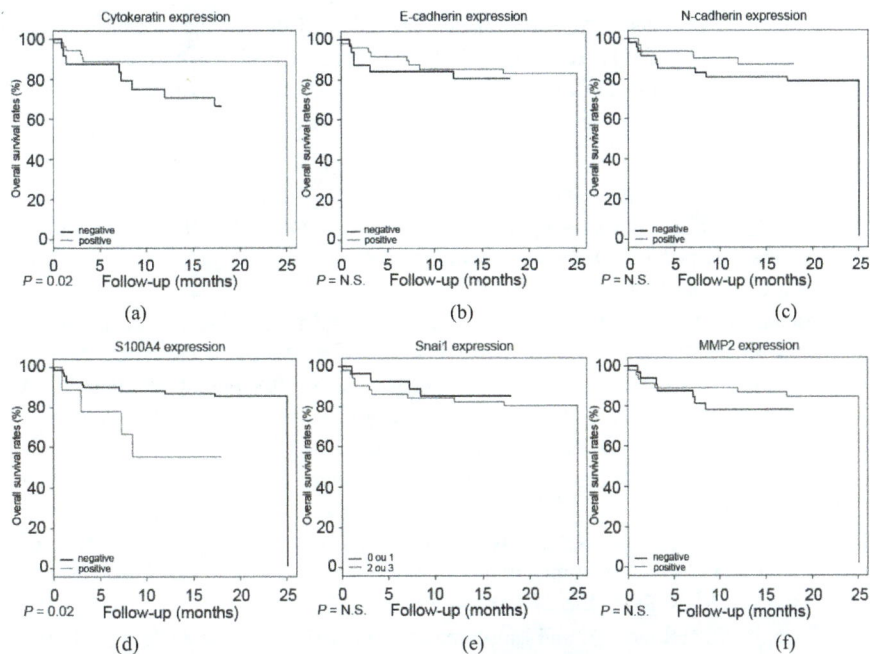

Figure 3. Survival curves using the Kaplan-Meier method by log rank test. (a) Cytokeratin expression; (b) E-cadherin expression; (c) N-cadherin expression; (d) S100A4 expression; (e) Snai-1 expression; (f) Matrix metalloproteinase 2 expression.

Another important aspect of EMT is the acquisition of mesenchymal protein markers, *i.e.* N-cadherin, Snai-1, S100A4, and MMP-2. In this study, the novel nuclear immunoexpression of S100A4 was significantly related with vascular invasion ($P = 0.0001$), features not previously demonstrated in dogs. Such S100A4 expression reveals it to be an interesting biomarker for evaluation of neoplastic progression in CMC, similarly to other authors' observations in humans. [12] [13] Additionally, it could be characterized as an independent predictive factor in multivariate analysis ($P = 0.01$; risk six times higher than in dogs that did not express nuclear S100A4), reinforcing its role as a useful biomarker for CMCs.

Novel Snai-1 expression was also detected and was related with E-cadherin loss ($P = 0.045$). These results indicate that EMT might also play an important role in the pathogenesis of CMCs. Previous studies in canine mammary tumors [9] did not reveal such relation in E-cadherin loss and Snai-1 expression, despite observing many EMT signs. This feature is supported by our finding of Snai-1 being highly expressed in the majority of CMCs, but not in benign tumors or non-neoplastic lesion. Since the loss of E-cadherin has already been documented as related to progression of non-infiltrating to highly infiltrating mammary carcinomas in dogs [14], consequently rising Snai-1 as a useful biomarker of neoplastic progression in CMCs.

Snai-1 was not consistently expressed in myoepithelial cells of non-neoplastic tissue and of simple carcinomas; however, we frequently observed expression of Snai-1 in myoepithelial cells from benign and malignant complex tumors, similarly to what was observed by other authors when analyzing metaplastic breast cancer in humans [15] [16]. These results suggest that Snai-1 may be important for the acquisition of a complete mesenchymal cell-like phenotype and possibly lead to metaplastic differentiation in myoepithelial cells. It is also plausible to think that the proliferation of myoepithelial cells in myoepithelium disorders of mammary tissue can possibly be triggered by Snai-1, since the overexpression of this zinc-finger protein is related to the activation of important intracellular signaling pathways that regulate cell proliferation and differentiation such as the Wnt pathway [17].

Despite the fact that no statistical significance was observed in relation to the expression of other EMT markers and pathological characteristics, changes in the expression patterns of such proteins were detected in neoplastic cells and can represent an important change in the phenotype of CMC cells during the neoplastic progression.

Acknowledgments

The National Council of Technological and Scientific Development, (CNPq), Brazil, provided financial support for Breno Salgado through the master research grant 130358/2010-0 and for Noeme Rocha through the research grant 479178/2010-0. The São Paulo Research Foundation (FAPESP) provided financial support for Noeme Rocha through the research grants 2008/57309-5 and 2010/51596-2. Additionally, the authors wish to thank Carlos Nascimento and Suely Nonogaki for their help with technical issues.

References

[1] Nerurkar, V.R., Chitale, A.R., Jalnakurpar, B.V., Naik, S. and Lalitha, V.S. (1989) Comparative Pathology of Canine Mammary Turmours. *Journal of Comparative Pathology*, **101**, 389-397. http://dx.doi.org/10.1016/0021-9975(89)90022-4

[2] Larue, L. and Bellacosa, A. (2005) Epithelial-Mesenchymal Transition in Development and Cancer: Role of Phosphatidylinositol 3' Kinase/AKT Pathways. *Oncogene*, **24**, 7443-7454. http://dx.doi.org/10.1038/sj.onc.1209091

[3] Jechlinger, M., Grunert, S., Tamir, I.H., Janda, E., Lüdermann, S., Waerner, T., Seither, P., Weith, A., Beug, H. and Kraut, N. (2003) Expression Profiling of Epithelial Plasticity in Tumor Progression. *Oncogene*, **22**, 7155-7169. http://dx.doi.org/10.1038/sj.onc.1206887

[4] Thiery, J.P. (2002) Epithelial-Mesenchymal Transitions in Tumour Progression. Nature Reviews *Cancer*, **2**, 442-454. http://dx.doi.org/10.1038/nrc822

[5] Gotzmann, J., Mikula, M., Eger, A., Schulte-Hermann, R., Foisner, R., Beug, H. and Mikulitis, W. (2004) Molecular Aspects of Epithelial Cell Plasticity: Implications for Local Tumor Invasion and Metastasis. *Mutation Research*, **566**, 9-20. http://dx.doi.org/10.1016/S1383-5742(03)00033-4

[6] Misdorp, W., Else, R.W., Hellmen, E. and Lipscomb, T.P. (1999) Histological Classification of Mammary Tumors of the Dog and Cat. Armed Forces Institute of Pathology, Washington.

[7] Elston, C.W. and Ellis, I.O. (1998) Assessment of Histological Grade. In: *Systemic Pathology*, 3rd Edition, Churchill Livingstone, London, 365-384.

[8] Bongiovanni, L., D'Andrea, A., Romanucci, M., Malatesta, D., Candolini, M., Salda, L.D., Mechelli, L., Sforna, M. and Brachelente, C. (2013) Epithelial-Mesenchymal Transition: Immunohistochemical Investigation of Related Molecules in Canine Cutaneous Epithelial Tumours. *Veterinary Dermatology*, **24**, 195-203. http://dx.doi.org/10.1111/j.1365-3164.2012.01116.x

[9] Im, K.S., Kim, J.H., Kim, N.H., Yu, C.H., Hur, T.Y. and Sur, J.H. (2012) Possible Role of Snail Expression as a Prognostic Factor in Canine Mammary Neoplasia. *Journal of Comparative Pathology*, **147**, 121-128. http://dx.doi.org/10.1016/j.jcpa.2011.12.002

[10] Willipinski-Stapelfeldt, B., Riethdorf, S., Assmann, V., Woefle, U., Rau, T., Sauter, G., Heukeshoven, J. and Pantel, K. (2005) Changes in Cytoskeletal Protein Composition of an Epithlelial-Mesenchymal Transition in Human Micrometastatic and Primary Breast Carcinoma Cells. *Clinical Cancer Research*, **11**, 8006-8014. http://dx.doi.org/10.1158/1078-0432.CCR-05-0632

[11] Karantza, V. (2011) Keratins in Health and Cancer: More than Mere Epithelial Cell Markers. *Oncogene*, **30**, 127-138. http://dx.doi.org/10.1038/onc.2010.456

[12] Rudland, S.S., Martin, L., Roshanlall, C., Winstanley, J., Leinster, S., Platt-Higgins, A., Carroll, J., West, C., Barraclough, R. and Rudland, P. (2006) Association of S100A4 and Osteopontin with Specific Prognostic Factors and Survival of Patients with Minimally Invasive Breast Cancer. *Clinical Cancer Research*, **12**, 1192-1200. http://dx.doi.org/10.1158/1078-0432.CCR-05-1580

[13] Ismail, N.I., Kaur, G., Hashim, H. and Hassan, M.S. (2008) S100A4 Overexpression Proves to Be Independent Marker for Breast Cancer Progression. *Cancer Cell International*, **8**, 12. http://dx.doi.org/10.1186/1475-2867-8-12

[14] Brunetti, B., Sarli, G., Preziosi, R., Monari, I. and Benazzi, C. (2005) E-cadherin and β-Catenin Reduction Influence Invasion But Not Proliferation and Survival in Canine Malignant Mammary Tumors. *Veterinary Pathology*, **42**, 781-787. http://dx.doi.org/10.1354/vp.42-6-781

[15] Nassar, A., Sookhan, N., Santisteban, M., Bryant, S.C., Boughey, J.C., Giorgadze, T. and Degnim, A. (2010) Diagnostic Utility of Snail in Metaplastic Breast Carcinoma. *Diagnostic Pathology*, **5**, 76. http://dx.doi.org/10.1186/1746-1596-5-76

[16] Gwin, K., Buell-Gutbrod, R., Tretiakova, M. and Montag, A. (2010) Epithelial-to-Mesenchymal Transition in Metaplastic Breast Carcinomas with Chondroid Differentiation: Expression of the E-Cadherin Repressor Snail. *Applied Immunohistochemistry and Molecular Pathology*, **19**, 526-531. http://dx.doi.org/10.1097/PAI.0b013e3181e8d54b

[17] Stremmer, V., de Crane, B., Berx, G. and Behrens, J. (2008) Snail Promotes Wnt Target Gene Expression and Interacts with β-Catenin. *Oncogene*, **27**, 5075-5080. http://dx.doi.org/10.1038/onc.2008.140

25

Migraine History and Breast Cancer Risk: A Systematic Review and Meta-Analysis

Shahab Rezaeian[1], Yousef Veisani[2*], Mohammad Ghorbani[3], Ali Delpisheh[4], Hedayat Abbastabar[3]

[1]Health Promotion Research Center, Zahedan University of Medical Sciences, Zahedan, Iran
[2]Student Research Committee, Ilam University of Medical Sciences, Ilam, Iran
[3]Department of Epidemiology, School of Health, Shiraz University of Medical Sciences, Shiraz, Iran
[4]Department of Clinical Epidemiology, Ilam University of Medical Sciences, Ilam, Iran
Email: shahab.rezayan@gmail.com, *yousefveisani@yahoo.com, ghorbani_epi@yahoo.com, alidelpisheh@yahoo.com, hedayat.abastabar@yahoo.com

Abstract

Objective: The relationship between migraine and breast cancer risk has been reported inconsistently across different epidemiological studies. This meta-analysis was performed to explore the overall effect of migraine on breast cancer risk. Method: An electronic search of different major databases was conducted, including PubMed, Scopus, ScienceDirect, and the Cochrane library until February 1st, 2015. Of 652 retrieved studies, six population-based studies including two cohort studies with 130,812 and four case-control studies with 14,396 people were included in the analysis. Results: There was an inverse relationship between migraine and breast cancer risk (OR = 0.77; 95% CI: 0.64, 0.92). Conclusion: The results of this meta-analysis showed that women with migraine history have a decreased risk of breast cancer. Further biological studies are needed to address the association.

Keywords

Migraine, Breast cancer, Meta-Analysis

1. Introduction

Gender and age-dependent prevalence of migraine was estimated by population based studies [1]-[2]. The prevalence rate of migraine varies in the general population and is more common in women [1] [3].

Breast cancer is the most common cancer as well as is the leading cause of cancer related mortality among

---

*Corresponding author.

woman worldwide [4]. Nevertheless, the etiology of breast cancer, as a momentous of public health problem, is not well known. Several studies have indicated that different risk factors including genetic, environmental, hormonal, lifestyle and physiological factors have an influence on the development of this malignancy [5]-[6].

Over the past decade numerous systematic review and meta-analysis studies were conducted to examine of an association between migraine and other diseases such as cardiovascular disease [7], ischemic stroke risk [8], and mortality [9]. On the other hand, there were also several population based studies which had extensively evaluated the relationship between migraine and female cancer, but with conflicting results. Some studies had reported that women with a history of migraine are at lower risk of breast cancer [10]-[14], whereas others reported no association [15]. In addition, no significant association was found between migraine history and risk of endometrial cancer [16].

We, therefore, aimed to explore the relationship between migraine history and breast cancer risk and to quantify the risk by conducting a meta-analysis. We also aimed to evaluate whether the associations varied by age at migraine diagnosis, histological subtype and hormone receptor status of breast cancer.

2. Methods

2.1. Search Strategies

We conducted a systematic search of all studies designed cohort and case-control studies addressing the association between migraine and breast cancer. A comprehensive literature search of numerous electronic databases including PubMed, Scopus, ScienceDirect and the Cochrane library was done up until February 1st, 2015.

A search strategy was conducted using the following search terms in the titles, abstract or key words: migraine, migraine disorder, breast, breast cancer, case-control studies, cohort studies, and observational studies. The citations and references listed in retrieved articles were also reviewed to identify additional related studies.

2.2. Inclusion Criteria

Two authors reviewed the retrieved studies independently to identify eligible studies by using the following criteria: 1) Study design: cohort or case-control study, 2) the breast cancer patients were confirmed by medical records 3) the migraine status was confirmed by medical records, 4) the numbers of case and control (in case-control studies) and exposed and non-exposed groups (in cohort studies) were reported or the relevant data was available to calculate the odds ratio (OR) or risk ratio(RR). Women with breast cancer were included regardless of age, race, menopausal and marital status.

2.3. Data Extraction and Quality Assessment

Two independent authors read full-text articles and the following information was extracted: name of the first author, publication year and location of study conduction, study design (cohort or case-control study), number of cases and controls or exposed and non-exposed, age at migraine diagnosis, histological subtype (ductal and lobular), and hormone (estrogen (ER) and progesterone (PR)) receptor status (ER+/PR+, ER+/PR−, ER−/PR−). The quality of studies was assessed according to the STROBE statement and the studies according with STROBE criteria were defined as high-quality studies [17].

2.4. Statistical Analysis

The pooled ORs with 95% confidence interval (CI) estimating the association between migraine and breast cancer were obtained using the random effect model. Cochran's Q test was used to identify the heterogeneity of results across studies and it was quantified using the I^2 statistic. Q statistic with p-value <0.10 or I^2 statistic >50% was considered as significant heterogeneity across studies. The between-study variance was estimated using tau-squared (t^2 or Tau^2) statistic [18]. We used Egger's linear regression test [19] to investigate publication bias (p < 0.05 set as significant level). Meta-analysis was performed by the comprehensive meta-analysis software version 2.0. The PRISMA statement was used as a guide in the reporting of this study [20].

3. Results

3.1. Description of Studies

Table 1 presents the characteristics of the studies included in the meta-analysis. Of 652 retrieved studies, we

Table 1. Characteristics of the studies included in the meta-analysis.

	Data source	Study type	Sampling	Cases	Control	Exposed	Non-exposed
Ghorbani *et al.* 2015 [14]	CR	Case-control		347	300	-	-
Lowry *et al.* 2014 [12]	SEER	Case-control	Population-based	715	376	-	-
Li *et al.* 2009 [11]	SEER	Case-control	Population-based	4568	4678	-	-
Mathes *et al.* 2008 [13]	CSS	Case-control	Population-based	1938	1474	-	-
Li *et al.* 2010 [10]	WHI	Cohort	Population-based	-	-	10464	80652
Winter *et al.* 2013 [15]	WHS	Cohort	Population-based	-	-	7318	32378

CR: Cancer Registry at the oncology center of Isfahan University of Medical Sciences, Iran; SEER: Surveillance Epidemiology and End Results cancer registry; CSS: Cancer Surveillance System; WHI: Women's Health Initiative; WHS: Women's Health Study.

eventually included 6 population-based studies in the meta-analysis including two cohort and four case-control studies involving 130812 and 14396 people, respectively. **Figure 1** presents the flowchart of the literature search process.

3.2. Summary and Subgroup Analyzed Results

Table 2 illustrates the summary effect sizes of breast cancer risk and migraine history by age at migraine diagnosis, histological subtype and hormone receptor status.

3.3. Association of Migraine History and Breast Cancer Risk

Summary results of six population-based studies (**Figure 2**) indicated that having any history of migraine was inversely associated with breast cancer risk (OR = 0.77; 95% CI: 0.64, 0.92).

3.4. Association of Age at Migraine Diagnosis and Breast Cancer Risk

We stratified the migraine history by the age at diagnosis (**Figure 3**). Pooled result from three studies showed that both age at migraine diagnosis < 20 years and over 20 years decreased the risk of breast cancer (OR = 0.66, 95% CI 0.48, 0.90 and OR = 0.68, 95% CI 0.47, 0.99, respectively). That means the women who reported a clinical diagnosis of migraine in age <20 or >20 years were significantly at lower risk of breast cancer.

3.5. Association of Migraine History and Breast Cancer Risk by Histological Subtype

The summary results of associations between migraine history and breast cancer risk showed that the association does not vary by histological type compared to non-migraineur women (**Figure 4**). That means women with a history of migraine had similarly reduced risks of both ductal and lobular carcinomas (OR = 0.84, 95% CI 0.70 - 1.01 and OR = 0.79, 95% CI 0.70, 0.90, respectively). Test for histological subgroup differences was not significant (p = 0.585). Overall, women with migraine history had a 19% reduced risk of breast cancer regardless of histological subgroup.

3.6. Association of Migraine History and Breast Cancer Risk by Hormone Receptor Status

Pooled result showed that women with migraine history had a 15% reduced risk of breast cancer regardless of hormone receptor status (OR = 0.85, 95% CI 0.77, 0.94). **Figure 5** shows the forest plot of OR estimates of association between migraine and breast cancer risk by hormone receptor status. We did not observe significant differences with regard to hormone receptor status (p = 0.253). On the other hand, migraineur women had a lower risk of ER+/PR+ (OR = 0.80, 95% CI 0.68, 0.93), ER+/PR− (OR = 0.82, 95% CI 0.67, 0.99), and ER−/PR− breast cancer (OR =0.97, 95% CI 0.80, 1.17).

3.7. Heterogeneity and Publication Bias

Significant heterogeneity between studies was noted in the studies. The results of Q-test showed that the studies

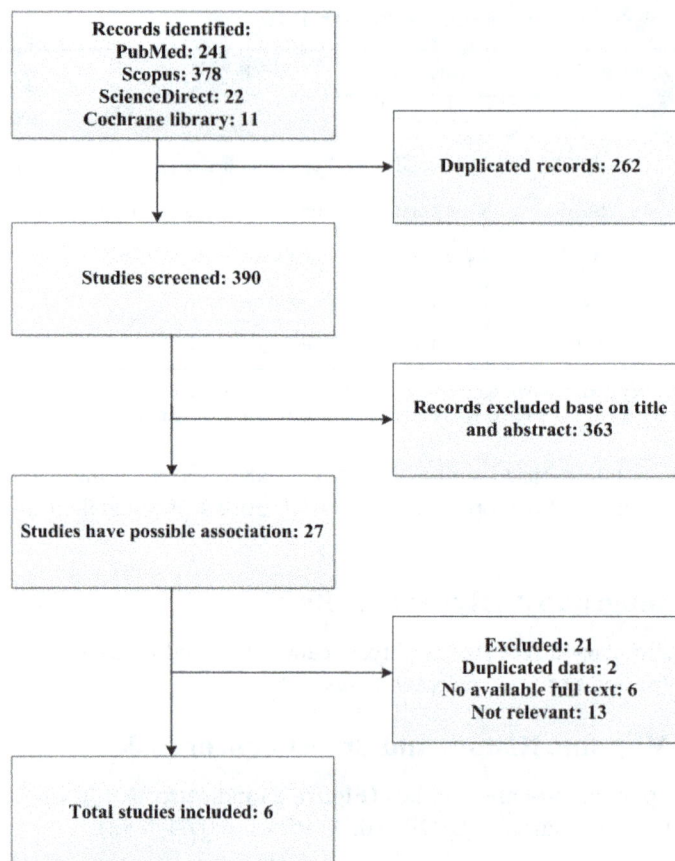

Figure 1. Flowchart of the literature search in the systematic review and meta-analysis.

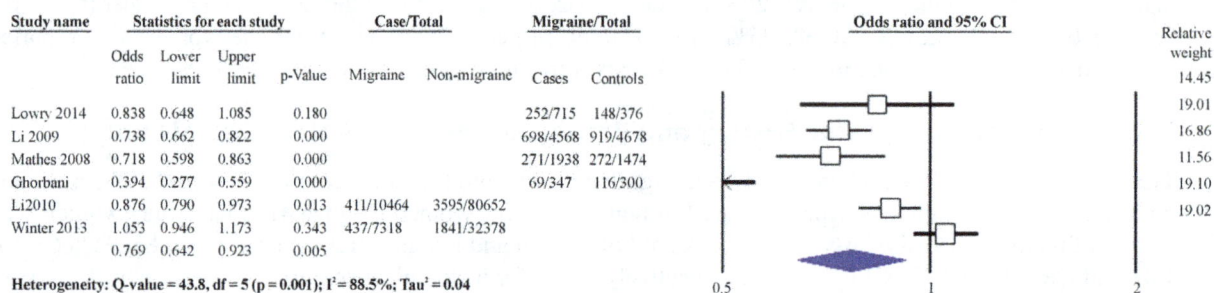

Figure 2. Forest plot of odds ratio estimate of association between migraine and breast cancer risk in the all studies.

were significantly heterogeneous (p < 0.001). The I^2 and tau statistics were 88.5% and 0.04, respectively (**Figure 2**). Of six included studies assessed the effect of migraine on breast cancer risk, five studies reported negative associations (four out of which were statistically significant) and one study reported non-significant positive association. The heterogeneity between studies with related statistics is shown in **Table 2**. We couldn't assess the publication bias using the funnel plot, because the number of included studies in the meta-analysis was relatively small. No publication bias was detected by Egger's regression (p = 0.647).

4. Discussion

The results of this meta-analysis revealed a significant negative relationship between migraine history and risk of breast cancer, women with migraine history have a 23% reduced risk of breast cancer. There was evidence of significant heterogeneity in the meta-analysis. We used the Q-test to detect of heterogeneity. Accordingly, this

Subgroup within study		Odds ratio	Lower limit	Upper limit	p-Value
Li 2009	<20 yr	0.84	0.68	1.04	0.103
Lowry 2014	<20 yr	0.54	0.36	0.81	0.003
Mathes 2008	<20 yr	0.56	0.39	0.80	0.001
		0.66	0.48	0.90	0.009
Li 2009	>20 yr	0.73	0.64	0.82	0.000
Lowry 2014	>20 yr	0.98	0.73	1.32	0.891
Mathes 2008	>20 yr	0.45	0.36	0.57	0.000
		0.68	0.47	0.99	0.042
Overall		0.67	0.52	0.85	0.001

Heterogeneity: Q-value = 24.6, df = 5 (p = 0.001); I^2 = 79.7%; Tau^2 = 0.05
Test for subgroup differences: Q-value = 0.02, df = 1 (p = 0.880)

Decreased Risk   Increased Risk

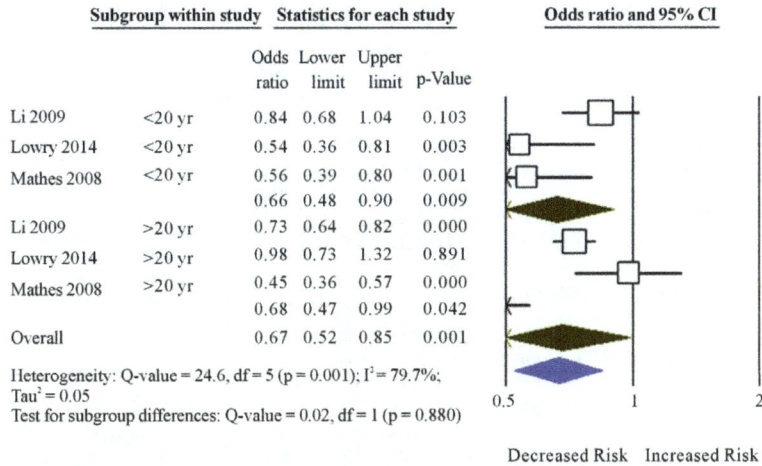

Figure 3. Forest plot of odds ratio estimates of breast cancer risk by age at migraine diagnosis.

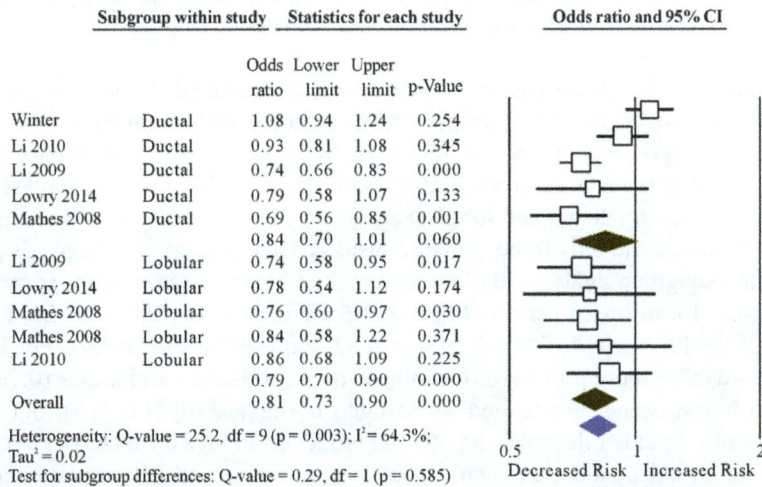

Subgroup within study		Odds ratio	Lower limit	Upper limit	p-Value
Winter	Ductal	1.08	0.94	1.24	0.254
Li 2010	Ductal	0.93	0.81	1.08	0.345
Li 2009	Ductal	0.74	0.66	0.83	0.000
Lowry 2014	Ductal	0.79	0.58	1.07	0.133
Mathes 2008	Ductal	0.69	0.56	0.85	0.001
		0.84	0.70	1.01	0.060
Li 2009	Lobular	0.74	0.58	0.95	0.017
Lowry 2014	Lobular	0.78	0.54	1.12	0.174
Mathes 2008	Lobular	0.76	0.60	0.97	0.030
Mathes 2008	Lobular	0.84	0.58	1.22	0.371
Li 2010	Lobular	0.86	0.68	1.09	0.225
		0.79	0.70	0.90	0.000
Overall		0.81	0.73	0.90	0.000

Heterogeneity: Q-value = 25.2, df = 9 (p = 0.003); I^2 = 64.3%; Tau^2 = 0.02
Test for subgroup differences: Q-value = 0.29, df = 1 (p = 0.585)

Decreased Risk   Increased Risk

Figure 4. Forest plot of odds ratio estimates of association between migraine and breast cancer risk by histological subtype.

Table 2. Summary effect sizes of breast cancer risk and migraine status by age at migraine diagnosis, histological subtype and hormone receptor status.

Subgroup	OR	95% CI		p value	No. of studies	Heterogeneity			
						Q-value	P for Q test	I-squared	Tau squared
<20 yr	0.66	0.48	0.90	0.009	3	5.88	0.053	66.0	0.05
>20 yr	0.68	0.47	0.99	0.042	3	18.61	0.001	89.3	0.09
ER−/PR−	0.97	0.80	1.17	0.754	4	5.61	0.132	46.5	0.02
ER+/PR−	0.82	0.67	0.99	0.043	4	3.78	0.287	20.6	0.01
ER+/PR+	0.80	0.68	0.93	0.003	4	10.23	0.017	70.7	0.02
Ductal	0.84	0.70	1.01	0.060	5	23.14	0.001	82.7	0.03
Lobular	0.79	0.70	0.90	0.001	5	0.99	0.912	0	0

Age at migraine diagnosis: <20 and >20 years; Histological subtype: ductal and lobular; Hormone receptor status: estrogen and progesterone receptor (ER+/PR+, ER+/PR− and ER−/PR−).

Study name	Subgroup within study	Odds ratio	Lower limit	Upper limit	p-Value
Li 2009	ER–/PR–	0.82	0.69	0.98	0.028
Mathes 2008	ER–/PR–	0.95	0.61	1.48	0.819
Winter 2013	ER–/PR–	1.01	0.76	1.34	0.948
Li 2004	ER–/PR–	1.22	0.91	1.63	0.179
		0.97	0.80	1.17	0.754
Li 2009	ER+/PR–	0.83	0.62	1.10	0.185
Mathes 2008	ER+/PR–	0.48	0.27	0.86	0.014
Winter 2013	ER+/PR–	0.89	0.64	1.24	0.498
Li 2010	ER+/PR–	0.90	0.65	1.23	0.503
		0.82	0.67	0.99	0.043
Li 2009	ER+/PR+	0.71	0.62	0.81	0.000
Mathes 2008	ER+/PR+	0.68	0.54	0.86	0.002
Winter 2013	ER+/PR+	0.95	0.82	1.10	0.501
Li 2010	ER+/PR+	0.84	0.72	0.98	0.025
		0.80	0.68	0.93	0.003
Overall		0.85	0.77	0.94	0.001

Heterogeneity: Q-value = 23.5, df = 11 (p = 0.015); I² = 53.3%;
Tau² = 0.02
Test for subgroup differences: Q-value = 2.75, df = 2 (p = 0.253)

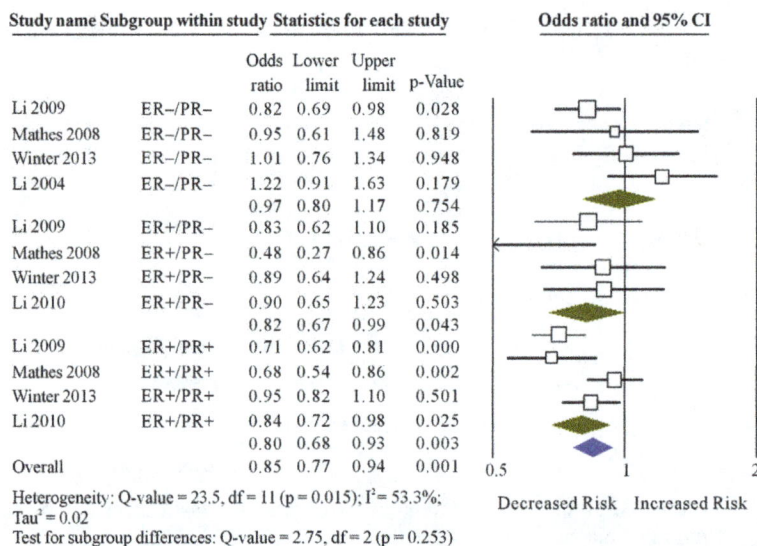

Figure 5. Forest plot of odds ratio estimates of association between migraine and breast cancer risk by hormone receptor status.

issue should be noted that the Q-test has low power when the included studies are small [18]. Therefore, some parts of the observed heterogeneity in the results can be attributed to the number of studies (including six studies) included in the meta-analysis. Subgroup meta-analyses by age at migraine diagnosis, histological subtype and hormone receptor status of breast cancer were also conducted (**Table 2**). Five included studies considered both histological subtype (including ductal and lobular) and hormone receptor status (including ER+/PR+, ER+/PR–, ER–/PR–) of breast cancer, and only three studies considered age at migraine diagnosis [11]-[13].

With regard to the subgroup analysis, the pooled results illustrate a significant correlation between migraine history and decreased risk of breast cancer (**Figures 3-5**). The summary estimate from the ER+/PR+ was more protective than in ER+/PR– or ER–/PR– (0.80 vs. 0.82 and 0.97, respectively). For histological subtype, the summary estimate was also more protective for lobular than for ductal carcinomas (0.79 vs. 0.84). Biologically, both migraine and breast cancer are related to estrogen hormone [10]-[11] [15], but the precise biology and hormonal pathways of migraine relevant to a potential reduction in breast cancer risk are poorly understood [13]. Prior studies showed an independent association between migraine and ER- breast cancer but reported a lower risk of ER+ [15]. Some studies mentioned this hypothesizes that migraine may be particularly associated with a reduced risk of hormone receptor positive tumors [21]. This association may be confounded by a factor entitled obesity. Previous epidemiological studies reported that obesity may be more strongly associated with ER+ postmenopausal breast cancer [22]-[26].

We stratified the migraine history by age at migraine diagnosis (<20 and >20 years). There was no significant difference between migraine and breast cancer by this variable suggesting that age is not strong confounder. One possible explanation for a lower risk of breast cancer in women with a history of migraine could be that such migraineur women are more likely to avoid migraine risk factors such as stress, cigarette smoking and alcohol. The findings of previous study were consistent with this hypothesis, in that alcohol and smoking were less common among migraineurs [27]. Another explanation about this lower risk may relate to specific migraine treatments [12].

Toward our understanding, this study represents the first systematic review of the relationship between migraine history and breast cancer risk. Other strengths of our study were subgroup analysis and all enrolled subject in primary studies was diagnosed based on clinical criteria for migraine and finally large overall sample size.

Following limitations of our study need to be considered. First, three of the included studies were case-control design and potential to recall bias. Second, because of lack of migraine classification according to clinical criteria in the enrolled studies, we could not perform the subgroup analysis based on this variable. Third, heterogeneity was significant and we could not specify source of heterogeneity in our study because of the limited number of available studies.

In conclusion, the results of this meta-analysis showed that women with migraine history have a decreased risk of breast cancer. Further biological studies are needed to address the association.

Acknowledgements

This research has not received any specific fund. The authors declare that there is no conflict of interest.

References

[1] Fernández-de-Las-Peñas, C., Palacios-Ceña, D., Salom-Moreno, J., López-de-Andres, A., Hernández-Barrera, V., Jiménez-Trujillo, I., *et al.* (2014) Has the Prevalence of Migraine Changed over the Last Decade (2003-2012)? A Spanish Population-Based Survey. *PLoS ONE*, **9**, e110530. http://dx.doi.org/10.1371/journal.pone.0110530

[2] Smitherman, T.A., Burch, R., Sheikh, H. and Loder, E. (2013) The Prevalence, Impact, and Treatment of Migraine and Severe Headaches in the United States: A Review of Statistics from National Surveillance Studies. *Headache: The Journal of Head and Face Pain*, **53**, 427-436. http://dx.doi.org/10.1111/head.12074

[3] Ramage-Morin, P.L. and Gilmour, H. (2014) Prevalence of Migraine in the Canadian Household Population. *Health Reports*, **25**, 10-16.

[4] Siegel, R., Ma, J., Zou, Z. and Jemal, A. (2014) Cancer Statistics. *CA: A Cancer Journal for Clinicians*, **64**, 9-29. http://dx.doi.org/10.3322/caac.21208

[5] WHO (2006) Guidelines for Management of Breast Cancer. Egypt.

[6] McPherson, K., Steel, C.M. and Dixon, J.M. (2000) ABC of Breast Diseases. Breast Cancer-Epidemiology, Risk Factors, and Genetics. *British Medical Journal*, **321**, 624-628. http://dx.doi.org/10.1136/bmj.321.7261.624

[7] Rist, P.M., Diener, H.C., Kurth, T. and Schürks, M. (2011) Migraine, Migraine Aura, and Cervical Artery Dissection: A Systematic Review and Meta-Analysis. *Cephalalgia*, **31**, 886-896. http://dx.doi.org/10.1177/0333102411401634

[8] Etminan, M., Takkouche, B., Isorna, F.C. and Samii, A. (2005) Risk of Ischaemic Stroke in People with Migraine: Systematic Review and Meta-Analysis of Observational Studies. *British Medical Journal*, **330**, 63. http://dx.doi.org/10.1136/bmj.38302.504063.8F

[9] Schürks, M., Rist, P.M., Shapiro, R.E. and Kurth, T. (2011) Migraine and Mortality: A Systematic Review and Meta-Analysis. *Cephalalgia*, **31**, 1301-1314. http://dx.doi.org/10.1177/0333102411415879

[10] Li, C.I., Mathes, R.W., Bluhm, E.C., Caan, B., Cavanagh, M.F., Chlebowski, R.T., *et al.* (2010) Migraine History and Breast Cancer Risk among Postmenopausal Women. *Journal of Clinical Oncology*, **28**, 1005-1010. http://dx.doi.org/10.1200/JCO.2009.25.0423

[11] Li, C.I., Mathes, R.W., Malone, K.E., Daling, J.R., Bernstein, L., Marchbanks, P.A., *et al.* (2009) Relationship between Migraine History and Breast Cancer Risk among Premenopausal and Postmenopausal Women. *Cancer Epidemiology, Biomarkers & Prevention*, **18**, 2030-2034. http://dx.doi.org/10.1158/1055-9965.EPI-09-0291

[12] Lowry, S.J., Malone, K.E., Cushing-Haugen, K.L. and Li, C.I. (2014) The Risk of Breast Cancer Associated with Specific Patterns of Migraine History. *Cancer Causes & Control*, **25**, 1707-1715. http://dx.doi.org/10.1007/s10552-014-0479-y

[13] Mathes, R.W., Malone, K.E., Daling, J.R., Davis, S., Lucas, S.M., Porter, P.L., *et al.* (2008) Migraine in Post-Menopausal Women and the Risk of Invasive Breast Cancer. *Cancer Epidemiology, Biomarkers & Prevention*, **17**, 3116-3122. http://dx.doi.org/10.1158/1055-9965.EPI-08-0527

[14] Ghorbani, A., Moradi, A., Gookizadeh, A., Jokar, S. and Sonbolestan, S.A. (2015) Evaluation of Relationship between Breast Cancer and Migraine. *Advanced Biomedical Research*, **4**, 14. http://dx.doi.org/10.4103/2277-9175.148297

[15] Winter, A.C., Rexrode, K.M., Lee, I.M., Buring, J.E., Tamimi, R.M. and Kurth, T. (2013) Migraine and Subsequent Risk of Breast Cancer: A Prospective Cohort Study. *Cancer Causes & Control*, **24**, 81-89. http://dx.doi.org/10.1007/s10552-012-0092-x

[16] Phipps, A.I., Anderson, G.L., Cochrane, B.B., Li, C.I., Wactawski-Wende, J., Ho, G.Y., *et al.* (2012) Migraine History, Nonsteroidal Anti-Inflammatory Drug Use, and Risk of Postmenopausal Endometrial Cancer. *Hormones and Cancer*, **3**, 240-248.

[17] von Elm, E., Altman, D.G., Egger, M., Pocock, S.J., Gøtzsche, P.C., Vandenbroucke, J.P., *et al.* (2007) Strengthening the Reporting of Observational Studies in Epidemiology (STROBE) Statement: Guidelines for Reporting Observational Studies. *British Medical Journal*, **335**, 806-808. http://dx.doi.org/10.1136/bmj.39335.541782.AD

[18] Borenstein, M., Hedges, L.V., Higgins, J.P.T. and Rothstein, H.R. (2009) Introduction to Meta-Analysis. John Wiley & Sons, Hoboken. http://dx.doi.org/10.1002/9780470743386

[19] Egger, M., Davey, S.G., Schneider, M. and Minder, C. (1997) Bias in Meta-Analysis Detected by a Simple, Graphical

Test. *British Medical Journal*, **315**, 629-634. http://dx.doi.org/10.1136/bmj.315.7109.629

[20] Liberati, A., Altman, D.G., Tetzlaff, J., Mulrow, C., Gøtzsche, P.C., Ioannidis, J.P., *et al.* (2009) The PRISMA Statement for Reporting Systematic Reviews and Meta-Analyses of Studies that Evaluate Healthcare Interventions: Explanation and Elaboration. *British Medical Journal*, **339**, b2700. http://dx.doi.org/10.1136/bmj.b2700

[21] Brandes, J.L. (2006) The Influence of Estrogen on Migraine: A Systematic Review. *The Journal of the American Medical Association*, **295**, 1824-1830. http://dx.doi.org/10.1001/jama.295.15.1824

[22] Suzuki, R., Orsini, N., Saji, S., Key, T.J. and Wolk, A. (2009) Body Weight and Incidence of Breast Cancer Defined by Estrogen and Progesterone Receptor Status—A Meta-Analysis. *International Journal of Cancer*, **124**, 698-712. http://dx.doi.org/10.1002/ijc.23943

[23] Vrieling, A., Buck, K., Kaaks, R. and Chang-Claude, J. (2010) Adult Weight Gain in Relation to Breast Cancer Risk by Estrogen and Progesterone Receptor Status: A Meta-Analysis. *Breast Cancer Research and Treatment*, **123**, 641-649. http://dx.doi.org/10.1007/s10549-010-1116-4

[24] Althuis, M.D., Fergenbaum, J.H., Garcia-Closas, M., Brinton, L.A., Madigan, M.P. and Sherman, M.E. (2004) Etiology of Hormone Receptor-Defined Breast Cancer: A Systematic Review of the Literature. *Cancer Epidemiology, Biomarkers & Prevention*, **13**, 1558-1568.

[25] Phipps, A.I., Malone, K.E., Porter, P.L., Daling, J.R. and Li, C.I. (2008) Body Size and Risk of Luminal, HER2-Overexpressing, and Triple-Negative Breast Cancer in Postmenopausal Women. *Cancer Epidemiology, Biomarkers & Prevention*, **17**, 2078-2086. http://dx.doi.org/10.1158/1055-9965.EPI-08-0206

[26] Munsell, M.F., Sprague, B.L., Berry, D.A., Chisholm, G. and Trentham-Dietz, A. (2014) Body Mass Index and Breast Cancer Risk According to Postmenopausal Estrogen-Progestin Use and Hormone Receptor Status. *Epidemiologic Reviews*, **36**, 114-136. http://dx.doi.org/10.1093/epirev/mxt010

[27] Rasmussen, B.K. (1995) Epidemiology of Migraine. *Biomedicine & Pharmacotherapy*, **49**, 452-455. http://dx.doi.org/10.1016/0753-3322(96)82689-8

26

Breast Cancer Survival in Cameroon: Analysis of a Cohort of 404 Patients at the Yaoundé General Hospital

Jean Dupont Kemfang Ngowa[1,2], Jean Marie Kasia[1,2], Jean Yomi[3], Achille Nkigoum Nana[1], Anny Ngassam[1], Irenée Domkam[4], Zacharie Sando[5], Paul Ndom[6]

[1]Department of Gynecology and Obstetrics, Yaoundé General Hospital, Faculty of Medicine and Biomedical Sciences, University of Yaounde I, Yaoundé, Cameroon
[2]Obstetrics and Gynecology Unit, Yaoundé General Hospital, Yaoundé, Cameroon
[3]Department of Radiation Therapy, Yaoundé General Hospital, Faculty of Medicine and Biomedical Sciences, University of Yaoundé I, Yaoundé, Cameroon
[4]Chantal Biya International Reference Centre for Research on HIV/AIDS Prevention and Management, Yaoundé, Cameroon
[5]Department of Morphological Sciences, Yaoundé General Hospital, Faculty of Medicine and Biomedical Sciences, University of Yaoundé I, Yaoundé, Cameroon
[6]Oncology Division, Yaoundé General Hospital, Yaoundé, Cameroon
Email: jdkemfang@yahoo.fr

Abstract

This study aimed to estimate the survival rate of breast cancer in a group of patients followed up at the Yaoundé General Hospital in Cameroon. A retrospective review of records of patients managed for breast cancer between 1995 and 2007 was carried out at the Yaoundé General Hospital. Survival analysis was carried out with survival defined as the time between the date of unequivocal diagnosis of cancer and the date of last follow-up or death. Survival curves were plotted in R.3.1.1 software. Mean age of the patients was 47.5 ± 12.36 years. Most of the patients (67.9%) presented with advanced breast cancer disease (stage III and IV). Overall patient survival rate was 30% at 5 years and 13.2% at 10 years. Median overall survival time was 2 (1.9 - 3) years. There was a correlation between survival and the stage of disease. The highest survival rates were recorded in stages I and II while the lowest rates were recorded in stage IV. There was no statistically significant difference in survival among the age groups (p = 0.15). Overall survival rates of breast cancer are 30% at 5 years and 13.2% at 10 years among Cameroonian patients and are lower compared with 90% and 82% respectively at 5 years and 10 years in some developed countries.

Keywords

Survival, Breast Cancer, Developing Countries

1. Introduction

Breast cancer is now the most frequent cancer of women worldwide with up to a million cases occurring annually [1]. In Cameroon, according to the Globocan 2010 estimation, breast cancer is the most frequent cancer in women before cervical cancer with an incidence of 27.9 per 100,000 women [2].

Lifestyle changes associated with urbanization and the concomitant loss of traditional protective factors appear to be associated with the rising incidence of breast cancer in African women [3] [4].

Although more than half of all new cases of breast cancer are diagnosed in the industrialized world (*i.e.* North America excluding Mexico and Western Europe), more than three quarters of breast cancer related deaths occur in the developing countries. This discordance in incidence and survival is largely related to the lack of organized mammographic screening in developing countries, the advanced stage at diagnosis (>60% of patients are diagnosed with stage III/IV breast cancer in the developing countries), poor access to care, and substandard treatment regimens [4]-[7].

Population-based survival represents the average prognosis of a cancer and is useful for assessing progress in cancer control, including the effect of early detection, diagnosis, treatment, and follow-up on cancer outcomes. The data are also helpful in making informed decisions to ensure improved and equitable cancer care [8].

Cancer survival statistics from developing countries are rare. The reasons for the paucity of information about cancer survival from developing countries are readily understandable. Cancer registries are a recent phenomenon in some developing countries, and do not exist at all in many others. Death registration in developing countries is often incomplete, not all deaths are registered, and the recorded cause of death may be inaccurate, or missing [9].

This study aimed to estimate the survival of a group of breast cancer patients followed up at the Yaoundé General Hospital (YGH) in Cameroon.

2. Patients and Methods

This was a retrospective study in which the medical records of breast cancer patients treated at the YGH between January 1995 and December 2007 were used. The end of the observation period of survival was the 31st of December 2013.

The YGH is one of the most specialized hospitals in the treatment of cancer in Cameroon. It has a number of services specialized in the treatment of cancers such as radiotherapy, medical oncology, anatomic pathology, nuclear medicine, gynecology and surgery. Breast cancer patients followed up at the YGH were most often referred from other health facilities and came from all parts of the country. The breast cancer treatment options offered in this institution are: radical mastectomy and breast conserving surgery; adjuvant and neoadjuvant chemotherapy with the use of the drug combination CAF (Cyclophosphamide: 500 mg/m^2, Adriamycin: 50 mg/m^2, 5-fluorouracil: 500 mg/m^2) every 21 days for 6 cycles; hormone therapy with Tamoxifen and radiotherapy delivered by a cobalt unit at the dose of 50 Gy over 5 weeks for post-mastectomy patients when indicated. However, in the case of breast conserving treatment, a dose of 50 Gy over 5 weeks with a boost dose of 15 Gy to the tumor site is administered.

Out of the 404 breast cancer patients registered in the YGH during the study period, 221 (54.75%) were included in our study. The patients excluded were those whose medical records were not found (139 cases) and those with no follow-up after diagnosis of breast cancer (44 cases).

The survival status of patients within 5 years or 10 years from the date of unequivocal diagnosis of cancer was obtained by active and passive methods. The passive assessment method of survival was based on medical records. Survival was calculated as the time between the date of diagnosis of cancer and the date of death from any cause or the date of loss to follow up or the date of last follow-up. The active measure undertaken to establish the survival status of patients without death information in their medical records was to contact the patient or their relatives by phone. The endpoint in this study was death, regardless of the cause. The socio-demographic information, disease characteristics and vital status of patients were collected.

Global and specific (by age, stage of disease, and treatment modalities) survival curves were estimated via the actuarial method. The equality of these curves was tested using a log-rank test. Analysis was done using R v3.1.0 (Statistical analysis system, GNU GPL).

3. Results

Between January 1995 and December 2007, 404 breast cancer patients were followed at the YGH. Of these, 221 patients who had a medical record found in the archives were included in this study. The socio-demographic characteristics of the patients are shown in **Table 1**. The mean age of the patients was 47.5 ± 12.36 years. The most represented age group was 40 - 49 years. Slightly more than half (56.10%) of the study population lived in rural areas and 51.13% of the patients were housewives.

Table 2 shows the clinical and histopathological aspects of breast cancer in the study population.

Consultation for the symptoms presented by the patient was the circumstance of breast cancer discovery in 61% of cases and screening mammography was the circumstance of discovery only in 9.5% of cases.

Invasive ductal carcinoma was the most represented histological type of breast cancer (79.63%) while invasive lobular carcinoma was found in 4.52% of cases. About the various treatment modalities in this study; 64.70% of patients underwent a radical mastectomy; 53.39% had neoadjuvant chemotherapy; 35.71% had adjuvant chemotherapy; 77.42% had radiotherapy and 19.0% had hormone therapy.

Table 1. Socio-demographic characteristics of breast cancer patients.

Variables	Patients n = 221 n (%)
Age groups (years)	
20 - 30 y	10 (4.5)
30 - 39 y	53 (24)
40 - 49 y	65 (29.4)
≥50 y	93 (42.1)
Marital status	
Married	83 (37.55)
Single	34 (15.38)
Widow	12 (5.42)
unknown	92 (41.62)
Profession	
Employed	97 (43.89)
Housewife	113 (51.13)
Unknown	11 (04.97)
Residential area	
Urban	92 (41.62)
Rural	124 (56.10)
Religion	
Christian	115 (52.03)
Muslim	14 (06.33)
Others	15 (06.78)
Unknown	77 (34.84)

Table 2. Clinical and histopathological aspects of breast cancer in the study population.

Variables	Patients n = 221 n (%)
Circumstance of breast cancer discovery	
Breast symptoms	135 (61.08)
Clinical breast examination	65 (29.41)
Mammography screening	21 (9.50)
Stage of breast cancer	
Stage I	4 (1.8)
Stage II	60 (27.14)
Stage III	123 (55.65)
Stage IV	27 (12.21)
Unknown stage	7 (3.16)
Histological subtype	
Ductal invasive carcinoma	176 (79.63)
Ductal *in situ* carcinoma	1 (0.45)
Lobular invasive carcinoma	10 (04.52)
Adenocarcinoma	23 (10.40)
Others	11 (4.97)
Therapeutic modalities	
Radical mastectomy	143 (64.70)
Breast conserving surgery	38 (17.19)
Neo adjuvant chemotherapy	118 (53.39)
Adjuvant chemotherapy	79 (35.74)
Radiotherapy	172 (77.82)
Hormone therapy	44 (19.90)

Figure 1 shows the overall survival curves for breast cancer over a period of 10 years. The overall median survival was 2 (1.9 - 3) years. Overall survival was 30% at 5 years and 13.2% at 10 years.

The specific survival curve according to the stage of disease is shown in **Figure 2**. The median survival was 5 (2.6 - 7.3) years at stage II; 3 (2.3 - 3.6) years at stage III and 1 (0.5 - 1.4) year at stage IV. All 4 patients in stage I were alive at the end of the observation period. There was a correlation between survival and the stage of disease. The highest survival rates were recorded in stages I and II and the lowest in stage IV. Furthermore, the difference between the survival curves at different stages of the disease was statistically significant ($p < 0.001$).

Figure 3 shows the survival curves for breast cancer with respect to age groups. There was no significant difference between these curves ($p = 0.15$).

Figure 4 shows the survival curves with respect to the type of surgery (**Figure 4(a)**) and treatment with radiotherapy or not (**Figure 4(b)**).

The median survival was 6 (2.8 - 9.1) years in patients who underwent breast conserving surgery and 2 (1.3 - 2.6) years for those who underwent radical mastectomy. Survival was significantly higher ($p = 0.01$) in the group of patients who underwent breast conserving surgery compared to those who underwent radical mastectomy.

On the other hand, there was no significant difference in survival ($p = 0.9$) between breast cancer patients who received radiotherapy and those who did not (**Figure 4(b)**). The median survival was 2 (1.4 - 2.5) years for patients who had radiotherapy and 2 (0.7 - 3.2) years for those who did not.

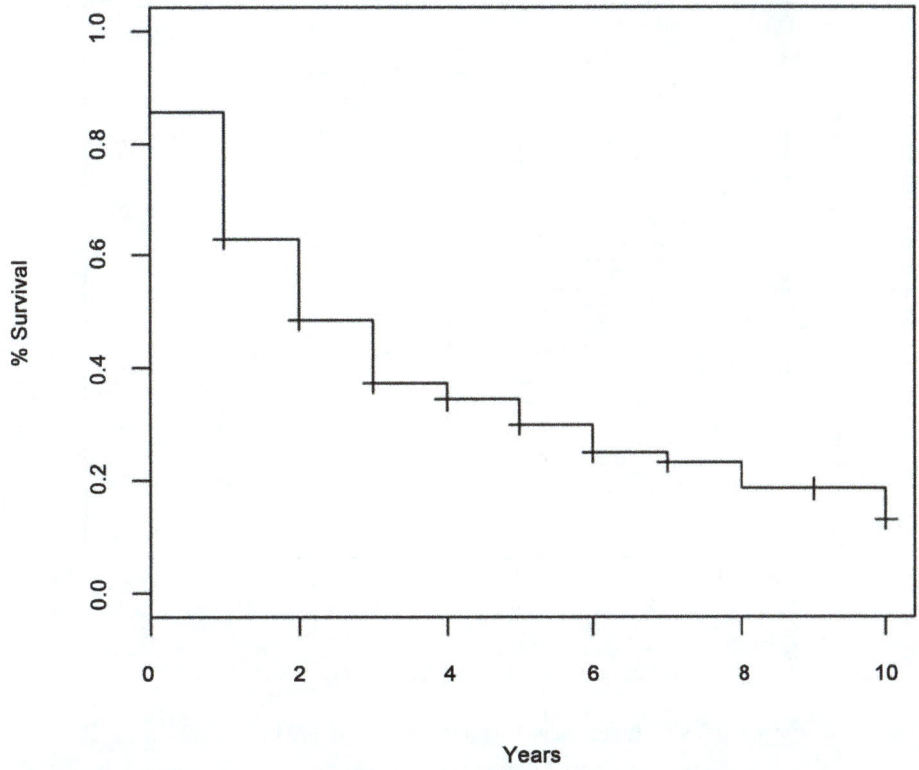

Figure 1. Overall survival curves for breast cancer over a period of 10 years.

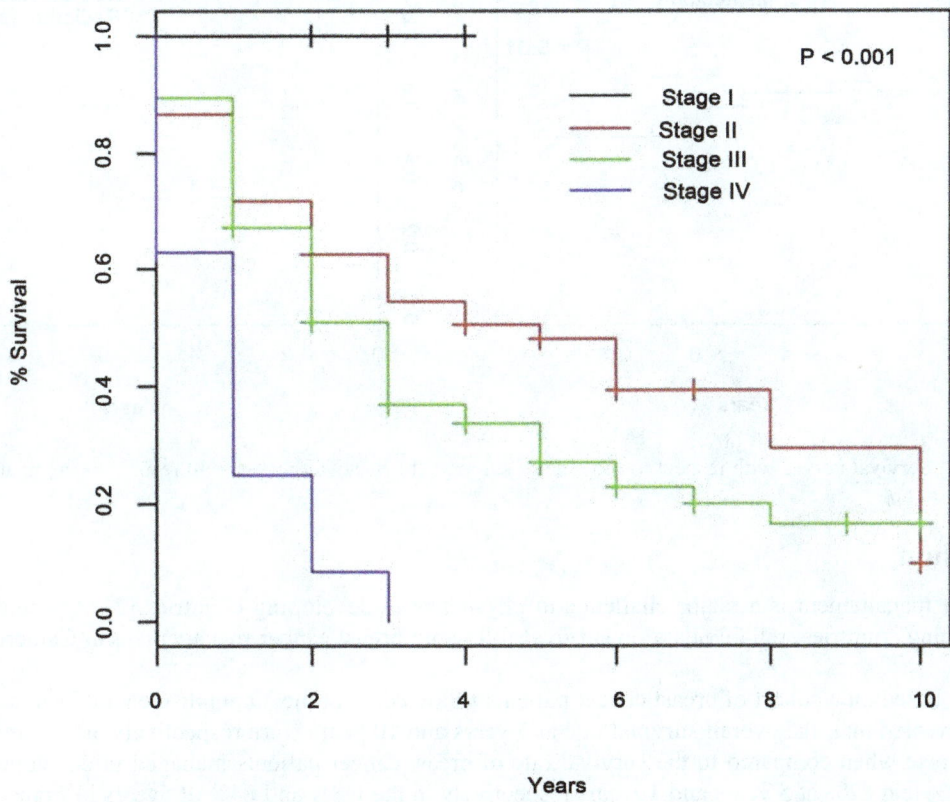

Figure 2. Specific survival curves according to the stage of disease.

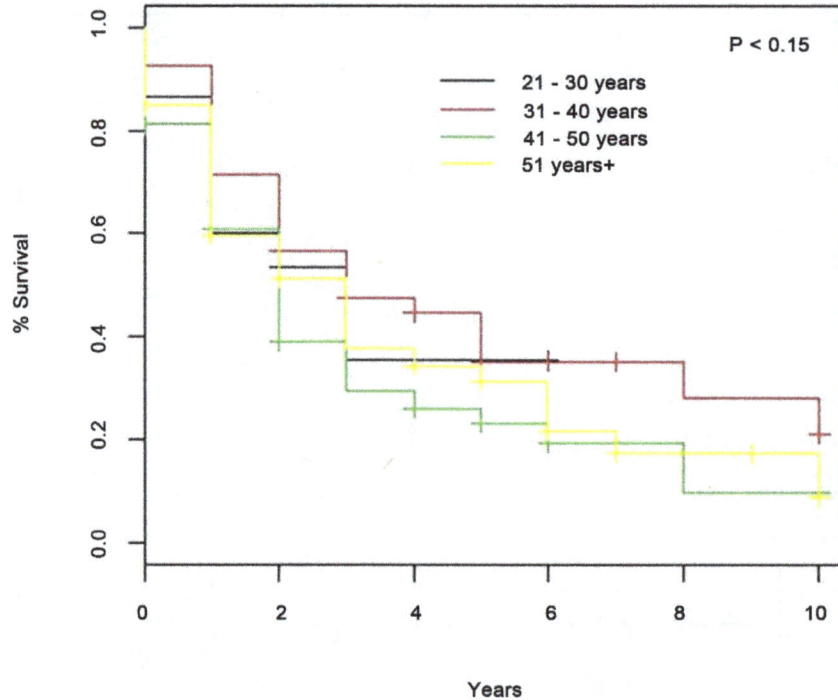

Figure 3. Survival curves for breast cancer with respect to age groups.

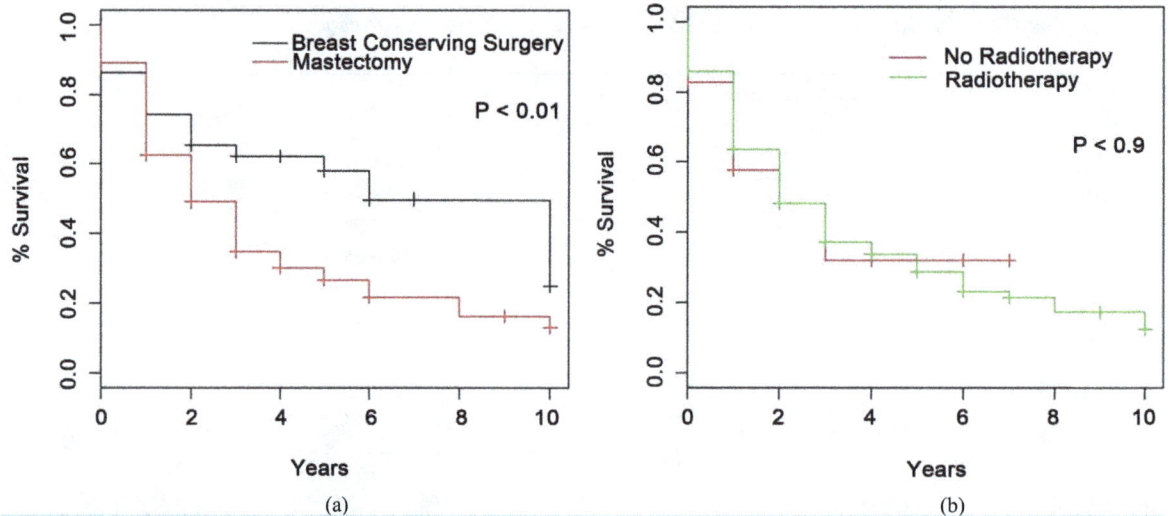

Figure 4. (a) Survival curves with respect to the type of surgery; (b) Survival curves with respect to the treatment with radiotherapy or not.

4. Discussion

Breast cancer management is a major challenge to physicians in developing countries [7]. As seen with many other developing countries, reliable data on survival following breast cancer management in Cameroon is lacking.

This study based on a cohort of breast cancer patients followed up at the Yaoundé General Hospital (YGH) in Cameroon revealed that, the overall survival rate at 5 years and 10 years were respectively 30% and 13.2%. Our results are worse when compared to the survival rate of breast cancer patients managed in developed countries which are 90% and 82% at 5 years and 10years respectively in the USA and 84% at 5years in France [10], [11]. This worse outcome of breast cancer patients in Cameroon is similar to that reported in Nigeria (25.6%), Tunisia

(50.5%), Uganda (46%) and Gambia (12%) at 5 years [8] [12] [13].

The poor survival from breast cancer in the developing countries when compared to some developed countries has been suggested to be related to the advanced stage at diagnosis and limited availability of adequate staging and therapy [3]. The later stage of disease at diagnosis in developing countries could be due to multiple factors like poverty, lack of screening programs low accessibility to diagnostic facilities, cultural beliefs constituting a barrier to early presentation [3]. The late stage of breast cancer (stage III, IV) represented 68% in this study confirming the data in the literature [12] [14]-[17].

Furthermore, the molecular and genetic differences in breast cancer may also contribute to geographic variations in survival. Insufficient data are currently available to define possible trends in different regions of the world [3]. In Cameroon, as in other developing countries, hormone receptors; HER2, p53, Ki 67 and BRCA1/BRCA2 expression could not be tested during the study period.

Overall survival varies according to the stage of breast cancer. Patients diagnosed with stage 0, I or II breast cancers tend to have higher overall survival rates than patients diagnosed with stage III or IV breast cancers [18].

Our results are similar to that of literature [18]. We observed a significant difference in survival between the different stages of breast cancer with the best survival being at stage I and II while the worse was at stage IV.

Breast cancer in young women compared to older women of 50 years and above is associated with a decreased survival [19]. As was seen in the study of Ben Gobrane *et al.* [20] at the Oncological Institute Salah Azaiez of Tunis, we found no significant difference in survival between the different age groups in our study. This could be due to a high proportion of advanced stage breast cancer in our study population which worsened the outcome, and to the low life expectancy in developing countries which could reduce considerably the survival of elderly women over 50 years. Internationally validated guidelines recommend adjuvant radiotherapy after breast conserving surgery and for patients with certain risk factors (T3/T4 or multicentricity) after mastectomy [21]. This strongly affects locoregional disease recurrence but has demonstrated a limited effect on long term survival [21]-[23].

In this study, there was no difference in survival between patients who underwent radiotherapy and those who did not probably due to high prevalence of advanced stage breast cancer.

Breast conserving surgery followed by adjuvant radiotherapy is an equivalent alternative to mastectomy for selected patients [22] [24] [25]. We found in this study significantly higher survival among patients who had breast conserving surgery when compared to those who had radical mastectomy. The difference in survival in these two groups could be due to the fact that breast conserving surgery is usually indicated for early breast cancer in contrast to mastectomy whose indications also include advanced stage disease.

The high proportion of loss to follow up because of unrecovered medical records is the main limitation of this study. This difficulty of archiving is very frequent in our hospitals and is a major challenge for research in developing countries. However, the results of this study provide an idea on breast cancer survival in our environment.

5. Conclusion

The overall survival rates of breast cancer are 30% at 5 years and 13.2% at 10 years among Cameroonian patients and are lower compared with 90% and 82% respectively at 5years and 10years in some developed countries [11]. Consistent to the literature, survival rates to the breast cancer in our study were correlated to stages of disease. These results challenge us to improve breast cancer care in our environment and especially to implement the breast cancer screening programs in our community in order to reduce the stage of disease at diagnosis. However, educational campaigns will be a first step because early detection cannot be successful if the population is unaware of the problem or has adverse misconceptions about the value of early detection.

Conflict of Interests

The authors declare that there is no conflict of interests regarding the publication of this paper.

References

[1]   Parkin, D.M., Bray, F., Ferlay, J. and Pisani, P. (2005) Global Cancer Statistics, 2002. *CA: A Cancer Journal for Clini-*

cians, **55**, 74-108. http://dx.doi.org/10.3322/canjclin.55.2.74

[2]   International Agency for Research on Cancer (2010) Globocan Cameroon Fact Sheets: Breast Cancer. Lyon, France. http://globocan.iarc.fr/

[3]   Hortobagyi, G.N., Salazar, J.G., Pritchard, K., *et al.* (2005) The Global Breast Cancer Burden: Variations in Epidemiology and Survival. *Clinical Breast Cancer*, **6**, 391-401. http://dx.doi.org/10.3816/CBC.2005.n.043

[4]   Porter, P. (2008) "Westernizing" Women's Risks? Breast Cancer in Lower-Income Countries. *New England Journal of Medicine*, **358**, 213-216. http://dx.doi.org/10.1056/NEJMp0708307

[5]   Walker, A.R.P., Adam, F.I. and Walker, B.F. (2014) Breast Cancer in Black African Women: A Changing Situation. *Journal of the Royal Society of Health*, **124**, 81-85. http://dx.doi.org/10.1177/146642400412400212

[6]   Vorobiof, D.A., Sitas, F. and Vorobiof, G. (2001) Breast Cancer Incidence in South Africa. *Journal of Clinical Oncology*, **19**, 125s-127s.

[7]   Anderson, O.B., Shyyan, R., Eniu, A., *et al.* (2006) Breast Cancer in Limited-Resource Countries: An Overview of the Breast Health Global Initiative 2005 Guidelines. *The Breast Journal*, **12**, S3-S15. http://dx.doi.org/10.1111/j.1075-122X.2006.00199.x

[8]   Sankaranarayanan, R., Swaminathan, R., Brenner, H., *et al.* (2010) Cancer Survival in Africa, Asia, and Central America: A Population-Based Study. *The Lancet Oncology*, **11**, 165-173. http://dx.doi.org/10.1016/S1470-2045(09)70335-3

[9]   Sankaranarayanan, R., Black, R.J., Swaminathan, R., *et al.* (1998) An Overview of Cancer Survival in Developing Countries. *IARC Scientific Pubications*, **145**, 135-173.

[10]   Bossard, N., Velten, M., Remontet, L., *et al.* (2007) Survival of Cancer Patients in France: A Population-Based Study from The Association of the French Cancer Registries (FRANCIM). *European Journal of Cancer*, **43**, 149-160.

[11]   American Cancer Society (2011) Breasts Cancer Facts Figures 2011-2012, Atlanta. American Cancer Society Inc. http://www.cancer.org/Research/CancerFactsfigures/BreastscancerFactsFigures/breast-cancer-facts-and-figures-2011-2012

[12]   Ahmed, B. (2002) Pronostic du cancer du sein chez les femmes tunisiennes: Analyse d'une série hospitalière de 729 patientes. *Santé Publique*, **14**, 231-241. http://dx.doi.org/10.3917/spub.023.0231

[13]   Popoola, A.O., Ogunleye, O.O., Ibrahim, N.A., Omodele, F.O. and Igwilo, A.I. (2012) Five Year Survival of Patients with Breast Cancer at the Lagos State University Teaching Hospital, Nigeria. *Online Journal of Medicine and Medical Science Research*, **1**, 24-31.

[14]   Kemfang, J.D., Yomi, J., Kasia, J.M., Mawamba, Y., Ekortah, A.C. and Vlastos, G. (2011) Breast Cancer Profile in a Group of Patients Followed up at the Radiation Therapy Unit of the Yaounde General Hospital, Cameroon. *Obstetrics and Gynecology International*, **2011**, Article ID: 143506.

[15]   Terfa, S.K., Odigie, V.I., Yusufu, L., Bidemi, O., Sani, M.S. and Kase, J.J. (2010) Pattern of Presentation and Survival of Breast Cancer in a Teaching Hospital in North Western Nigeria. *Oman Medical Journal*, **25**, 104-107. http://dx.doi.org/10.5001/omj.2010.29

[16]   Anyanwu, S.N. (2000) Survival Following Treatment of Primary Breast Cancer in Eastern Nigeria. *East African Medical Journal*, **77**, 539-543.

[17]   Essiben, F., Foumane, P., Mboudou, E.T., Dohbit, J.S., Mve Koh, V. and Ndom, P. (2013) Diagnostic et traitement du cancer du sein au Cameroun. A propos de 65 cas. *Mali Medical*, **28**, 38-42.

[18]   Wilkinson, G.S., Edgerton, F., Wallace Jr., H.J., Reese, P., Patterson, J. and Priore, R. (1979) Delay, Stage of Disease and Survival from Breast Cancer. *Journal of Chronic Disease*, **32**, 365-373. http://dx.doi.org/10.1016/0021-9681(79)90078-X

[19]   Fowble, B.L., Schultz, D.J., Overmoyer, B., Solin, L.J., Fox, K., Jardines, L., *et al.* (1994) The Influence of Young Age on Outcome in Early Stage Breast Cancer. *International Journal of Radiation Oncology*Biology*Physics*, **30**, 23-33. http://dx.doi.org/10.1016/0360-3016(94)90515-0

[20]   Gobrane, H.B., Fakhfakh, R., Rahal, K., *et al.* (2007) Pronostic du cancer du sein à l'institut de carcinologique Salah Azaiez de Tunis. *Eastern Mediteranean Health Journal*, **13**, 309-318.

[21]   Wolters, R., Regierer, A.C., Schwentner, L., *et al.* (2012) A Comparison of International Breast Cancer Guidelines—Do the National Guidelines Differ in Treatment Recommendations? *European Journal of Cancer*, **48**, 1-11. http://dx.doi.org/10.1016/j.ejca.2011.06.020

[22]   Wöckel, A., Wolters, R., Wiegel, T., *et al.* (2014) The Impact of Adjuvant Radiotherapy on the Survival of Primary Breast Cancer Patients: A Retrospective Multicenter Cohort Study of 8935 Subjects. *Annals of Oncology*, **25**, 628-632. http://dx.doi.org/10.1093/annonc/mdt584

[23]   Whelan, T.J., Julian, J., Wright, J., Jadad, A.R. and Levine, M.L. (2000) Does Locoregional Radiation Therapy Im-

prove Survival in Breast Cancer? A Meta-Analysis. *Journal of Clinical Oncology*, **18**, 1220-1229.

[24] Fisher, B., Anderson, S., Bryant, J., *et al.* (2002) Twenty-Year Follow-Up of a Randomized Trial Comparing Total Mastectomy, Lumpectomy, and Lumpectomy Plus Irradiation for the Treatment of Invasive Breast Cancer. *New England Journal of Medicine*, **347**, 1233-1241. http://dx.doi.org/10.1056/NEJMoa022152

[25] Veronesi, U., Cascinelli, N., Mariani, L., *et al.* (2002) Twenty-Year Follow-Up of a Randomized Study Comparing Breast-Conserving Surgery with Radical Mastectomy for Early Breast Cancer. *New England Journal of Medicine*, **347**, 1227-1232. http://dx.doi.org/10.1056/NEJMoa020989

27

Study of the Effect of Silymarin on Viability of Breast Cancer Cell Lines

Saieh Hajighasemlou[1,2], Mohammadmorad Farajollahi[2,3]*, Mahmoud Alebouyeh[1], Hossein Rastegar[1], Mojgan Taghizadeh Manzari[1], Milad Mirmoghtadaei[4], Behjat Moayedi[5], Maryam Ahmadzadeh[6], Mansure Kazemi[7], Farzad Parvizpour[8], Safoora Gharibzadeh[9]

[1]Iran Foods and Drug Organization, Tehran, Iran
[2]Department of Biotechnology, Iran University of Medical Sciences, Tehran, Iran
[3]Alborz Food and Drug Laboratory, Fardis, Iran
[4]School of Medicine, Tehran University of Medical Sciences, International Campus (TUMS-IC), Tehran, Iran
[5]Isfahan University of Medical Sciences, Isfahan, Iran
[6]Department of Pharmaceutical Biotechnology, School of Pharmacy, Shahid Beheshti University of Medical Sciences, Tehran, Iran
[7]Department of Tissue Engineering, School of Medical Advanced of Technologies in Medicine, Tehran University of Medical Sciences, Tehran, Iran
[8]Department of Applied Cell Sciences, School of Medical Advanced of Technologies in Medicine, Tehran University of Medical Sciences, Tehran, Iran
[9]Department of Epidemiology and Biostatistics, School of Public Health, Tehran University of Medical Sciences, Tehran, Iran.
Email: *mahdiy@yahoo.com

Abstract

Background: Breast cancer is the most prevalent cancer and results in 14% of cancer-related deaths among women worldwide. The aim of this study is to investigate the anticancer effects of Silymarin on two breast cancer cell lines (BT-474, SK-BR-3). Methods and Material: Two breast cancer cell lines—SK-BR-3 and BT-474—were incubated for 24 hours in standard conditions before adding 100, 200, 400, 800, 1600 µM Silymarin to each well. Alamar blue was then added to the wells after 24, 48 and 72 hours of incubation and cell viability was determined using fluorescence reader to detect the optical density. Results were analyzed using generalized estimating equations (GEE) method in STATA 12.0. Results: we demonstrated the *Silybum marianum* inhibition of two-cell lines SK-BR-3 and BT-474 growth at different concentrations after 24, 48 and 72 hours. Silymarin increased cell death in both cell lines. Conclusion: Silymarin can be combined with other anti-neoplastic agents to obtain better results.

*Corresponding author.

Keywords

Silymarin, Breast Cancer, SK-BR-3, BT-474

---

1. Introduction

Silybum marianum (milk thistle) is a plant of the Asteraceae family that grows naturally in some parts of Europe, Asia (including Iran) and the United States [1]. Silymarin is a complex mixture of polyphenolic molecules, including seven closely related flavonolignans (silybin A, silybin B, isosilybin A, isosilybin B, silychristin, isosilychristin, silydianin) and one flavonoid (taxifolin); the active ingredient is Silibinin which has long been used in traditional medicine and shows antioxidant, anti-inflammatory and anti-cancer properties and can induce apoptosis in some cells [2] [3]. Anti-neoplastic properties of Silymarin have been demonstrated in cancers of prostate [4]-[6], Ovaries, lung, skin, bladder and breast [7]-[11].

Although the exact mechanisms involved in antineoplastic effects of silymarin in breast cancer have not been identified, possible underlying explanations include induction of G1 arrest and apoptosis through inhibiting cyclin-dependent kinases activity and epidermal growth factor receptor signaling, and increasing Cip1/p21 and p27 [9] [12]-[16].

Breast cancer is a major health problem more commonly seen in the developed countries. Breast cancer is the leading cause of death in women 40 - 59 years and more than a million new cases are detected annually [17] [18]. In Iran breast cancer is the commonest cancer among women comprising 21.4% of all cancers among females. Studies indicate that breast cancer presents about one decade earlier in Iranian women than in developed countries [19]-[21].

In present study, we examine the *in vitro* effect of different Silymarin concentrations on two breast cancer cell lines: SK-BR-3 and BT-474 by determining cell viability after 24, 48 and 72 hours of incubation with alamar blue using fluorescent reader.

2. Materials and Methods

Silymarin powder (Sigma) solution in Dimethyl Sulfoxide (DMSO, Sigma) was prepared as stock at the concentration of 30,000 μL/mL and kept at −20°C. During the test required concentrations using phosphate buffered saline (PBS) were prepared from this stock solution. Cell culture medium (Gibco®) consisted of RPMI1640 and DMEM, trypsin, antibiotics, fresh bovine serum (FBS) and anti-mycoplasma. Alamar blue fluorescence reagent from Invitrogen and cell lines SK-BR-3 and BT-474 were purchased from Cell Bank of Iran, Pasteur Institute. Cells were cultured at standard conditions (temperature of 37°C, humidity of 95% and 5%CO_2 gas pressure) and the culture was replaced at 48 and 72-hour intervals.

A suspension of 25,000 cells were added to each well and incubated for 24 hours at 37°C to stick to the bottom of the wells. 10 wells were assigned for each concentration (100, 200, and 400, 800 and 1600 mM) and 10 wells without Silymarin as our controls. The DMSO concentration in the controls wells was adjusted to be the same as the test wells.

After incubation the wells for 24, 48 and 72 hours, 25 μl Alamar blue was added to each well and the plates were incubated for an additional 3 hours. Absorbance was measured at 530 and 590 nm using a fluorescence reader.

3. Results

Results of the effect of *Silybum marianum* were evaluated on two cell lines BT-474 and SK-BR-3 are summarized in the **Figure 1** and **Figure 2**.

Time trends of cells were examined using generalized estimating equations (GEE) that account for correlation between samples. For BT-474 cell line we found significant difference between samples of different incubation periods (P-value < 0.001). We then compared the control group with different silymarin concentrations of different incubation periods (one to three days). **Table 1** shows the significance difference between the control and silymarin groups. This difference remains significant but declines after Day 1.

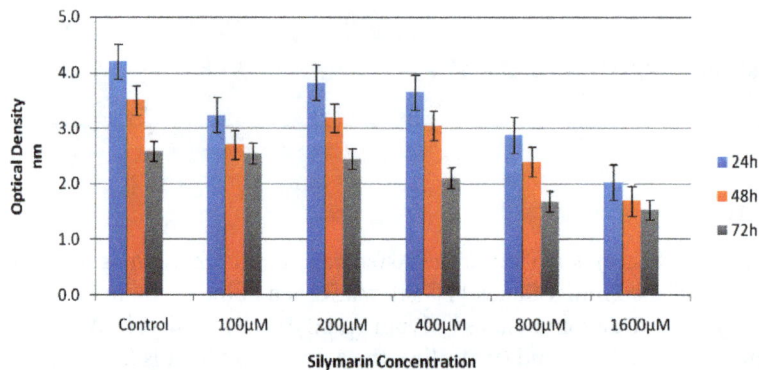

Figure 1. Silymarin effect on the BT-474 cell line after 24, 48 and 72 hours of incubation: Cell viability was significantly reduced compared to control for all concentrations at 24 and 48 hours and for concentrations of ≥400 μM at 72 hours.

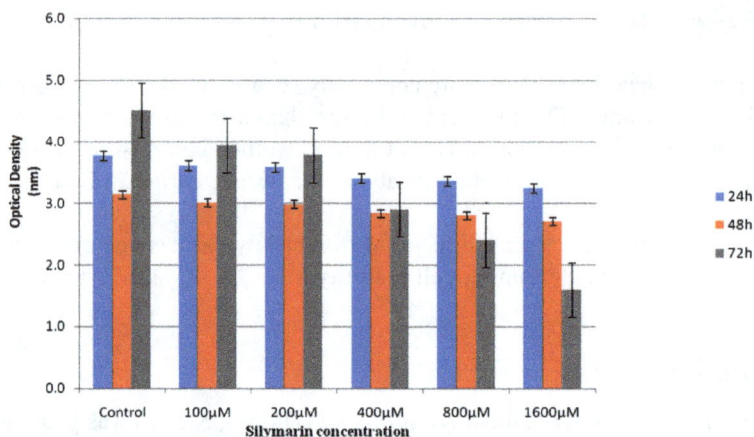

Figure 2. The effect of Silymarin on the SK-BR-3 cell line after 24, 48 and 72 hours: Cell viability differed significantly at all concentrations only after 72 hours; the difference was not significant at any concentration after 24 or 48 hours of incubation.

Table 1. Comparisons of different concentrations with control group.

| | BT-474 | | | |
	Day 1	Day 2	Day 3	P-value
100 μM	−966.72	−805.6	−47.8	<0.001
200 μM	−380.88	−317.4	−143.3	<0.001
400 μM	−551.64	−459.7	−478.9	<0.001
800 μM	−1326.72	−1105.6	−905	<0.001
1600 μM	−2177.76	−1814.8	−1053.3	<0.001

For SK-BR-3 cell line we also found a significant interaction between incubation period (days) and different concentrations, which suggests a varying degree of silymarin effect at the same concentration but in different incubation periods; we could not however detect any pattern for such decline.

4. Discussion

Anti-growth and anti-tumor effects of *Silybum marianum* have been noted in many cancers over recent years. This study was the first to employ Alamar blue in order to detect cell viability which is more sensitive than the conventional MTT assay [22].

In the present study, cell viability was significantly reduced in comparison to the controls. This effect increased over the time course from 24 - 72 hours, and also from lower to higher concentrations of Silymarin from 0 - 1600 μM. Our data are in consistent with that of Gharagozloo and colleagues showed that *Silybum marianum* has an inhibitory effect on HepG2 cell line growth [23]. It would be compatible with the research by Singh who has studied the effect of *Silybum marianum* on human endothelial cell line and has showed that this drug is able to inhibit cell proliferation [24], also compatible with the research by Li and colleagues that examined the effect of *Silybum marianum* on cell Anip973 line (lung cancer), and showed that *Silybum marianum* inhibited cell proliferation and activates apoptosis via the mitochondrial pathway [25]. Sigh and colleagues in other study, the effect of *Silybum marianum* on Hairless SKH-1 mice, demonstrated that it has a strong protective effect against photocarcinogen and inhibitory effects on inflammatory responses and angiogenesis [26]. Similarly, Rajamanickam and colleagues examined the effect of *Silybum marianum* on colorectal cancer in a mouse model of APC (min/+) and showed that it had anticancer effects in this model of cancer that is consistent with the findings from this study [27]. The results would be compatible with the results of the study by Kim and colleagues in 2011, showed that Silymarin could reduce the ligand-induced EGFR and metalloproteinase 9 (MMP-9) in both cell lines SK-BR-3 and BT-474 [28]. Our results are compatible with research by Provinciali that showed antitumor effects of the *silybin*-phosphatidylcholine *complex (IdB* 1016) *on the development of mammary tumors in HER-2/neu transgenic mice* [29].

Here we suggest that a similar mechanism is involved as has been proposed for silymarin effect on prostate cancer: G1 phase cell cycle arrest most probably through inhibition of cyclin-dependent kinases (CDK) activity and epidermal growth factor receptor (erbB2) signaling [9] [12]-[14].

As showed above *in vitro* and *in vivo* studies and the results of the present study, all confirmed antioxidant and anticancer properties of these drugs. The highest concentration of Silymarin used in this study was the 1600 μM; higher doses are suggested to achieve the optimum dose. The highest level of cell apoptosis observed in the present study at 72-hour incubation proposed that long-term incubation of cells with the drug may increase efficiency of its action on the cancer cells. Both cell lines studied here were Her2 positive, a similar study on Her2 negative cell lines would be valuable.

5. Conclusion

We demonstrated the *Silybum marianum* inhibition of two cell lines SK-BR-3 and BT-474 growth at different concentrations, and increased cell death in both cell lines. Silymarin can be combined with other anti-neoplastic agents to obtain better results.

Acknowledgements

We would like to thank all our study participants for their commitment to this study. Iran University of Medical Science and Iran Food and Drug Organization (IRI.FDO) provided financial support.

Conflict of Interest

This research sponsored by Iran Food and Drug Organization and Iran University of Medical Sciences.

References

[1] Osuchowski, M., Johnson, V., He, Q. and Sharma, R. (2004) Alterations in Regional Brain Neurotransmitters by Silymarin, a Natural Antioxidant Flavonoid Mixture, in BALB/c Mice. *Pharmaceutical Biology*, **42**, 384-389. http://dx.doi.org/10.1080/13880200490519712

[2] Kroll, D.J., Shaw, H.S. and Oberlies, N.H. (2007) Milk Thistle Nomenclature: Why It Matters in Cancer Research and Pharmacokinetic Studies. *Integrative Cancer Therapies*, **6**, 110-119. http://dx.doi.org/10.1177/1534735407301825

[3] Davis-Searles, P.R., *et al.* (2005) Milk Thistle and Prostate Cancer: Differential Effects of Pure Flavonolignans from *Silybum marianum* on Antiproliferative end Points in Human Prostate Carcinoma Cells. *Cancer Research*, **65**, 4448-4457. http://dx.doi.org/10.1158/0008-5472.CAN-04-4662

[4] Kiruthiga, P.V., Beema Shafreen, R., Karutha Pandian, S. and Pandima Devi, K. (2007) Silymarin Protection against Major Reactive Oxygen Species Released by Environmental Toxins: Exogenous H2O2 Exposure in Erythrocytes. *Ba-*

sic Clinical Pharmacology Toxicology, **100**, 414-419. http://dx.doi.org/10.1111/j.1742-7843.2007.00069.x

[5]   Manna, S.K., Mukhopadhyay, A., Van, N.T. and Aggarwal, B.B. (1999) Silymarin Suppresses TNF-Induced Activation of NF-Kappa B, c-Jun N-terminal Kinase, and Apoptosis. *Journal of Immunology*, **163**, 6800-6809.

[6]   Li, L.H., *et al.* (2007) Silymarin Enhanced Cytotoxic Effect of Anti-Fas Agonistic Antibody CH11 on A375-S2 Cells. *Journal of Asian Natural Products Research*, **9**, 593-602. http://dx.doi.org/10.1080/10286020600882502

[7]   Singh, R.P. and Agarwal, R. (2006) Prostate Cancer Chemoprevention by Silibinin: Bench to Bedside. *Molecular Carcinogenesis*, **45**, 436-442. http://dx.doi.org/10.1002/mc.20223

[8]   Singh, R.P. and Agarwal, R. (2004) A Cancer Chemopreventive Agent Silibinin, Targets Mitogenic and Survival Signaling in Prostate Cancer. *Mutation Research*, **555**, 21-32. http://dx.doi.org/10.1016/j.mrfmmm.2004.05.017

[9]   Zi, X., Grasso, A.W., Kung, H.J. and Agarwal, R. (1998) A Flavonoid Antioxidant, Silymarin, Inhibits Activation of erbB1 Signaling and Induces Cyclin-Dependent Kinase Inhibitors, G1 Arrest, and Anticarcinogenic Effects in Human Prostate Carcinoma DU145 Cells. *Cancer Research*, **58**, 1920-1929.

[10]   Scambia, G., *et al.* (1996) Antiproliferative Effect of Silybin on Gynaecological Malignancies: Synergism with Cisplatin and Doxorubicin. *European Journal of Cancer*, **32A**, 877-882. http://dx.doi.org/10.1016/0959-8049(96)00011-1

[11]   Sharma, G., Singh, R.P., Chan, D.C. and Agarwal, R. (2003) Silibinin Induces Growth Inhibition and Apoptotic Cell Death in Human Lung Carcinoma Cells. *Anticancer Research*, **23**, 2649-2655.

[12]   Zi, X., Feyes, D.K. and Agarwal, R. (1998) Anticarcinogenic Effect of a Flavonoid Antioxidant, Silymarin, in Human Breast Cancer Cells MDA-MB 468: Induction of G1 Arrest through an Increase in Cip1/p21 Concomitant with a Decrease in Kinase Activity of Cyclin-Dependent Kinases and Associated Cyclins. *Clinical Cancer Research*, **4**, 1055-1064.

[13]   Deep, G., Oberlies, N.H., Kroll, D.J. and Agarwal, R. (2007) Isosilybin B and Isosilybin A Inhibit Growth, Induce G1 Arrest and Cause Apoptosis in Human Prostate Cancer LNCaP and 22Rv1 Cells. *Carcinogenesis*, **28**, 1533-1542. http://dx.doi.org/10.1093/carcin/bgm069

[14]   Roy, S., Kaur, M., Agarwal, C., Tecklenburg, M., Sclafani, R.A. and Agarwal, R. (2007) p21 and p27 Induction by Silibinin Is Essential for Its Cell Cycle Arrest Effect in Prostate Carcinoma Cells. *Molecular Cancer Therapeutics*, **6**, 2696-2707.

[15]   Kaur, M., *et al.* (2009) Silibinin Suppresses Growth and Induces Apoptotic Death of Human Colorectal Carcinoma LoVo Cells in culture and Tumor Xenograft. *Molecular Cancer Therapeutics*, **8**, 2366-2374. http://dx.doi.org/10.1158/1535-7163.MCT-09-0304

[16]   Zhu, W., Zhang, J.S. and Young, C.Y. (2001) Silymarin Inhibits Function of the Androgen Receptor by Reducing Nuclear Localization of the Receptor in the Human Prostate Cancer Cell Line LNCaP. *Carcinogenesis*, **22**, 1399-1403. http://dx.doi.org/10.1093/carcin/22.9.1399

[17]   Jemal, A., *et al.* (2011) Global Cancer Statistics. *CA: A Cancer Journal for Clinicians*, **61**, 69-90. http://dx.doi.org/10.3322/caac.20107

[18]   Ferlay, J., Soerjomataram, I., Ervik, M., Dikshit, R., Eser, S., Mathers, C., Rebelo, M., Parkin, D.M., Forman, D. and Bray, F. (2013) GLOBOCAN 2012 v1.0, Cancer Incidence and Mortality Worldwide: IARC Cancer Base No. 11 [Internet]. Lyon, France: International Agency for Research on Cancer. http://globocan.iarc.fr

[19]   Mousavi, S.M., *et al.* (2007) Breast Cancer in Iran: An Epidemiological Review. *The Breast Journal*, **13**, 383-391. http://dx.doi.org/10.1111/j.1524-4741.2007.00446.x

[20]   Noroozi, A., Jomand, T. and Tahmasebi, R. (2011) Determinants of Breast Self-Examination Performance among Iranian Women: An Application of the Health Belief Model. *Journal of Cancer Education*, **26**, 365-374. http://dx.doi.org/10.1007/s13187-010-0158-y

[21]   Bidgoli, S.A., Ahmadi, R. and Zavarhei, M.D. (2010) Role of Hormonal and Environmental Factors on Early Incidence of Breast Cancer in Iran. *Science of the Total Environment*, **408**, 4056-4061. http://dx.doi.org/10.1016/j.scitotenv.2010.05.018

[22]   Deep, G. and Agarwal, R. (2007) Chemopreventive Efficacy of Silymarin in Skin and Prostate Cancer. *Integrative Cancer Therapies*, **6**, 130-145. http://dx.doi.org/10.1177/1534735407301441

[23]   Gharagozloo, M. and Amirghofran, Z. (2007) Effects of Silymarin on the Spontaneous Proliferation and Cell Cycle of Human Peripheral Blood Leukemia T Cells. *Journal of Cancer Research and Clinical Oncology*, **133**, 525-532. http://dx.doi.org/10.1007/s00432-007-0197-x

[24]   Singh, R.P., *et al.* (2005) Silibinin Strongly Inhibits Growth and Survival of Human Endothelial Cells via Cell Cycle Arrest and Downregulation of Survivin, Akt and NF-kappaB: Implications for Angioprevention and Antiangiogenic Therapy. *Oncogene*, **24**, 1188-1202. http://dx.doi.org/10.1038/sj.onc.1208276

[25]   Li, W., *et al.* (2011) Molecular Mechanism of Silymarin-Induced Apoptosis in a Highly Metastatic Lung Cancer Cell

Line Anip973. *Cancer Biotherapy and Radiopharmaceuticals*, **26**, 317-324. http://dx.doi.org/10.1089/cbr.2010.0892

[26] Gu, M., Singh, R.P., Dhanalakshmi, S., Agarwal, C. and Agarwal, R. (2007) Silibinin Inhibits Inflammatory and Angiogenic Attributes in Photocarcinogenesis in SKH-1 Hairless Mice. *Cancer Research*, **67**, 3483-3491. http://dx.doi.org/10.1158/0008-5472.CAN-06-3955

[27] Rajamanickam, S., Velmurugan, B., Kaur, M., Singh, R.P. and Agarwal, R. (2010) Chemoprevention of Intestinal Tumorigenesis in APCmin/+ Mice by Silibinin. *Cancer Research*, **70**, 2368-2378. http://dx.doi.org/10.1158/0008-5472.CAN-09-3249

[28] Kim, S., *et al.* (2011) Silibinin Suppresses EGFR Ligand-Induced CD44 Expression through Inhibition of EGFR Activity in Breast Cancer Cells. *Anticancer Research*, **31**, 3767-3773.

[29] Provinciali, M., *et al.* (2007) Effect of the Silybin-Phosphatidylcholine Complex (IdB 1016) on the Development of Mammary Tumors in HER-2/Neu Transgenic Mice. *Cancer Research*, **67**, 2022-2029. http://dx.doi.org/10.1158/0008-5472.CAN-06-2601

28

Lack of Association between Polymorphisms in rs2981582, rs2420946, rs17102287, rs1219648, rs2981578, and rs17542768 Sites of *FGFR*2 Gene with Breast Cancer in the Population of Kazakhstan

Timur S. Balmukhanov*, Alexandra K. Khanseitova, Victoria G. Nigmatova, Alena S. Neupokoeva, Daria A. Sharafutdinova, Nagima A. Aitkhozhina

Department of Structural and Functional Genomics, M. Aitkhozhin Institute of Molecular Biology and Biochemistry, Almaty, Republic of Kazakhstan
Email: *imbbtimur@mail.ru

Abstract

Worldwide, breast cancer (BC) is the most common invasive cancer in women. Fibroblast growth factor receptor 2 (FGFR2) is a tyrosine kinase receptor that is a member of the family of individually distinct fibroblast growth factor receptors involved in tumorigenesis. *FGFR*2 gene is amplified and over expressed in breast cancer (1 - 3). The aim of the study was to determine whether polymorphisms in rs2981582, rs2420946, rs17102287, rs1219648, rs2981578, and rs17542768 in *FGFR*2 gene are associated with breast cancer susceptibility in the population of Kazakhstan. The statistically significant associations between SNPs analyzed and breast cancer risk according χ^2 and $p < 0.05$ criterions were not evaluated. The information describing the association of SNPs in *FGFR*2 with BC risk in the world populations could not be unambiguously used for Kazakhstan population.

Keywords

Fibroblast Growth Factor Receptor 2 (FGFR2), Single Nucleotide Polymorphism (SNP), Association, Breast Cancer (BC), Kazakhstan

---

*Corresponding author.

1. Introduction

Worldwide, breast cancer (BC) is the most common invasive cancer in women. Fibroblast growth factor receptor 2 (FGFR2) is a tyrosine kinase receptor that is a member of the family of individually distinct fibroblast growth factor receptors involved in tumorigenesis. *FGFR2* gene is amplified and overexpressed in breast cancer [1]-[3].

A meta-analysis of 37 studies of rs2981582, rs2420946, rs17102287, rs1219648, rs2981578, and rs17542768 polymorphisms demonstrated that these *FGFR2* SNPs are a risk factor associated with increased BC susceptibility, but these associations vary significantly in different racial and ethnic groups [4].

Significant associations between breast cancer risk and SNPs in rs11200014, rs2981579, rs1219648, rs2420946 of *FGFR2* (P_{trend} for all SNPs < 0.0001) were found in Jewish and Arab Israeli population [5].

Kazakhstan is situated in the middle of Central Asia. The multinational population of Kazakhstan totaled 17.2 million in 2013 with the major ethnic groups represented by mongoloid Asian Kazakhs (65%) and Caucasian Russians (22%), according to the Agency of the Republic of Kazakhstan on Statistics data [6].

The aim of the present work was to determine the association of individual SNPs in rs2981582, rs2420946, rs17102287, rs1219648, rs2981578, and rs17542768 sites of *FGFR2* with BC in Kazakh and Russian ethnic groups of Kazakhstan.

In studies performed in Russia, the associations of *FGFR2*'s SNPs with BC risk were shown for rs1219648, especially in combination with polymorphisms in *TP53* [7]; rs2981582 in the population of West Siberia [8]; and rs2981582, particularly in genetically-enriched BC patients versus elderly tumor-free women [9]. In Kazakhstan the presented research devoted to the evaluation of association of SNPs of *FGFR2* with BC is performed at a first time.

2. Materials and Methods

2.1. Patients and Controls

Informed consent was received from all individuals prior to study inclusion. Ethical permissions were obtained from the ethical committees of the medical organizations listed below. Venous blood samples (5 ml) were collected from 495 women of Asian Kazakh (311 Kazakh) and Russian Caucasian (184 Russian) descent with diagnosed and histologically confirmed BC from the Kazakh Research Institute of Oncology and Radiology and Regional Oncological Dispensary (Almaty, Kazakhstan). Samples obtained from 190 healthy Kazakh and 170 Russian female blood donors (Almaty City Blood Center) without clinical symptoms or family history of cancer according to a questionnaire were used as a control. The average age of BC patients was 49.58 ± 8.70 (Kazakhs) and 53.40 ± 9.97 (Russians) years, while that of control donors was 49.84 ± 6.09 (Kazakhs) and 50.43 ± 6.56 (Russians) years old.

2.2. DNA Extraction and Genotyping

Genomic DNA was isolated from blood using commercially available DNA Blood & Tissue extraction kits (Qiagen, USA) according to the manufacturer's instructions. Genotyping was performed by restriction fragment length polymorphism (RFLP) analysis of polymerase chain reaction (PCR) products. Deoxyribonucleoside triphosphates (dNTP), restriction endonucleases, and *Taq*DNA-polymerase were purchased from SibEnzyme (Russia).The PCR reaction mixture (10 μl total volume) contained 67 mM Tris-HCl, (pH 8.8), 16.6 mM $(NH_4)_2SO_4$, 2 mM $MgCl_2$, 0.01% Tween-20, 0.15 mg/ml bovine serum albumin, 2 pM primers, 0.25 mM dNTPs, 100 ng template DNA, and 1 unit of *Taq*DNA-polymerase using a Mastercycle gradient (Eppendorf, Germany). PCR-amplified products were separated by 8% polyacrylamide gel electrophoresis at 50 mA and 300 V for 2 - 3 h. RFLP products were visualized by 0.05% ethidium bromide staining and analyzed using GelDoc-Imager (BioRad, USA). Primers were designed by Primer3 (v. 0.4.0) [10], and *FGFR2* nucleotide sequences of interest were obtained from the Ensemble data base [11]. Amplification conditions and primers for each FGFR2 nucleotide sequence are presented in **Table 1**.

Each PCR product was digested with the appropriate restriction endonuclease according the manufacturer's recommendations (SibEnzyme, Russia). PCR fragment and restriction product sizes and endonucleases used are presented in **Table 2**.

Table 1. Sites analyzed, primers sequences, amplification conditions.

Site	Primers	Amplification conditions
rs2981582	F 5'-CAGGCACCAGGTGGACTC-3' R 5'-CGAGGACTACATGAGGCTGA-3'	95°C - 5 min, 35 cycles (95°C - 30 s, 64.5°C - 30 s, 72°C - 40 s), 72°C - 5 min
rs2420946	F 5'-AAGCCCTCAGACGACAGAAA-3' R 5'-CTGCTCAACCTGGGATCTGT-3'	94°C - 7 min, 35 cycles (94°C - 30 s, 57°C - 30 s, 72°C - 40 s), 72°C - 7 min
rs17102287	F 5'-CCTCTGCTGGTGCCCTATAA- 3' R 5'-TGGCTTTGTGCAATATCGTATC-3'	95°C - 3 min, 35 cycles (95°C - 30 s, 63°C - 35 s, 72°C - 35 s), 72°C - 5 min
rs1219648	F 5'-CACGCCTATTTTACTTGACACGC-3' R 5'-ATTTGTATGTGGTAGCTGACTTC-3'	95°C - 2 min, 35 cycles (95°C - 30 s, 58°C - 30 s, 72°C - 30 s), 72°C - 5 min
rs2981578	F 5'-AATGCTGCTTTGGAGGATTG-3' R 5'-CCAGAGGACTGAAACCCACA-3'	95°C - 4 min, 35 cycles (95°C - 30 s, 56.8°C - 35 s, 72°C - 40 s), 72°C - 5 min
rs17542768	F 5'-CAGACCCCCAGAGGAATCTT-3' R 5'-CTGGGTGGGCTTGTAGGTAG-3'	95°C - 3 min, 36 cycles (95°C - 30 s, 60°C - 40 s, 72°C - 30 s), 72°C - 5 min

Table 2. Sites analyzed, PCR product size, restriction fragments size, restriction endonucleases.

Site	PCR product size, bp	Restriction fragments size	Endonuclease
rs2981582	233	T allele - 233 bp, C allele - 211 bp, 22 bp	*BspAC*I
rs2420946	269	T allele - 269 bp, C allele - 244 bp, 25 bp	*AspLE*I
rs17102287	237	T allele - 237 bp, C allele - 212 bp, 25 bp	*Fat*I
rs1219648	133	A allele - 133 bp,G allele - 109 bp, 24 bp	*BstHH*I
rs2981578	173	A allele - 173 bp, G allele - 89 bp, 84 bp	*BspAC*I
rs17542768	206	A allele - 206 bp,G allele - 159 bp, 47 bp	*BstC*8I

Table 3. The allele frequencies and genotypes distribution of *FGFR*2 gene rs2420946, rs2981578, rs1219648, rs1281582, rs17102287, rs17542768 polymorphic sites in Kazakh ethnic groups of patients (cases) and controls.

Alleles/genotypes	Cases % (n)	Controls % (n)	P	χ^2	OR (95% CI)
		Kazakhs			
rs2420946					
C	59.2 (366)	54.4 (196)	0.14	2.13	1.22 (0.93 - 1.58)
T	40.8 (252)	45.6 (164)			0.82 (0.63 - 1.07)
CC	34.0 (105)	26.7 (48)			1.42 (0.94 - 2.12)
TC	50.5 (156)	55.6 (100)	0.24	2.85	0.82 (0.56 - 1.18)
TT	15.5 (48)	17.8 (32)			0.85 (0.52 - 1.39)
rs2981578					
A	45.4 (334)	46.4 (231)	0.73	0.12	0.96 (0.76 - 1.21)
G	54.6 (402)	53.6 (267)			1.04 (0.83 - 1.31)
AA	19.0 (70)	23.3 (58)			0.77 (0.52 - 1.15)
AG	52.7 (194)	46.2 (115)	0.24	2.83	1.30 (0.94 - 1.79)
GG	28.3 (104)	30.5 (76)			0.90 (0.63 - 1.28)
rs1219648					
A	59.4 (366)	60.3 (216)	0.78	0.08	0.96 (0.74 - 1.26)
G	40.6 (250)	39.7 (142)			1.04 (0.80 - 1.36)
AA	34.7 (107)	36.3 (65)			0.93 (0.64 - 1.37)
AG	49.4 (152)	48.0 (86)	0.94	0.12	1.05 (0.73 - 1.52)
GG	15.9 (49)	15.6 (28)			1.02 (0.62 - 1.69)
rs1281582					
C	61.8(465)	61.2(350)	0.81	0.06	1.03 (0.82 - 1.28)
T	38.2(287)	38.8(222)			0.97 (0.78 - 1.22)
CC	38.6(145)	35.3(101)			1.15 (0.84 - 1.58)
CT	46.5(175)	51.7(148)	0.41	1.81	0.81 (0.60 - 1.10)
TT	14.9(56)	12.9(37)			1.18 (0.75 - 1.84)
rs17102287					
T	75.3 (521)	76.7 (437)	0.57	0.32	0.93 (0.72 - 1.20)
C	24.7 (171)	23.3 (133)			1.08 (0.83 - 1.40)
TT	56.1 (194)	57.2 (163)	0.63	0.92	0.96 (0.70 - 1.31)

Continued

TC	38.4 (133)	38.9 (111)			0.98 (0.71 - 1.35)
CC	5.5 (19)	3.9 (11)			1.45 (0.68 - 3.09)
rs17542768					
A	92.3 (696)	89.5 (501)	0.07	3.20	1.41 (0.97 - 2.07)
G	7.70 (58)	10.5 (59)			0.71 (0.48 - 1.03)
AA	84.6 (319)	78.9 (221)			1.47 (0.98 - 2.19)
AG	15.4 (58)	21.1 (59)	0.17	3.55	0.68 (0.46 - 1.02)
GG	0 (0)	0 (0)			0.74 (0.01 - 37.56)

P—Fisher's exact test p-value; OR—Odds Ratio; CI—Confidence Interval.

Table 4. The allele frequencies and genotypes distribution of *FGFR2* gene rs2420946, rs2981578, rs1219648, rs1281582, rs17102287, rs17542768 polymorphic sites in Russian ethnic group of patients (cases) and controls.

Alleles/genotypes	Cases % (n)	Controls % (n)	P	χ^2	OR (95% CI)
			Russian		
rs2420946					
C	60.9 (223)	60.2 (200)	0.85	0.03	1.03 (0.76 - 1.39)
T	39.1 (143)	39.8 (132)			0.97 (0.72 - 1.32)
CC	32.2 (59)	34.3 (57)			0.91 (0.58 - 1.42)
TC	57.4 (105)	51.8 (86)	0.4948	1.48	1.25 (0.82 - 1.91)
TT	10.4 (19)	13.9 (23)			0.72 (0.38 - 1.38)
rs2981578					
A	56.4 (246)	55.5 (234)	0.77	0.08	1.04 (0.79 - 1.36)
G	43.6 (190)	44.5 (188)			0.96 (0.73 - 1.26)
AA	31.2 (68)	31.3 (66)			1.00 (0.66 - 1.50)
AG	50.5 (110)	48.3 (102)	0.85	0.33	1.09 (0.75 - 1.59)
GG	18.3 (40)	20.4 (43)			0.88 (0.54 - 1.42)
rs1219648*					
A	64.0 (233)	64.1 (209)	0.98	0	1.00 (0.73 - 1.36)
G	36.0 (131)	35.9 (117)			1.00 (0.74 - 1.37)
AA	37.4 (68)	41.1 (67)			0.85 (0.55 - 1.32)
AG	53.3 (97)	46.0 (75)	0.33	2.21	1.34 (0.88 - 2.05)
GG	9.30 (17)	12.9 (21)			0.70 (0.35 - 1.37)
rs1281582					
C	63.5 (284)	62.0 (306)	0.63	0.23	1.07 (0.82 - 1.39)
T	36.5 (162)	38.0 (188)			0.94 (0.72 - 1.22)
CC	39.2 (87)	38.6 (95)			1.02 (0.71 - 1.49)
CT	48.6 (108)	46.7 (115)	0.73	0.63	1.08 (0.75 - 1.55)
TT	12.2 (27)	14.6 (36)			0.81 (0.47 - 1.38)
rs17102287					
T	83.6 (373)	80.5 (401)	0.21	1.54	1.24 (0.88 - 1.73)
C	16.4 (73)	19.5 (97)			0.81 (0.58 - 1.13)
TT	69.1 (154)	65.1 (162)			1.20 (0.82 - 1.76)
TC	29.1 (65)	30.9 (77)	0.31	2.36	0.92 (0.62 - 1.36)
CC	1.8 (4)	4.00 (10)			0.44 (0.13 - 1.41)
rs17542768					
A	84.2 (401)	87.3 (433)	0.17	1.86	0.78 (0.54 - 1.12)
G	15.8 (75)	12.7 (63)			1.29 (0.90 - 1.85)
AA	69.7 (166)	75.4 (187)			0.75 (0.50 - 1.12)
AG	29.0 (69)	23.8 (59)	0.36	2.03	1.31 (0.87 - 1.96)
GG	1.30 (3)	0.8 (2)			1.57 (0.26 - 9.48)

P—Fisher's exact test p-value; OR—Odds Ratio; CI—Confidence Interval.
*In the group of patients alleles frequencies did not corresponded to Hardy-Weinberg equilibrium.

2.3. Statistical Analysis

The Pearson χ^2 and Fisher's exact tests were used to compare differences between allele frequencies and genotypes distribution between groups of BC patients and control. Cancer risk associated with genotype was calculated with odds ratios (ORs) and 95% confidence intervals (CI). All BC cases and controls were tested to be in Hardy-Weinberg equilibrium. Statistical analyses were performed using STATISTICA v. 5.0 software (StatSoft, USA). Fisher's exact test and Chi-square criterion were estimated using Free Statistics Calculator v. 3.0 [12].

3. Results and Discussion

To investigate whether SNPs in rs2981582, rs2420946, rs17102287, rs1219648, rs2981578, and rs17542768 of *FGFR*2 gene are associated with BC in Kazakhstan population, we performed PCR-RFLP based assay. The results of genotyping in Kazakh ethnic group (311 BC patients and 190 controls) are presented in **Table 3** and the results of genotyping in Russian ethnic group (184 BC patients and 170 controls) are presented in **Table 4**. Allele frequencies in all groups corresponded to Hardy-Weinberg equilibrium with the exception of site rs1219648 in the group of BC patients. The differences neither in allele's frequency nor in genotypes distribution were evaluated in both Kazakh and Russian ethnic groups.

The information describing the association of SNPs in *FGFR*2 with BC risk in the world populations could not be unambiguously used for Kazakhstan population.

References

[1] Grose, R. and Dickson, C. (2005) Fibroblast Growth Factor Signaling in Tumorigenesis. *Cytokine & Growth Factor Reviews*, **16**, 179-186. http://dx.doi.org/10.1016/j.cytogfr.2005.01.003

[2] Moffa, A.B. and Ethier, S.P. (2007) Differential Signal Transduction of Alternatively Spliced FGFR2 Variants Expressed in Human Mammary Epithelial Cells. *Journal of Cellular Physiology*, **210**, 720-731. http://dx.doi.org/10.1002/jcp.20880

[3] Moffa, A.B., Tannheimer, S.L. and Ethier, S.P. (2004) Transforming Potential of Alternatively Spliced Variants of Fibroblast Growth Factor Receptor 2 in Human Mammary Epithelial Cells. *Molecular Cancer Research*, **2**, 643-652.

[4] Wang, H., Yang, Z. and Zhang, H. (2013) Assessing Interaction between the Associations of Fibroblast Growth Receptor 2 Common Gene Variants and Hormone Receptor Status with Breast Cancer Risk. *Breast Cancer Research and Treatment*, **137**, 511-522. http://dx.doi.org/10.1007/s10549-012-2343-7

[5] Raskin, L., Pinchev, M., Arad, C., Lejbkowicz, F., Tamir, A., Rennert, H.S., Rennert, G. and Gruber, S.G. (2008) FGFR2 Is a Breast Cancer Susceptibility Gene in Jewish and Arab Israeli Populations. *Cancer Epidemiology, Biomarkers & Prevention*, **17**, 1060-1065. http://dx.doi.org/10.1158/1055-9965.EPI-08-0018

[6] Agency of the Republic of Kazakhstan on Statistics Data. (2013) http://www.stat.gov.kz

[7] Cherdyntseva, N.V., Denisov, E.V., Litvakov, N.V., Maksimov, V.N., Malinovskaya, E.A., Babyshkina, N.N., Slonimskaya, E.M., Voevoda, M.L. and Choinzonov, E.L. (2012) Crosstalk between the FGFR2 and TP53 Genes in Breast Cancer: Data from an Association Study and Epistatic Interaction Analysis. *DNA and Cell Biology*, **31**, 306-311. http://dx.doi.org/10.1089/dna.2011.1351

[8] Boyarskikh, A.U., Zarubina, N.A., Biltueva, J.A., Sinkina, T.V., Voronina, E.N., Lazarev, A.F., Petrova, V.D., Aulchenko, Y.S. and Filipenko, M.L. (2009) Association of FGFR2 Gene Polymorphisms with the Risk of Breast Cancer In Population of West Siberia. *European Journal of Human Genetics*, **17**, 1688-1691.

[9] Gorodnova, T.V., Kuligina, E.Sh., Yanus, G.A., Katanugina, A.S., Abysheva, S.N., Togo, A.V. and Imvanitov, E.N. (2010) Distribution of *FGFR*2, *MAP3K*1, *LSP*1, and 8q24 Alleles in Genetically Enriched Breast Cancer Patients versus Elderly Tumor-Free Women. *Cancer Genetics and Cytogenetics*, **199**, 69-72. http://dx.doi.org/10.1016/j.cancergencyto.2010.01.020

[10] http://bioinfo.ut.ee/primer3-0.4.0/

[11] http://www.ensembl.org

[12] http://www.danielsoper.com/statcalc3

Permissions

All chapters in this book were first published in ABCR, by Scientific Research Publishing; hereby published with permission under the Creative Commons Attribution License or equivalent. Every chapter published in this book has been scrutinized by our experts. Their significance has been extensively debated. The topics covered herein carry significant findings which will fuel the growth of the discipline. They may even be implemented as practical applications or may be referred to as a beginning point for another development.

The contributors of this book come from diverse backgrounds, making this book a truly international effort. This book will bring forth new frontiers with its revolutionizing research information and detailed analysis of the nascent developments around the world.

We would like to thank all the contributing authors for lending their expertise to make the book truly unique. They have played a crucial role in the development of this book. Without their invaluable contributions this book wouldn't have been possible. They have made vital efforts to compile up to date information on the varied aspects of this subject to make this book a valuable addition to the collection of many professionals and students.

This book was conceptualized with the vision of imparting up-to-date information and advanced data in this field. To ensure the same, a matchless editorial board was set up. Every individual on the board went through rigorous rounds of assessment to prove their worth. After which they invested a large part of their time researching and compiling the most relevant data for our readers.

The editorial board has been involved in producing this book since its inception. They have spent rigorous hours researching and exploring the diverse topics which have resulted in the successful publishing of this book. They have passed on their knowledge of decades through this book. To expedite this challenging task, the publisher supported the team at every step. A small team of assistant editors was also appointed to further simplify the editing procedure and attain best results for the readers.

Apart from the editorial board, the designing team has also invested a significant amount of their time in understanding the subject and creating the most relevant covers. They scrutinized every image to scout for the most suitable representation of the subject and create an appropriate cover for the book.

The publishing team has been an ardent support to the editorial, designing and production team. Their endless efforts to recruit the best for this project, has resulted in the accomplishment of this book. They are a veteran in the field of academics and their pool of knowledge is as vast as their experience in printing. Their expertise and guidance has proved useful at every step. Their uncompromising quality standards have made this book an exceptional effort. Their encouragement from time to time has been an inspiration for everyone.

The publisher and the editorial board hope that this book will prove to be a valuable piece of knowledge for researchers, students, practitioners and scholars across the globe.

List of Contributors

Áine Gorman, Michael Sugrue, Zuhair Ahmed and Alison Johnston
Donegal Clinical and Research Academy, Breast Centre North West, Letterkenny Hospital, Donegal, Ireland

Ana Fátima Fernandes, Amanda Cruz, Camila Moreira, Míria Conceição Santos and Tiago Silva
Department of Nursing, Federal University of Ceará, Fortaleza, Brazil

Damien Mikael Hansra, Orlando Silva, Ashwin Mehta and Eugene Ahn
Department of Hematology and Oncology, Sylvester Comprehensive Cancer Center at the University of Miami, Miami, USA

Rodrigo dos Santos Horta, Gleidice Eunice Lavalle, Rúbia Monteiro de Castro Cunha, Larissa Layara de Moura and Roberto Baracat de Araújo
Veterinary School, Universidade Federal de Minas Gerais-UFMG, Belo Horizonte, Brazil

Geovanni Dantas Cassali
Biological Sciences Institute, Universidade Federal de Minas Gerais-UFMG, Belo Horizonte, Brazil

Abduelmula R. Abduelkarem, Fatima Khalifa Saif, Salma Saif and Talal Ali Alshoaiby
College of Pharmacy, University of Sharjah, Sharjah, UAE

Javier Encinas Méndez and Josep Verge Schulte-Eversum
Consorci Sanitari Garraf. H. Sant Camil, Sant Pere de Ribes, Spain

Joan Francesc Julián Ibáñez, Manel Cremades Pérez, Jordi Navinés and Manel Fraile López-Amor
Hospital Germans Trias i Pujol, Badalona, Spain

Manel Armengol Carrasco
H. U. Vall d' Hebron, Barcelona, Spain

Ahmed Abbas, Ali Al-Zaher, Ali El Arini and Ikram Chaudhry
Department of Surgery, King Fahad Specialist Hospital, Dammam, KSA

Fadak S. Alshayookh, Howayda M. Ahmed, Ibrahim A. Awad and Saddig D. Jastaniah
Department of Diagnostic Radiology, Faculty of Applied Medical Sciences, King Abdulaziz University, Jeddah, KSA

T. M. Allweis and G. Yahalom
Kaplan Medical Center, Rehovot, Israel

L. Strauss, Z. Malyutin, A. Bassein Kapov-Kagan, I. Novikov and B. Piura
Eventus Diagnostics (Israel) LTD, Ora, Israel

T. B. Bevers
University of Texas, MD Anderson Cancer Center, Houston, USA

S. Iacobelli
Media Pharma Srl, Chieti, Italy

M. T. Sandri
Laboratory Medicine Division, Istituto Europeo di Oncologia, Milan, Italy

A. Bitterman
Carmel Medical Center, Surgery A, Haifa, Israel

P. Engelman
Zvulun Breast Center, Clalit Organization, Kiryat Bialik, Israel

M. Rosenberg
Eventus Diagnostics Inc., Miami, USA

Laith R. Sultan, Ghizlane Bouzghar, Benjamin J. Levenback, Nauroze A. Faizi, Emily F. Conant and Chandra M. Sehgal
Department of Radiology, University of Pennsylvania, Philadelphia, USA

Santosh S. Venkatesh
Department of Electrical Engineering, University of Pennsylvania, Philadelphia, USA

Reham G. Garout, Howayda M. Ahmed, Saddig D. Jastaniah and Ibrahim A. Awad
Department of Diagnostic Radiology, Faculty of Applied Medical Sciences, King Abdulaziz University, Jeddah, KSA

Ahmed Majeed Al-Shammari, Nahi Y. Yaseen and Ayman Hussien
Experimental Therapy Department, Iraqi Center for Cancer and Medical Genetic Research, Al-Mustansiriyah University, Baghdad, Iraq

Worod Jawad Kadhim Allak and Mahfoodha Umran
Biotechnology Department, Collage of Science, Baghdad University, Baghdad, Iraq

Breno S. Salgado and Noeme S. Rocha
Departamento de Patologia, Faculdade de Medicina de Botucatu, Universidade Estadual Paulista, Campus de Botucatu, Botucatu, Brazil

Breno S. Salgado and Fátima Gärtner
Instituto de Ciências Biomédicas Abel Salazar, Universidade do Porto (Intitute of Biomedical Sciences Abel Salazar of University of Porto), Oporto, Portugal

Suely Nonogaki and Rafael M. Rocha
Fundação Antônio Prudente, Hospital A.C. Camargo, São Paulo, Brazil

Luisa M. Soares and Noeme S. Rocha
Departamento de Clínica Veterinária, Faculdade de Medicina Veterinária e Zootecnia, Universidade Estadual Paulista, UNESP,. Botucatu, Brazil

Angela Akamatsu, Cristiano R. N. da Silva, Thiago P. Anacleto and Rodolfo Malagó
Hospital Escola de Medicina Veterinária, Fundação de Ensino e Pesquisa de Itajubá—FEPI, Itajubá, Brazil

Muhittin Yaprak, Ayhan Mesci, Ayhan Dınckan, Okan Erdogan and Cumhur Arici
Department of General Surgery, Akdeniz University School of Medicine, Antalya, Turkey

Gülgün Erdogan
Department of Pathology, Akdeniz University School of Medicine, Antalya, Turkey

Gulbin Aricic
Department of Anesthesiology, Akdeniz University School of Medicine, Antalya, Turkey

Barıs Ozcan
Department of General Surgery, Medstar Antalya Hospital, Antalya, Turkey

Ellen G. Engelhardt, Matti A. Rookus and Marjanka K. Schmidt
Division of Psychosocial Research and Epidemiology, Netherlands Cancer Institute, Amsterdam, The Netherlands

Mieke Kriege, Maartje J. Hooning and Caroline Seynaeve
Family Cancer Clinic, Department of Medical Oncology, Erasmus MC-Daniel den Hoed Cancer Centre, Rotterdam, The Netherlands

Rob A. E. M. Tollenaar
Department of Surgery, Leiden University Medical Centre, Leiden, The Netherlands

Christina J. van Asperen
Department of Clinical Genetics, Leiden University Medical Centre, Leiden, The Netherlands

Margreet G. E. M. Ausems
Department of Medical Genetics, University Medical Centre Utrecht, Utrecht, The Netherlands

Lonneke V. van de Poll-Franse
Eindhoven Cancer Registry, Comprehensive Cancer Centre South, Eindhoven, The Netherlands

Stella Mook
Department of Radiation Oncology, Netherlands Cancer Institute, Amsterdam, The Netherlands

Senno Verhoef
Family Cancer Clinic, Netherlands Cancer Institute, Amsterdam, The Netherlands

HEBON Collaborators
Hereditary Breast and Ovarian Cancer Netherlands (HEBON) Collaborators (see end of article for full list of HEBON collaborators and affiliations)

Marjanka K. Schmidt
Division of Molecular Pathology, Netherlands Cancer Institute, Amsterdam, The Netherlands

Anja Brügmann
Institute of Pathology, Aalborg Hospital, Aalborg, Denmark

E. Nexo, B. S. Sorensen and Anja Brügmann
Department of Clinical Biochemistry, Aarhus University Hospital, Aarhus, Denmark

V. Jensen
Institute of Pathology, Aarhus University Hospital, Aarhus, Denmark

J. P. Garne
Department of Breast Surgery, Aalborg Hospital, Aalborg, Denmark

Ketan Vagholkar
Department of Surgery, Dr. D. Y. Patil Medical College, Navi Mumbai, India

Basem Battah and Jumana Saleh
Faculty of Pharmacy, Damascus University, Damascus, Syria

Marroan Bachour and Maher Salamoon
Al Bairouni University Hospital, Damascus, Damascus, Syria

Abdul Hameed Baloch and Jamil Ahmad
Department of Biotechnology and Informatics, BUITEMS, Quetta, Pakistan

Shakeela Daud
Center for Advanced Molecular Biology (CAMB), Lahore, Pakistan

Jameela Shuja, Fateh Ali and Mohammad Akram
CENAR, Quetta, Pakistan

Adeel Ahmad
Institute of Biochemistry and Biotechnology (IBBt), UVAS, Lahore, Pakistan

Dost Mohammad Baloch
Lasbela University of Agriculture, Water and Marine Sciences, Balochistan

Abdul Majeed Cheema
Institute of Molecular Biology and Biotechnology, The University of Lahore, Pakistan

Mohammad Iqbal
Bolan Medical College/Hospital (BMC) Quetta

Wisit Tangkeangsirisin and Ginette Serrero
A&G Pharmaceutical Inc., Columbia, USA

Wisit Tangkeangsirisin
Present Address: Department of Biopharmacy, Faculty of Pharmacy, Silpakorn University, Nakhon Pathom, Thailand

Ginette Serrero
Program in Oncology, Greenebaum Cancer Center of the University of Maryland, Baltimore, USA

Alison Johnston, Sharon Curran and Michael Sugrue
Breast Centre North West, Letterkenny Hospital, Donegal Clinical Research Academy, Donegal, Ireland

Alberto Testori, Valentina Errico, Edoardo Bottoni, Emanuele Voulaz, Roberto Travaglini and Marco Alloisio
General and Thoracic Surgery, IRCCS Humanitas Research Hospital, Via Manzoni, Rozzano (Milan), Italy

Stefano Meroni
Breast Imaging Division, European Institute of Oncology, Via Ripamonti, Milan, Italy

Ryan Sugrue, Katherine McGowan, Cillian McNamara and Michael Sugrue
Department of Breast Surgery and Radiology Letterkenny and Donegal Clinical Research Academy, National University of Ireland, Galway, Ireland

Breno S. Salgado and Noeme S. Rocha
Departamento de Patologia, Faculdade de Medicina de Botucatu, Universidade Estadual Paulista (UNESP), Botucatu, Brazil

Noeme S. Rocha
Laboratório de Patologia Investigativa e Comparada, Departamento de Clínica Veterinária, Faculdade de Medicina Veterinária e Zootecnia, Universidade Estadual Paulista (UNESP), Botucatu, Brazil

Rafael M. Rocha and Fernando A. Soares
Departamento de Anatomia Patológica, Hospital A. C. Camargo, Fundação Antônio Prudente, São Paulo, Brazil

Fátima Gärtner
Institute of Pathology and Molecular Immunology (IPATIMUP), Oporto, Portugal

Shahab Rezaeian
Health Promotion Research Center, Zahedan University of Medical Sciences, Zahedan, Iran

Yousef Veisani
Student Research Committee, Ilam University of Medical Sciences, Ilam, Iran

Mohammad Ghorbani and Hedayat Abbastabar
Department of Epidemiology, School of Health, Shiraz University of Medical Sciences, Shiraz, Iran

Ali Delpisheh
Department of Clinical Epidemiology, Ilam University of Medical Sciences, Ilam, Iran

Jean Dupont Kemfang Ngowa, Jean Marie Kasia, Achille Nkigoum Nana and Anny Ngassam
Department of Gynecology and Obstetrics, Yaoundé General Hospital, Faculty of Medicine and Biomedical Sciences, University of Yaounde I, Yaoundé, Cameroon

Jean Dupont Kemfang Ngowa and Jean Marie Kasia
Obstetrics and Gynecology Unit, Yaoundé General Hospital, Yaoundé, Cameroon

Jean Yomi
Department of Radiation Therapy, Yaoundé General Hospital, Faculty of Medicine and Biomedical Sciences, University of Yaoundé I, Yaoundé, Cameroon

Irenée Domkam
Chantal Biya International Reference Centre for Research on HIV/AIDS Prevention and Management, Yaoundé, Cameroon

Zacharie Sando
Department of Morphological Sciences, Yaoundé General Hospital, Faculty of Medicine and Biomedical Sciences, University of Yaoundé I, Yaoundé, Cameroon

Paul Ndom
Oncology Division, Yaoundé General Hospital, Yaoundé, Cameroon

Saieh Hajighasemlou, Mahmoud Alebouyeh, Hossein Rastegar and Mojgan Taghizadeh Manzari
Iran Foods and Drug Organization, Tehran, Iran

Mohammadmorad Farajollahi and Saieh Hajighasemlou
Department of Biotechnology, Iran University of Medical Sciences, Tehran, Iran

Mohammadmorad Farajollahi
Alborz Food and Drug Laboratory, Fardis, Iran

Milad Mirmoghtadaei
School of Medicine, Tehran University of Medical Sciences, International Campus (TUMS-IC), Tehran, Iran

Behjat Moayedi
Isfahan University of Medical Sciences, Isfahan, Iran

Maryam Ahmadzadeh
Department of Pharmaceutical Biotechnology, School of Pharmacy, Shahid Beheshti University of Medical Sciences, Tehran, Iran

Mansure Kazemi
Department of Tissue Engineering, School of Medical Advanced of Technologies in Medicine, Tehran University of Medical Sciences, Tehran, Iran

Farzad Parvizpour
Department of Applied Cell Sciences, School of Medical Advanced of Technologies in Medicine, Tehran University of Medical Sciences, Tehran, Iran

Safoora Gharibzadeh
Department of Epidemiology and Biostatistics, School of Public Health, Tehran University of Medical Sciences, Tehran, Iran

Timur S. Balmukhanov, Alexandra K. Khanseitova, Victoria G. Nigmatova, Alena S. Neupokoeva, Daria A. Sharafutdinova and Nagima A. Aitkhozhina
Department of Structural and Functional Genomics, M. Aitkhozhin Institute of Molecular Biology and Biochemistry, Almaty, Republic of Kazakhstan

www.ingramcontent.com/pod-product-compliance
Lightning Source LLC
Chambersburg PA
CBHW080522200326
41458CB00012B/4300